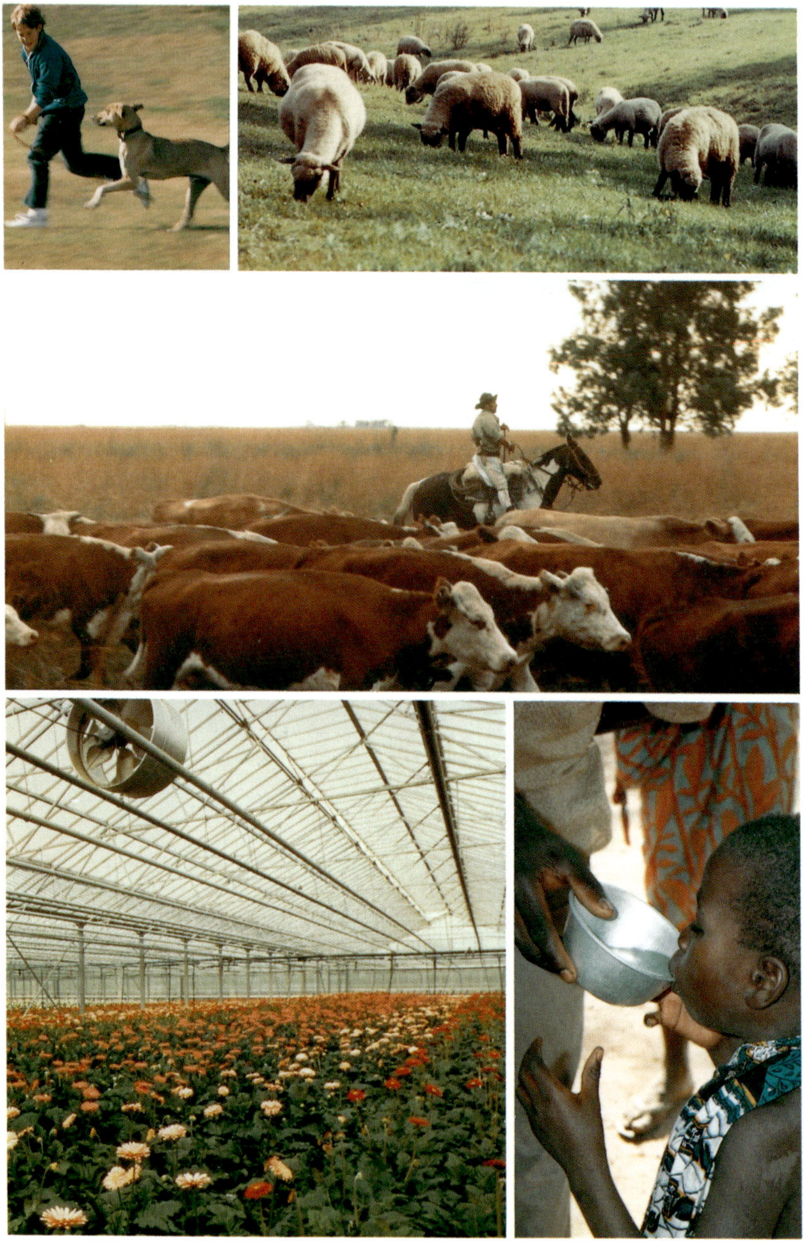

Ivermectin and abamectin are used to control parasites and pests of livestock, pets, plants, and people.

Ivermectin and Abamectin

William C. Campbell
Editor

Ivermectin and Abamectin

With 66 Illustrations

Springer-Verlag
New York Berlin Heidelberg
London Paris Tokyo

William C. Campbell
Merck Institute for Therapeutic Research
Rahway, N.J. 07065

Library of Congress Cataloging-in-Publication Data
Ivermectin and abamectin / edited by William C. Campbell.
p. cm.
Includes index.
ISBN 0-387-96944-6
1. Ivermectin. 2. Abamectin. I. Campbell, William C. (William Cecil), 1930–
SF918.I83I94 1989
636.089'6964061—dc20 89-6254
CIP

Typeset by TCSystems, Inc., Shippensburg, PA.
Printed and bound by RR Donnelley & Sons, Harrisonburg, VA.
Printed in the United States of America

9 8 7 6 5 4 3 2 1

ISBN 0-387-96944-6 Springer-Verlag New York Berlin Heidelberg
ISBN 3-540-96944-6 Springer-Verlag Berlin Heidelberg New York

Dedicated

to the memory of the late Mr. Robert K. Hartman and the late Mr. Robert E. Ormond, who contributed to the discovery of the avermectins, and to the late Dr. Mohammed A. Aziz, who directed the clinical evaluation of ivermectin in humans.

Preface

Ivermectin was introduced to the marketplace as an antiparasitic drug in 1981, and abamectin was introduced as an agricultural pesticide (and as an antiparasitic drug) in 1985. They are both members of the avermectin family of compounds, and their impact has been enormous. The efficacy of ivermectin against nematode and arthropod parasites is unprecedented in potency and breadth of spectrum. Its worldwide acceptance in livestock production and in the health care of companion animals has made it a major commercial success. Its efficacy in human onchocerciasis (river blindness) has made it a promising candidate for the control of one of the most insidious and intractable of tropical diseases. Abamectin is in commercial use as an agricultural pesticide, and its applications are continuing to expand. Most striking of all, perhaps, is the intense scientific activity triggered by the discovery of the avermectin compounds. In the fields of chemistry, microbiology, parasitology, entomology, biochemistry, pharmacology, and the clinical and agricultural sciences, interest in the avermectins has evolved rapidly, and a considerable bibliography has already been amassed. Chemicals that are widely used raise correspondingly wide concerns about safety—and the ongoing evaluation of the avermectins thus far has included not only studies on the safety of the compounds for the animals, plants, and people in which they are used but also studies on their safety for the people who make and apply them, safety for the people who eat the plants and animals to which these agents have been applied, and safety for the environment which is exposed, one way or another, to their effects. Given the intense industrial and scientific interest in ivermectin and abamectin, and the likelihood that they will be the forerunners of an expanding family of relatives and descendants, it seems timely to take stock of what we have learned about them so far.

With few exceptions, the authors of this book are members of the scientific staff of the Merck Sharp & Dohme Research Laboratories; and there were reasons for this. In certain disciplines, such as toxicology and fermentation technology, most of the available information on the avermectins has been obtained by MSDRL scientists, and they are therefore in a good position to review the data. The toxicological and environmental safety data that have been accumulated within our laboratories have been made available to governmental regulatory agencies and other interested parties in the form of official reports, but have seldom appeared in the scientific literature. In other disciplines, much information already has appeared in the scientific literature; but here, too, a large proportion of the research has been carried out by, or in collaboration with, our own scientists—and the names of those individuals inevitably came to mind as prospective authors of review chapters. There was, moreover, a practical advantage in the preponderance of MSDRL authors: the chapters could be prepared synchronously. The editor knows, from hard-won experience, the difficulty of getting manuscripts from far-flung scribes with no obligation other than a cheerfully and hastily given promise to write a chapter for a particular volume. In some multiauthored books, a chapter written by a conscientious contributor may be older by many months, or even by a few years, than one written by some hopelessly delinquent contributor. In the present case, the editor has been blessed with colleagues who have been willing to make an extraordinary effort to bring their labors to fruition at the same time. This book, then, comes close to the objective of capturing a likeness of its subject at one instant in time.

Except in the context of synthetic and microbiological chemistry (which must of necessity deal with structural diversity), this volume deals almost exclusively with ivermectin and abamectin—not with the extended family of the avermectins or with the related family known as milbemycins.

The expression of dosage in terms of micrograms (μg) per kilogram of body weight has become commonplace in accounts of the efficacy of these compounds, and this form is generally used in this book. Toxicological studies, however, usually deal with multiples of milligrams, rather than fractions, and in that context dosages are expressed in terms of milligrams (mg) per kilogram of body weight.

The chapters of the book have been arranged in three groups. The first deals with the basic chemical, biochemical, and microbiological aspects; the second deals with pharmacological, safety, and environmental aspects; and the third covers practical use of the compounds as antiparasitic and pesticidal agents. In the case of human application, however, the available safety data have emerged from the clinical experience, and are to be found in Part III.

William C. Campbell

Acknowledgments

The editor thanks Dr. Harold D. Hafs, Vice-President of Animal Science Research, Merck, Sharp & Dohme Research Laboratories, and Dr. Mark Licker, Executive Editor, Springer-Verlag, for their support and counsel throughout the preparation of this volume. He is indebted to Dr. M.H. Fisher for preparation of the introductory statement on Nomenclature and Physical Properties and to Dr. Dennis J. Underwood for the computer-generated structural models that appear on the cover.

Contents

Contributors

G.W. Benz, Ph.D.
Department of Animal Science Research, Merck Sharp & Dohme Research Laboratories, Rahway, New Jersey 07065

K.R. Brown, M.D.
Department of Clinical Research, Merck Sharp & Dohme Research Laboratories, West Point, Pennsylvania 19486

Barry C. Buckland, Ph.D.
Department of Biochemical Process Research and Development, Merck Sharp & Dohme Research Laboratories, Rahway, New Jersey 07065

R.W. Burg, Ph.D.
Department of Basic Microbiology, Merck Institute for Therapeutic Research, Rahway, New Jersey 07065

William C. Campbell, Ph.D.
Department of New Drug Discovery, Merck Institute for Therapeutic Research, Rahway, New Jersey 07065

S.T. Chen, Ph.D.
Department of Fermentation Microbiology, Merck Sharp & Dohme Research Laboratories, Rahway, New Jersey 07065

Shuet-Hing Lee Chiu, Ph.D.
Department of Animal Drug Metabolism, Merck Sharp & Dohme Research Laboratories, Rahway, New Jersey 07065

J.L. Cox, Ph.D.
Department of Animal Science Research, Merck Sharp & Dohme Research Laboratories, Rahway, New Jersey 07065

J. Di Netta, J.D.
Department of Regulatory Affairs, Merck Sharp & Dohme Research Laboratories, Rahway, New Jersey 07065

George V. Downing, Ph.D.
Department of Analytical Research, Merck Sharp & Dohme Research Laboratories, Rahway, New Jersey 07065

R.A. Dybas, Ph.D.
Department of Agricultural Research, Merck Sharp & Dohme Research Laboratories, Three Bridges, New Jersey 08887

David W. Fink, Ph.D.
Department of Animal Formulation Development, Merck Sharp & Dohme Research Laboratories, Rahway, New Jersey 07065

M.H. Fisher, Ph.D.
Department of Synthetic Chemistry Research, Merck Sharp & Dohme Research Laboratories, Rahway, New Jersey 07065

Lea R. Gordon, D.V.M., Ph.D.
Department of Safety Assessment, Merck Sharp & Dohme Research Laboratories, West Point, Pennsylvania 19486

B.M. Greene, M.D.
Division of Geographic Medicine, School of Medicine, University of Alabama at Birmingham, Birmingham, Alabama 35205

S.J. Gross, Ph.D.
Department of Animal Science Research, Merck Sharp & Dohme Research Laboratories, Rahway, New Jersey 07065

L.S. Grosso, Ph.D.
Department of Agricultural Research, Merck Sharp & Dohme Research Laboratories, Three Bridges, New Jersey 08887

B.A. Halley, Ph.D.
Department of Animal Drug Metabolism, Merck Sharp & Dohme Research Laboratories, Rahway, New Jersey 07065

O.D. Hensens, Ph.D.
Department of Natural Product Chemistry, Merck Sharp & Dohme Research Laboratories, Rahway, New Jersey 07065

LOUIS KAPLAN, Ph.D.
Department of Fermentation Microbiology, Merck Sharp & Dohme Research Laboratories, Rahway, New Jersey 07065

GEORGE R. LANKAS, Ph.D.
Department of Safety Assessment, Merck Sharp & Dohme Research Laboratories, West Point, Pennsylvania 19486

W.H.D. LEANING, B.V.Sc.
Department of Technical Services, MSD AGVET, Rahway, New Jersey, 07065

A.Y.H. LU, Ph.D.
Department of Animal Drug Metabolism, Merck Sharp & Dohme Research Laboratories, Rahway, New Jersey 07065

H. MROZIK, Ph.D.
Department of Synthetic Chemistry Research, Merck Sharp & Dohme Research Laboratories, Rahway, New Jersey 07065

M. NALLIN OMSTEAD, Ph.D.
Department of Fermentation Microbiology, Merck Sharp & Dohme Research Laboratories, Rahway, New Jersey 07065

R.J. NESSEL, Ph.D.
Department of Regulatory Affairs, Merck Sharp & Dohme Research Laboratories, Rahway, New Jersey 07065

ARTURO G. PORRAS, Ph.D.
Department of Drug Metabolism, MerSharp & Dihme Research Laboratories, West Point, Pennsylvania 19486

J.M. PRESTON, B.V.M.S., Ph.D.
Department of Animal Science Research, Merck Sharp & Dohme Research Laboratories, Rahway, New Jersey 07065

J.D. PULLIAM, D.V.M., Ph.D.
Department of Animal Science Research, Merck Sharp & Dohme Research Laboratories, Rahway, New Jersey 07065

S.F. RICKARD, Ph.D.
Department of Agricultural Research, Merck Sharp & Dohme Research Laboratories, Three Bridges, New Jersey 08887

R.A. Roncalli, D.V.M.
Department of Animal Science Research, Merck Sharp & Dohme Research Laboratories, Rahway, New Jersey 07065

J.M. Schaeffer, Ph.D.
Department of Biochemical Parasitology, Merck Sharp & Dohme Research Laboratories, Rahway, New Jersey 07065

M.D. Schulman, Ph.D.
Department of Fermentation Microbiology, Merck Sharp & Dohme Research Laboratories, Rahway, New Jersey 07065

R.L. Seward, D.V.M.
Department of Animal Drug Evaluation, Merck Sharp & Dohme Research Laboratories, Rahway, New Jersey 07065

M.D. Soll, B.V.Sc.
Department of Animal Science Research, Merck Sharp & Dohme Research Laboratories, Rahway, New Jersey 07065

E.O. Stapley, Ph.D.
Department of Basic Microbiology, Merck Institute for Therapeutic Research, Rahway, New Jersey 07065

H.R. Taylor, M.D.
Dana Center for Preventive Ophthalmology, The Wilmer Institute, The Johns Hopkins University, Baltimore, Maryland 21205

M.J. Turner, Ph.D.
Department of Biochemical Parasitology, Merck Sharp & Dohme Research Laboratories, Rahway, New Jersey 07065

P.G. Wislocki, Ph.D.
Department of Agricultural Research, Merck Sharp & Dohme Research Laboratories, Three Bridges, New Jersey 08887

NOMENCLATURE AND PHYSICAL PROPERTIES

NATURAL AVERMECTINS

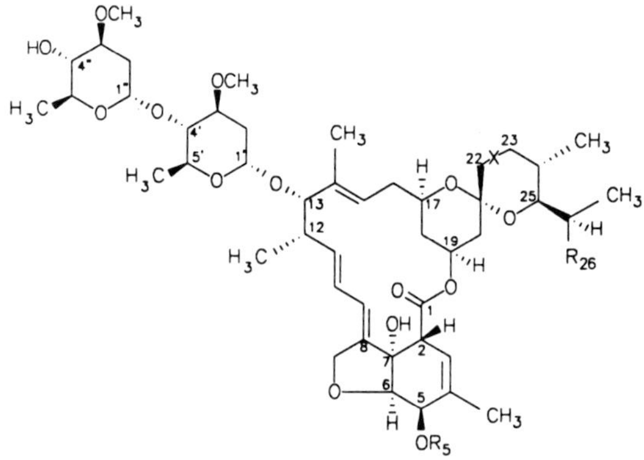

components A : $R_5 = CH_3$ components 1 : X = -CH=CH-

components B : $R_5 = H$ components 2 : X = $-CH_2\overset{OH}{CH}-$

components a : $R_{26} = C_2H_5$

components b : $R_{26} = CH_3$

ABAMECTIN

Synonyms: Avermectin B_1; AVM; C-076; MK-936.

Trade names: AVID® AGRI-MEK® VERTIMEC® AVOMEC®

Abamectin contains at least 80% of avermectin B_{1a} and not more than 20% of avermectin B_{1b}.

Avermectin B_{1a}

$C_{48}H_{72}O_{14}$; mol wt: 872. off-white powder; $[\alpha]_D + 55.7 \pm 2°$ (c = 1.06 in chloroform); uv max (methanol): 237, 243, 252 nm (ϵ 29, 120; 31,850; 20,510).

Avermectin B_{1b}

$C_{47}H_{70}O_{14}$ mol. wt. 858.

IVERMECTIN

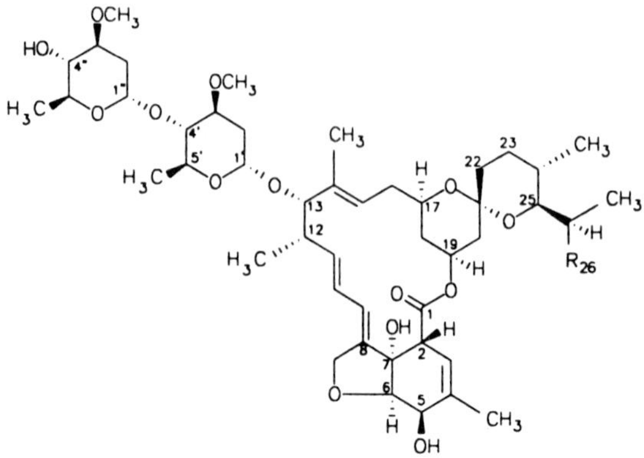

Synonyms: 22,23-Dihydroavermectin B_1; 22,23-dihydro C-076B_1; MK-933;

Trade names: HEARTGARD 30®; CARDOMEC®; EQVALAN®; IVOMEC.®; ZIMECTERIN®; MECTIZAN®

Semisynthetic derivative of the avermectins, q.v. Ivermectin contains at least 80% of 22,23-dihydroavermectin B_{1a} and less than 20% of 22,23-dihydroavermectin B_{1b}. Off-white powder; $[\alpha]_D + 71.5 \pm 3°$ (c = 0.755 in chloroform); uv max (methanol): 238, 245 nm (ϵ 27,100; 30,100).

Component B_{1a} (MK-932)

$C_{48}H_{74}O_{14}$ mol. wt. 874

5-O-Demethyl-22,23-dihydroavermectin A_{1a}; 22,23-dihydroavermectin B_{1a}; 22,23-dihydro C-076B_{1a}

$R = C_2H_5$

Crystals from ethanol/water, m.p. 1545 − 157°C

Component B_{1b}

$C_{47}H_{72}O_{14}$ mol. wt. 860

5-0-Demethyl-25-de(l-methylpropyl)-22,23-dihydro-25-(1-methylethyl)avermectin A_{1a}; 22,23-dihydroavermectin B_{1b}

$R = CH_3$

CHAPTER 1

Chemistry

M.H. Fisher and H. Mrozik

I. Structures of the Naturally Occurring Avermectins

The avermectin structures are closely related complex 16-membered macrocyclic lactones. Although they share structural features with the antibacterial macrolides and the antifungal macrocyclic polyenes, the avermectins are not usually grouped with those compounds. Avermectins have neither antibacterial nor antifungal activities and do not inhibit protein or chitin syntheses as do the other two groups. In the avermectins the macrocycle is a backbone for further substitution with a spiroketal unit (C-17 to C-28), a hexahydrobenzofuran unit (C-2 to C-8a), and a disaccharide substituent at C-13 (Fisher and Mrozik 1984, Davies and Green 1986). The milbemycins are structurally related but are missing the C-13 disaccharide substituent (Takiguchi *et al.* 1980). Although the milbemycins and their potent miticidal and acaricidal properties were discovered shortly before the avermectins, their anthelmintic properties became known only after the discovery of the avermectins.

Fermentation of the actinomycete *Streptomyces avermitilis* produces 4 homologous pairs of closely related compounds: avermectin A_1, A_2, B_1, and B_2, originally also called compounds C-076 A_1 through B_2. The A-compounds have a 5-methoxy, whereas the B-compounds have a 5-hydroxy substituent; and the 1-compounds have a 22,23-double bond which is formally obtained by dehydration of the axial 23-hydroxy group of the 2-compounds. The 4 pairs are further divided into the major components A_{1a}, A_{2a}, B_{1a}, B_{2a}—with a secondary butyl sidechain at carbon position 25—and the minor components (usually present in amounts of 1% to 20%) A_{1b}, A_{2b}, B_{1b}, B_{2b}—with an isopropyl substi-

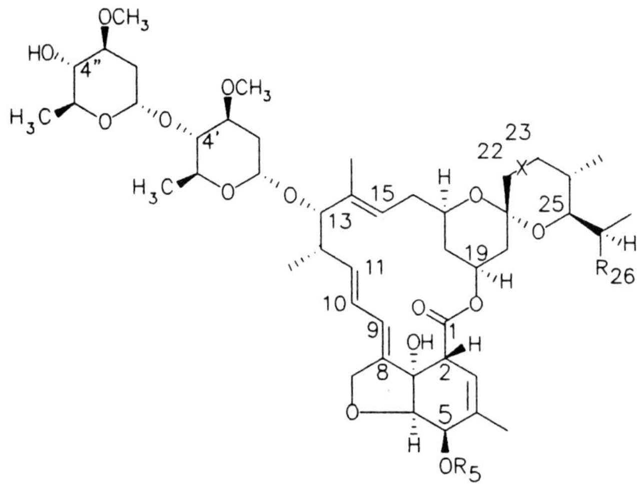

Avermectin	R_5	R_{26}	C_{22}–X–C_{23}
A_{1a}	CH_3	C_2H_5	$-CH{=}CH-$
A_{1b}	CH_3	CH_3	$-CH{=}CH-$
B_{1a}	H	C_2H_5	$-CH{=}CH-$
B_{1b}	H	CH_3	$-CH{=}CH-$
A_{2a}	CH_3	C_2H_5	$-CH_2-\overset{OH}{CH}-$
A_{2b}	CH_3	CH_3	$-CH_2-\overset{OH}{CH}-$
B_{2a}	H	C_2H_5	$-CH_2-\overset{OH}{CH}-$
B_{2b}	H	CH_3	$-CH_2-\overset{OH}{CH}-$
Ivermectin	H	>80% C_2H_5 <20% CH_3	$-CH_2-CH_2-$

FIGURE 1.1. Avermectin structures.

tuent at C-25 (Figure 1.1). Three of these—A_{2a}, B_{1a}, and B_{2a}—are produced in quantity in the fermentation. Avermectin B_{1a} is the most important because it has high potency against a broad spectrum of endo- and ectoparasites of farm animals and many agricultural mite and insect pests. It also serves as starting material for the semisynthetic 22,23-dihydro analog, which is used almost exclusively under the generic name ivermectin for both prevention and cure of parasitic infections of animals.

Because the separation of the major 25-secondary-butyl components A_{1a} through B_{2a} from the minor 25-iso-propyl components A_{1b} through B_{1b} is very tedious and impractical on a large scale, and because the biological activities of the two homologs are practically identical, the avermectin components are often used as a mixture of these two homologs. In such cases they are just defined as A_1, A_2, B_1, and B_2, which means a mixture of not less than 80% of components "a" (and not more than 20% of components "b"), and the antiparasitic agent ivermectin (22,23-dihydroavermectin B_1) is marketed as such a mixture.

Avermectin B_{1a} contains 5 double bonds, 2 of which are conjugated as an 8,9,10,11-diene function. This results in a strong UV absorption at 245 nm, an advantageous property for analytical detection. Of the 3 remaining double bonds, the two 3,4- and 14,15-enes are trisubstituted and the 22,23-ene (occurring only in the 1-components) is cisdisubstituted. Avermectin B_{1a} has 3 free hydroxy groups, a very reactive secondary allylic C-5, a somewhat less reactive secondary C-4″, and a relatively unreactive tertiary allylic C-7 hydroxygroup. The compound also has many ether bonds, of which the 2 glycosydic ones at C-1′ and C-1″ of the 2-deoxy sugars are particularly interesting: they are responsible for the ease of acidic alcoholyses and hydrolyses of the disaccharide to the monosaccharides and aglycones.

The avermectin structures were determined by spectral means (Albers-Schönberg *et al.* 1981) and shown to be closely related to the milbemycins (Mishima *et al.* 1975). Final confirmation of the structure as well as relative and absolute stereochemistry was achieved by X-ray crystallography of avermectin B_{2a} aglycone and of avermectin B_{1a} (Springer *et al.* 1981). Isolation of more than 1 mole of L-oleandrose served as reference for the absolute stereochemistry and proved that the disaccharide was made up of 2 identical sugars. Extensive mass spectral fragmentation patterns (Figure 1.2) and high field ^{1}H- and ^{13}C-NMR assignments (Tables 1.1 and 1.2) for avermectin B_{1a}, 22,23-dihydroavermectin B_{1a} (main component of ivermectin) and many derivatives have been described and serve as ready references for the identification of newly obtained derivatives. A detailed ^{1}H NMR study suggests that the conformation of avermectin B_{1a} in solution is very closely related to its conformation in the crystal structure.

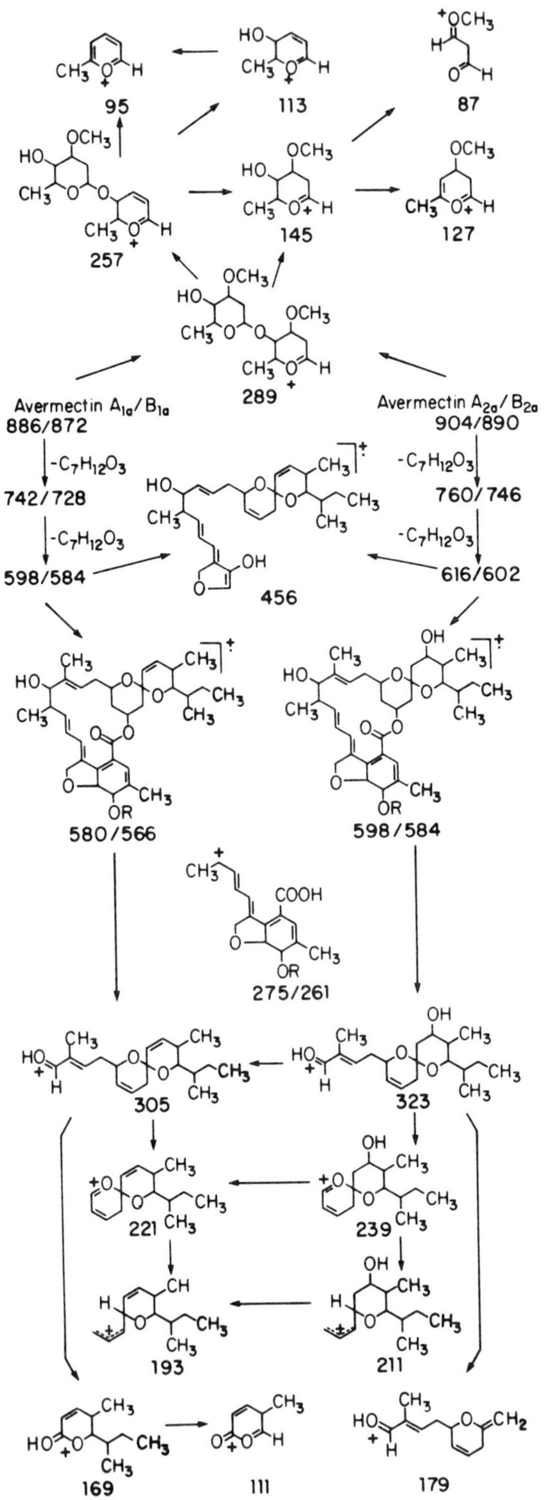

FIGURE 1.2. Mass fragments of avermectins. (G. Albers-Schönberg, B.H. Arison, J.C. Chabala, A.W. Douglas, P. Eskola, M.H. Fisher, A. Lusi, H. Mrozik, J.L. Smith and R.L. Tolman, J. Am. Chem. Soc. 103, 4216 [1981]).

TABLE 1.1. ^{1}H NMR Data for ivermectin and avermectin B_{1a}.

H	Ivermectin δ (ppm)	Avermectin B_{1a} δ (ppm)
C_2H	3.30 (q, 2.0)	3.33
C_3H	5.44 (q, ~1)	5.46
C_4CH_3	1.88 (s)	1.90
C_5OH	unassigned	2.38
C_5H	4.31 (t, 7.0)	4.34 (t, 6.0)
C_6H	3.99 (d, 6.0)	4.08 (d, 6.0)
C_7OH	4.16 (s)	4.01
$C_{8a}H_2$	4.69 (d,d, ~14.2, ~2.0)	4.74 (d,d, 16.0, 2.0)
	4.71 (d,d, ~14.2, ~2.0)	4.72 (d,d, 16.0, 2.0)
C_9H	~5.88 (m)	5.91 (m)
$C_{10}H$	~576 (m)	5.78 (m)
$C_{11}H$	~5.76 (m)	5.78 (m)
$C_{12}CH_3$	1.17 (d)	1.18 (d)
$C_{12}H$	2.54 (m)	2.55
$C_{13}H$	3.96 (broad s)	3.98
$C_{14}CH_3$	1.50 (s)	1.50
$C_{15}H$	5.00 (d, 10.0)	5.03 (d,d, 10.0, 4.0)
$C_{16}CH_2$	2.35 (m)	2.2–2.4
$C_{17}H$	~3.65 (m)	3.90 (m)
$C_{18}H_2$	ax ~0.85 (q)	0.88 (q 12)
	eq ~1.78 (d)	1.80 (br.d 12)
$C_{19}H$	5.38 (t,t,5.0,5.0)	5.44 (m)
$C_{20}H_2$	unassigned	eq. 2.09 (dd 12, 4)
		ax 1.50–1.65
$C_{22}H_2/C_{22}H$	unassigned	5.82 (dd 10, 1.7)
$C_{23}H_2/C_{23}H$	unassigned	5.60 (dd 10, 2)
$C_{24}H$	unassigned	unassigned
$C_{24}CH_3$	0.79 (d)	0.93
$C_{25}H$	3.59 (d,11.0)	3.52 (d, 9)
$C_{26}H$	unassigned	1.50–1.65
$C_{26}CH_3$	0.86 (d)	0.92
$C_{27}CH_2$	unassigned	1.50–1.65
$C_{28}CH_3$	0.94 (t)	0.95
C_1H	4.8 (d, ~3.0)	4.82 (d,3)
$C_2'H_2$	unassigned	2.2–2.4
$C_3'H$	~3.3 or 3.6	3.66 (ddd 12,7,4)
$C_3'OCH_3$	3.44 or 3.45	3.46 or 3.44
$C_4'H$	3.26 (t, 9.0)	3.28 (t, 9.0)
$C_5'H$	3.84 (d,q,9.2,9.0)	3.88 (d, q, 9, 6)
$C_5'CH_3$	1.28 or 1.25 (d)	1.27
$C_1''H$	5.42 (d, 3.0)	5.44 (d, 3.5)
$C_2''CH_2$	unassigned	2.2–2.4
$C_3''H$	~3.6 or 3.81	3.52 (m)
$C_3''CH_3$	3.44 or 3.45	3.46 or 3.44
$C_4''OH$	2.52 (d,1.9)	2.52
$C_4''OH$	3.18 (d,t,1.9,9.0)	3.20 (t,9.5)
$C_5''H$	3.78 (d,q,9.5,7.0)	3.81 (d, q, 9.5, 6.5)
$C_5''CH_3$	1.28 or 1.25 (d)	1.30

Courtesy Dr. Byron Arison, Merck & Co.

TABLE 1.2. ^{13}C NMR Data for avermectin B_{1a} and ivermectin.

C	Shifts (ppm) B_{1a}	Shifts (ppm) IVM
28	12.0	12.1
26a	12.9	12.4
14a	15.1	15.1
24a	16.4	17.4
6′	17.7	17.7
6″	18.4	18.4
4a	19.9	19.9
12a	20.2	20.2
ΣCH_3	8	
27	27.5	27.3
24	30.6	31.2
16	~34.3	34.5
2′	~34.3	34.2
2″	~34.3	34.2
26	35.2	35.5
18	36.6	36.9
12	39.8	39.7
20	40.5	41.2
2	45.7	45.7
$-CH_2-$	6	
>CH–	4	
$\Sigma(CH_2/CH)$	10	
3′a	56.4	56.4
3″a	56.4	56.5
$\Sigma(OCH_3)$	2	
5′	67.3	67.2
5	67.8	67.7
19	~68.2	68.7
8a	~68.2	68.4
17	~68.4	67.2
5″	~68.4	68.1
25	75.0	76.7
4″	76.1	76.0
3″	78.3	78.2
3′	79.4	79.2
6	79.4	79.4
4′	80.5	80.4
7	80.5 (s)	80.4
13	82.0	81.8
CH_2O	1	
CH–O	12	
C–O	1	
$R(CH_xO)$	14	
1′	95.0	94.8
21	95.8	97.5
1″	98.5	98.5

TABLE 1.2. *Continued.*

C	Shifts (ppm) B_{1a}	IVM
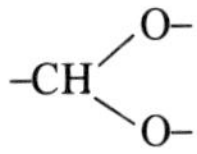	2	
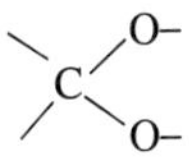	1	
$\Sigma(CH_XO_2)$	3	
15	1118.1	118.1
3	118.4	118.3
9	120.4	120.4
10	124.8	124.7
23	127.9	28.1
14	135.2	135.0
22	136.2	35.7
4	137.9	137.8
11	−138.0	138.0
8	139.7	139.6
–*C*H = C	7	
>*C* = C	3	
$\Sigma(CH_X = C)$	10	
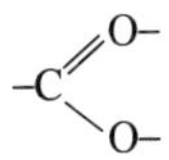	173.6	173.8
$\Sigma(CO_2)$	1	
overall Σ	48	

II. Chemical Properties

Avermectins are highly lipophilic substances and dissolve in most organic solvents, such as chloroform, methylene chloride, acetone, alcohols, toluene, cyclohexane, dimethylformamide, dimethylsulfoxide, and tetrahydrofuran. Their solubility in water is correspondingly low—only .006 to .009 ppm (= mg/l).

Chemical stability studies are easy to monitor by silicagel thin-layer chromatography (TLC) or by high-performance liquid chromatography (HPLC), most advantageously using a reverse-phase C_{18} coated column (Miller *et al.* 1979). HPLC peaks or TLC spots are visualized by their UV absorption at 245 nm; the TLC spots can also be detected by ceric sulfate or phosphomolybdic acid staining.

The well-known acid lability of 2-deoxy-glycosides predicts that the avermectins are acid-sensitive. They are stable in anhydrous glacial acetic acid solution at room temperature, but aqueous AcOH and more rapidly stronger acids such as dilute HC1, H_2SO_4, and p-toluenesulfonic acid in methanol solution cleave off the first sugar. Much stronger concentrations of methanolic or aqueous acids are necessary to hydrolyze off the second sugar to give the aglycone. Although the 5,7-dihydroxy-3,4-cyclohexene part of the molecule might be expected to be subject to dehydration to an aromatic derivative, this does not occur very readily, thus allowing the preparation of monosaccharides and aglycones in good yields.

The avermectins contain an acidic proton at the asymmetric C-2 next to the lactone carbonyl group. Treatment with a strong base such as methanolic potassium hydroxide, sodium methoxide, or 1,8-diazabicyclo [5.4.0] undec -7-ene (DBU) causes epimerization at that center and shifts the beta-gamma double bond into conjugation with the lactone carbonyl (Figure 1.3; from Pivnichny *et al.* 1983, 1988). Prolonged base treatment leads to aromatization of the 6-membered ring, opening of the lactone ring, and further degradation to a gross mixture of unidentified products. Anhydrous pyridine, however, even at temperatures up to 100° C, is without effect. Strongly basic conditions must be avoided during reactions of avermectins, but, consequently, strong alkali can be used to destroy avermectin residues for safe disposal.

UV light below 280 nm rapidly isomerizes the E (trans) 8,9 and 10,11 double bonds to the 8,9- and 10,11-Z isomers. Prolonged irradiation leads to a large number of unidentified decomposition products which lack any UV absorption (Figure 1.4; from Mrozik *et al.* 1988). Solutions of

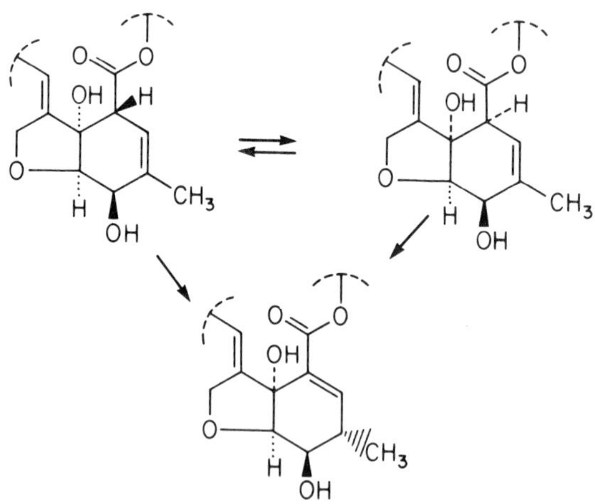

FIGURE 1.3. Treatment of ivermectin with methanolic potassium hydroxide solution. Adapted from J. Pivnichny et al. Copyright 1983 by The American Pharmaceutical Association. (Reprinted by permission of the copyright owner.)

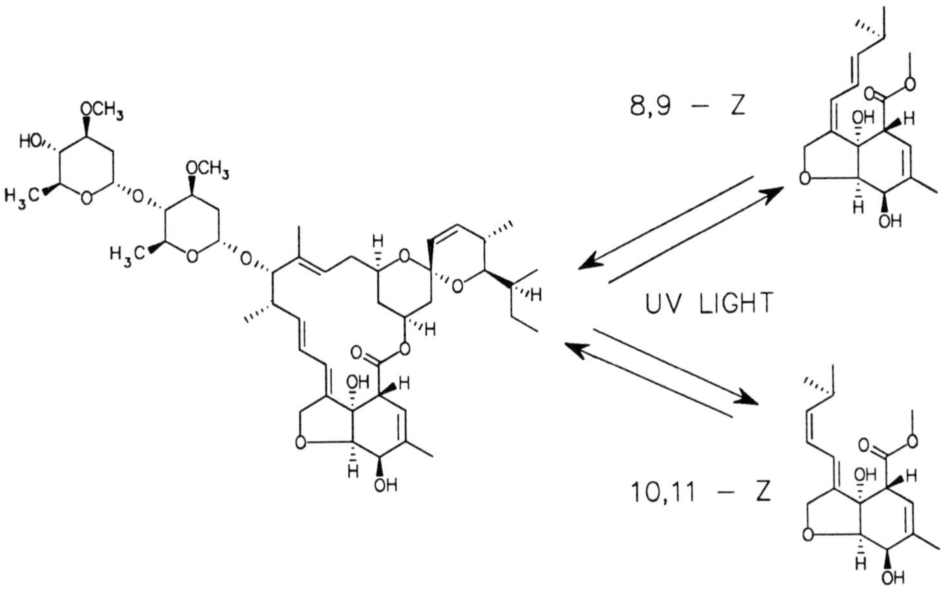

FIGURE 1.4. Photoisomerization of Avermectins. (Adapted from Mrozik et al. 1988.)

avermectins in pyrex flasks are generally stable because the glass excludes UV light.

III. Chemistry

A. Hydroxy Group Characteristics

Avermectin B_1 and ivermectin each contain 2 secondary and 1 tertiary hydroxy group. The 2 secondary alcohols are readily acetylated with acetic anhydride in pyridine, although at 0° C, the reaction yields a fair amount of the 4″- but not the 5-monoacetate. With more reactive acid chlorides, however, it is not possible to obtain the 4″-monoacyl derivative; moreover, it is necessary to protect the 5-OH as a 5-O-tertiary butyldimethysilyl (TBDMS) derivative, which can be prepared selectively due to the hindered C-4″ position (Mrozik *et al.* 1982a). Removal of the 5-protecting group is accomplished with p-toluenesulfonic acid monohydrate (p-TsOH × H_2O) in MeOH (1%, room temperature for 20 to 30 minutes; longer reaction times generate substantial amounts of monosaccharide) or with an HF-pyridine-THF mixture (Bliard *et al.* 1987). It is sometimes possible to prepare 5-monoacyl derivatives directly from unprotected ivermectin by careful use of 1 equivalent of acylation reagent, particularly when the latter is bulky (e.g., bis-trichloroethoxy phosphoryl chloride). Many 4″-O-substituted derivatives have been prepared, as they retain considerable bioactivities; whereas 5-O-substitution products lose most anthelmintic activities. Other protecting groups used advantageously include phenoxyacetyl (reversed by NaOMe in MeOH or NH_3 in MeOH) (Gallo *et al.* 1983) or trichloroethylcarbonate (reversed by zinc-AcOH reduction).

Because the avermectins exhibit unprecedented potency, they are used at unusually low doses of 6 to 300 μg/kg, which makes the detection and isolation of residues and metabolites from animal tissue a new challenge. For this reason a very sensitive analytical assay required a derivative suitable for detection at levels down to 1/10 or 1/100 of one ppm. Ivermectin and avermectin B_1 are therefore converted into an aromatic derivative which allows detection via fluorescence absorbance. For this purpose avermectin B_1, ivermectin, or their derivatives were heated with acetic anhydride (Ac_2O) in pyridine at 100° C for 24 hours (Tolan *et al.* 1980). The reaction time can be reduced to 1 hour by using N-methyl imidazole as a catalyst (Tway, Wood, and Downing 1981). The resultant 4″-O-acetyl-2,5,6,7-bisdehydro analog is detected after HPLC separation and characterized by a distinct retention time. Using a C_2-extraction cartridge, with 22,23-dihydro avermectin B_{1a} monosaccharide as an internal standard, it is possible to detect as little as 1 ng/ml of ivermectin in plasma or milk (Chiou, Stubbs, and Bayne 1987). This procedure was adapted as a confirmatory assay by hydrolysis of the avermectin derivatives to aglycone, monosaccharide, and parent disaccharide (vide infra), subsequent aromatization, and, finally, detection of 3 distinct HPLC peaks corresponding to the acetylated bisdehydro aglycone, monosaccharide, and parent compound peaks via fluorescence detection. A procedure using chemical ionization mass spectrometry/mass spectrometry (MS/MS) was developed for a confirmatory assay of ivermectin tissue residues in cattle (Tway *et al.* 1984). It is also possible to determine avermectins directly after extraction, using a synthetically isomerized avermectin derivative as internal standard for HPLC with UV detection (Pivnichny, Shim, and Zimmerman 1983). A HPLC-reverse isotope dilution assay is available for the determination of ivermectin residues in animal tissue (Chiu *et al.* 1985). A similar fluorescent derivative containing a 5-phenol group obtained by dehydration of the 5-keto derivative of ivermectin with ammonium acetate was also reported (Stong 1987).

B. Monosaccharides and Aglycones

The macrocyclic lactone of all avermectins has at carbon 13 an α-L-oleandrosyl-α-L-oleandrosyloxy substituent which is a 2-deoxy sugar glycoside; and as such it is relatively sensitive to acid hydrolysis or alcoholysis. A solution of ivermectin in methanol containing a strong acid such as 1% sulfuric acid readily gives a good yield of the aglycone after 16 to 24 hours at room temperature. When isopropanol is substituted for methanol in this reaction, a good yield of the monosaccharide is obtained, as the bulkier isopropanol preferentially attacks the sterically less hindered 1″-position over the 1'-position, which is attached directly to the C-13 of the macrocycle, which in turn is flanked on either side by the C-12 and C-14 methyl groups respectively (Figure 1.5; from Chabala *et al.* 1980). These procedures readily yield the monosaccharides of ivermectin and avermectin B_1 and the aglycone of ivermectin. The preparation of the aglycone of avermectin B_1, however, is complicated: under the reaction conditions, addition of methanol to the 22,23-double bond occurs, yielding mainly the 2 epimeric 22,23-dihydro-23-methoxy monosaccharides and/or aglycones. The aglycone of avermectin B_1 therefore must be prepared with aqueous acid; it can be obtained as a 1 : 1 mixture of aglycone and monosaccharide using 10% sulfuric acid in aqueous THF solution (Mrozik *et al.* 1982b).

Removal of the 13-hydroxy group from avermectin aglycones gives 13-deoxyavermectin aglycones which are closely related to certain milbe-

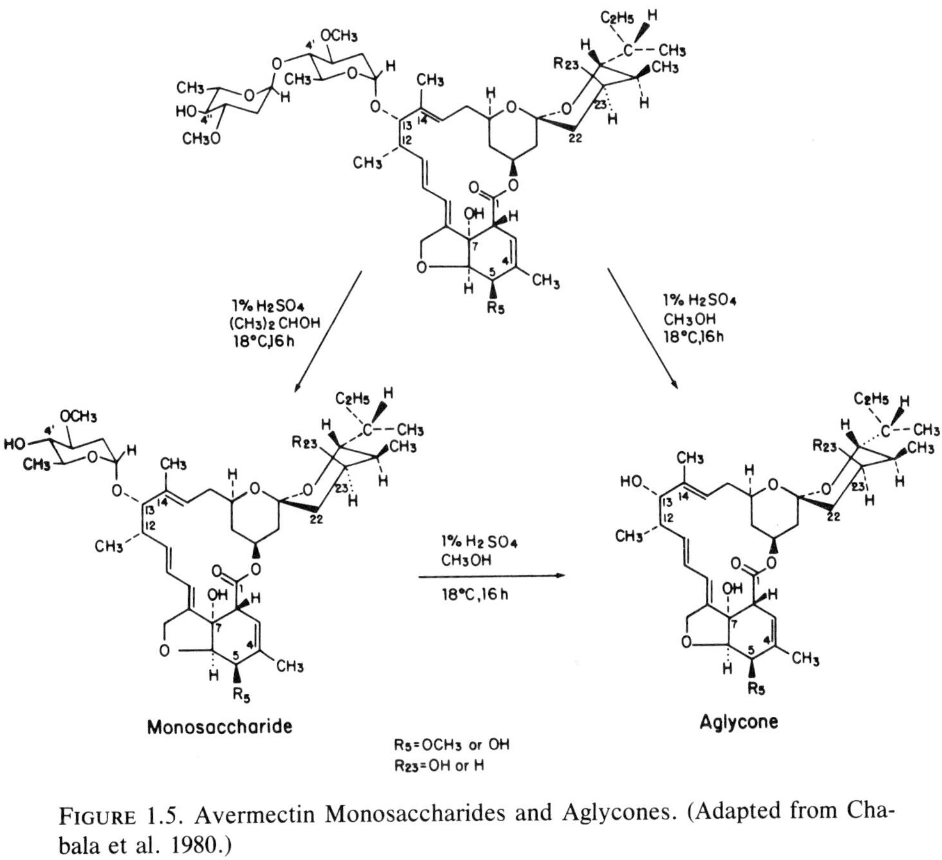

FIGURE 1.5. Avermectin Monosaccharides and Aglycones. (Adapted from Chabala et al. 1980.)

mycins. For example, ivermectin was converted into its aglycones (22,23-dihydroavermectin B_{1a} and B_{1b} aglycones): the 5-hydroxy group was then protected as an O-tert-butyldimethylsilyl group; then the 13-hydroxy group was substituted by chloro; the 13-chloro group was removed by reduction; C-5-OH deprotected; and, finally, the C-25 B_{1a} and B_{1b} homologs were separated into 13-deoxy-23,23-dihydroavermectin B_{1a} and B_{1b} aglycones (Mrozik *et al.* 1983). Interestingly, the latter was subsequently also obtained from a milbemycin fermentation and given the name milbemycin B41-D.

C. Oxidations

Avermectin B_1 and ivermectin have 2 secondary hydroxy groups susceptible to oxidation to the corresponding ketones. Due to the allylic nature of the C-5 hydroxy group, its selective oxidation to 5-oxoavermectin is readily accomplished with manganese dioxide (Chabala, Rosegay, and Walsh 1981). Although tautomerisation to the enol and elimination of the remaining tertiary C-7 hydroxy group leads to a phenol (Stong 1987), the 5-oxo derivatives are nonetheless stable enough to allow further chemical reactions. Particularly important is the stereospecific reduction with $NaBH_4$ to the 5-β alcohol with natural configuration, which is used to prepare tritiated avermectin derivatives (vide infra). Reaction with trifluoroacetic anhydride, however, gives the 2,5,6,7-tetradehydro phenol analog. Use of mild oxidation procedures such as oxalyl chloride-DMF (Swern oxidation) gives 4″,5-dioxo avermectin derivatives or—after protection of the C-5 hydroxy group as a tert-butyldimethylsilyl derivative—5-O-tert-butyldimethylsilyl-4″-oxoavermectins, which are valuable intermediates for further 4″-modified analogs. Sodium borohydrate reduction of the 4″-keto function gives a mixture of 4″-epimeric hydroxy compounds, with the unnatural axial 4″-hydroxy group the major product and the natural epimer the minor one. Reductive amination with $NaCNBH_3$ and NH_4OAc likewise yields an epimeric mixture of 4″-amino derivatives with interesting biological properties (Mrozik 1984a).

The avermectins also possess a number of allylic positions that are susceptible to oxidative modification. In particular the 8a methylene group—which is both allylic and α to an ether oxygen—is susceptible to radical oxidation. The primary product is the 8a-hydroperoxide, which has been isolated occasionally as an impurity of an avermectin B_1 reaction (such as the catalytic hydrogenation of avermectin B_1 with Wilkinson's rhodium chloride-triphenylphosphine catalyst to obtain ivermectin). An 8a-hydroxy derivative can also be detected occasionally as a metabolite (Bull *et al.* 1984) or as an impurity arising presumably by air oxidation. An 8a-oxo-derivative can be obtained by oxidizing 5-O-protected avermectins with pyridinium dichromate (Mrozik and Waksmunski 1985). This also can arise by treating the 8a-hydroperoxide with base.

The allylic 4a-methyl group can be oxidized with SeO_2-catalyzed tert-butylhydroperoxide to a 4a-hydroxy analog (Mrozik 1984b).

The double bonds of avermectins react with m-chloroperbenzoic acid to give 3,4-, 8,9-, and 14,15-epoxides. The 8,9-epoxide is the major product and can be isolated in good yield (Mrozik 1985a). The 8,9-oxide was opened by aqueous acids to the 8,9-diol (Figure 1.6; from Smith and Thompson 1985). The 3,4-diol can be obtained readily and regiospecifically by osmium tetroxide oxidation. Neither peracids nor OsO_4 will attack the 22,23-double bond. The 10,11-double bond can be oxidized selectively with N-bromacetamide to the 11,10-bromohydrin.

D. Reductions Including Ivermectin

Reductions of avermectin B_1 containing 5 double bonds with Pd or Pt catalysts proceed at almost comparable rates at the 2 disubstituted 10,11- and 22,23-double bonds to give a mixture of 10,11- and 22,23-dihydro derivatives. Further hydrogenation leads to 10,11,22,23-tetrahydro and 3,4,10,11,22,23-hexahydro derivatives; exhaustive hydrogenation leads to 3,4,8,9,10,11,22,23-octahydro analogs. Under no circumstances is the 14,15-double bond hydrogenated. For the preparation of ivermectin (22,23-dihydro avermectin B_1), Wilkinson's homogeneous $(Ph_3P)_3RhCl$ catalyst was employed for the regiospecific hydrogenation of avermectin B_1's 22,23-double bond, which is the only disubstituted cis double bond (Figure 1.7; from Chabala *et al.* 1980). To prepare 10,11-dihydro avermectin B_1, the regioselective reaction with N-bromacetamide was used to make a 11,10-bromohydrin, which can then be dehalogenated and deoxygenated to the desired product.

E. Radiolabeled Derivatives

Because ivermectin (= 22,23-dihydroavermectin B_1) is obtained by catalytic reduction of avermectin B_1 (vide infra), the same procedure using tritium gas conveniently affords tritiated ivermectin (22,23-^{3}[H]-

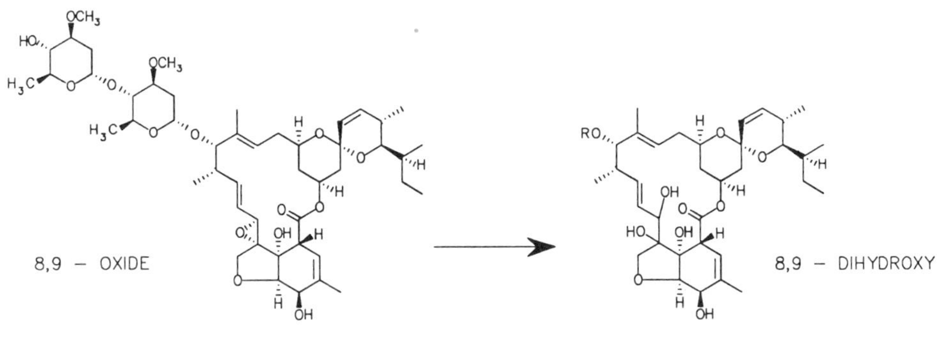

FIGURE 1.6. Avermectin B_1 8,9-oxide and its hydrolysis to the 8,9-diol. (Adapted from Smith 1985.)

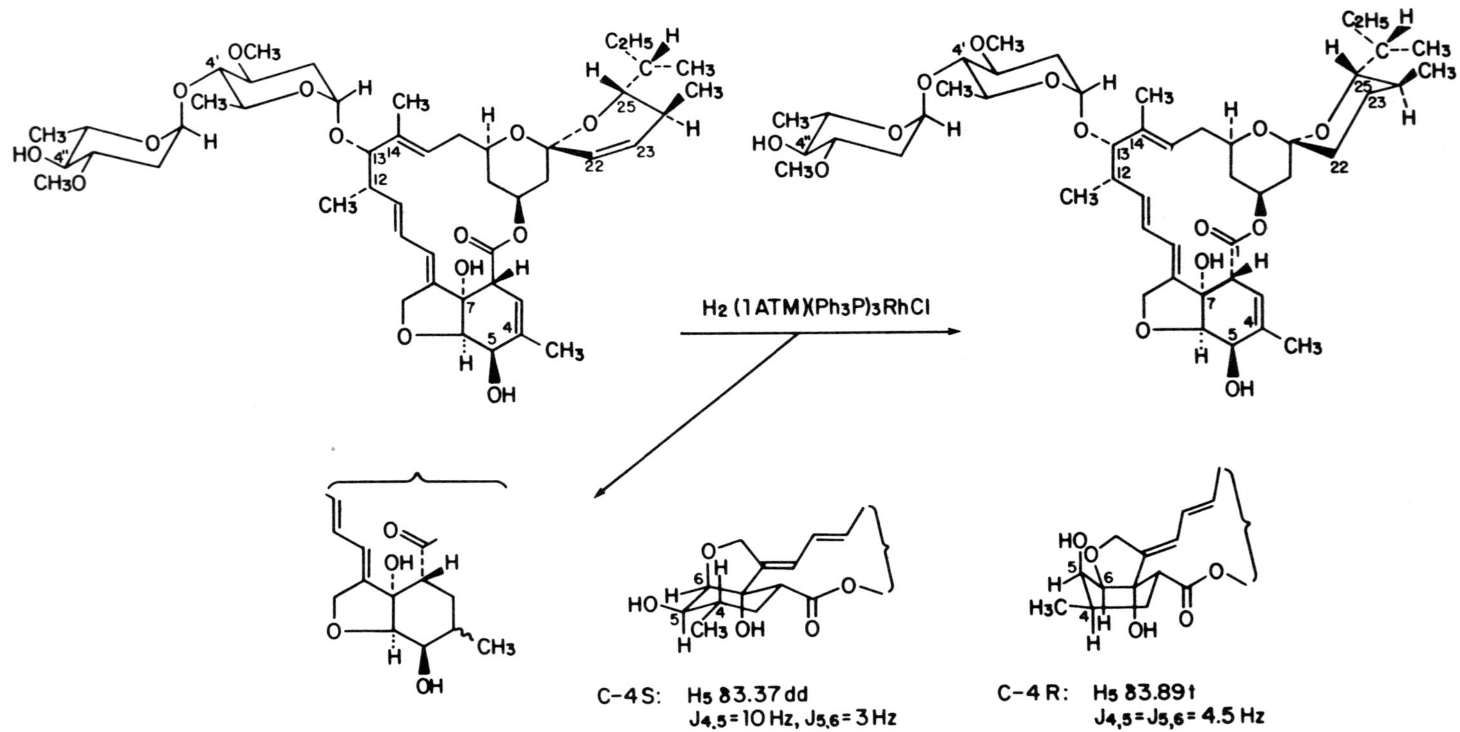

FIGURE 1.7. Synthesis of ivermectin by selective hydrogenation of avermectin B_1. (Adapted from Chabala et al. 1980.)

22,23-dihydroavermectin B_1). The preparation of a tritiated derivative containing a 22,23-double bond starts with the readily available 5-ketone, which is reduced with ^{3}[H]-sodiumborohydride stereospecifically to a 5-^{3}[H]-derivative (Chabala, Rosegay, and Walsh 1981). Carbon-14-labeled avermectins can be obtained by a biosynthetic process using sodium (1-^{14}C)propionate as labeled precurser (Ku and Hwang 1985).

F. Alkylations

Because avermectins are sensitive to strong base, alkylations are difficult. In the presence of silver oxide, however, the more reactive alkylating reagents (such as methyl iodide) react readily at the 5-hydroxy group, and more slowly at the remaining hydroxy groups (including the tertiary 7-hydroxy) (Fisher, Lusi, and Tolman 1980).

G. Interconversions of Avermectins

Methylation of avermectins B_1 and B_2 leads to the corresponding derivatives of the A series. A procedure involving the oxidation of the 5-methoxy group with mercuric acetate and NaBH4 reduction of the 5-keto-intermediate allows the conversion of the A to the B components (Mrozik, Eskola, and Fisher 1986). The 23-hydroxy group of the "2" components—after selective protection of the other secondary hydroxy groups—is converted to a thionocarbonate, which can be eliminated to give the 22,23-double bond of the "1" components; alternatively, it can be reduced with tributyltin hydride to the 22,23-dihydro derivatives (= ivermectins) (Mrozik, Eskola, and Fisher 1982).

H. Glycoside Syntheses

Avermectin aglycones, monosaccharides, and the naturally occurring disaccharides themselves have been further modified by attaching various sugars to the different hydroxy groups. Most of these methods have used 1-bromo sugars via the Königs-Knorr procedure (Fisher and Tolman 1979, 1980). More recently, the use of 1-phenylthio and 1-fluoro sugars has resulted in better yields of those glycosides (Nicolaou *et al.* 1984). There are also derivatives of avermectin B_1 containing fluoro groups in the sugars (Bliard *et al.* 1987). A mixture of the two anomeric methyl glycosides of oleandrose is obtained by acid methanolysis of avermectins, and these have been converted to L-oleandrose (Els, Celmer, and Murai 1958) and the 1-phenylthio glycoside (Nicolaou *et al.* 1984). The 4-α-L-oleandrosyl-L-oleandrose disaccharide was obtained through an oxidative degradation of avermectin B_1 (Hanessian *et al.* 1987). L-Oleandrose and the 4-alfa-L-oleandrosyl-L-oleandrose disaccharide was also obtained by total synthesis (Wuts and Bigelow 1983; Danishefsky *et al.* 1987).

IV. Structure–Activity

The avermectins, when administered orally to sheep, demonstrate activity against gastrointestinal parasites. A study was done to compare the anthelminitic activities of the principal naturally occurring avermectins, the monosaccharides and aglycones, and some reduced derivatives (Chabala *et al.* 1980). The data are shown in Table 1.3.

In general, compounds of the B-series, containing a 5-hydroxy group, are more potent than those of the A-series, containing a 5-methoxy group. The 1-series and 2-series have similar potency against many parasites, but the 2-series compounds showed some important deficiencies which made them less interesting. For example, avermectin B_2 was inactive against adult *Haemonchus contortus* in sheep at 0.1 mg/kg per os. Reduction of the 22,23-olefin had only a small effect on potency but conferred sufficient overall improvement in spectrum and safety that 22,23-dihydro avermectin B_1 was selected for commercial development under the nonproprietary name ivermectin. The monosaccharides were two to fourfold less active than the disaccharide, and dihydroavermectin B_1 aglycone was thirtyfold less potent.

A study of the activities of various acylated avermectins against *Trichostronglyus colubriformis* in gerbils is shown in Tables 1.4 and 1.5 (Mrozik *et al.* 1982a).

The 4″-O-acetates have the same potencies as the unsubstituted com-

TABLE 1.3. Activity of avermectin derivatives against adult gastrointestinal helminths of experimentally infected sheep on oral administration.

		Efficacy[a]					
Structure[b]	Dose, mg/kg	H.c.[c]	O.c.	T.a.	T.c.[a]	C.spp	O.c.
A_1	0.1	2	2	0	0	2	0
A_2	0.1	3	3	3	3	0	3
B_1	0.05	3	3	3	3	3	3
B_2	0.1	0	3	3	3	3	3
H_2A_1	0.3	3	2	0	1	0	3
H_2B_1	0.1	3	3	3	3	3	3
B_1MS	0.15	2	2	3	3	3	0
B_2MS	0.2	1	1	3	3	3	3
H_2B_1MS	0.3	3	3	3	3	2	3
H_2B_1AG	3.0	1	2	3	3	1	3
H_4B_1	0.2	0	0	1	0	0	3

[a] O = <50%, 1 = 50–74%, 2 = 75–90%, 3 = > 90% efficacy. Abbreviations used: *H.c., Haemonchus contortus; O.c., Ostertagia circumcinta; T.a., Trichostrongylus axei; T.c., Trichostrongylus colubriformis; C.spp., Cooperia spp; O.c., Oesophagostomum columbianum.*

[b] MS = monosaccharide, AG = aglycone, H_2 = 22,23-dihydro derivative, H_4 = 3,4,22,23-tetrahydro derivative. [c] Benzimidazole resistant.

TABLE 1.4. Derivatives of avermectin A_{2a} and B_{2a} and anthelmintic activity against *trichostrongylus colubriformis* in gerbils.

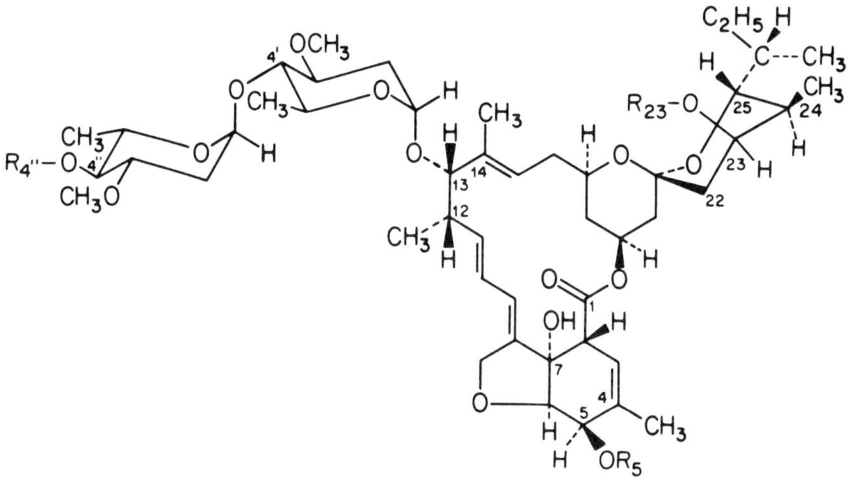

No.	R_4''	R_2	R_{23}	Anthelmintic act.[a]
1	H	CH_3	H	0.005
3	H	H	H	0.0125
4	CH_3CO	CH_3	H	0.0625
5	H	CH_3	CH_3CO	0.25
6	CH_3CO	CH_3	CH_3CO	0.5
10	CH_3CO	CH_3CO	CH_3CO	0.5

Reprinted from H. Mrozik *et al.* 1982a, by permission of The American Chemical Society.

pounds, whereas 5- and 23-acylation are generally detrimental to activity. In particular the 5-hydroxy group is essential for good anthelmintic activity, as illustrated by the diminished activity of the 5-methoxy and 5-O-t-butyldimethylsilyl derivatives.

The efficacy of acylated avermectins was also investigated against a broad spectrum of parasites in sheep as shown in Table 1.6 (Mrozik *et al.* 1982a).

The *T. colubriformis* sheep results closely parallel the relative potencies in gerbils.

The activities of avermectin B_1, its 2-epimer, and the conjugatively stabilized Δ^2 isomer were compared against the two-spotted spider mite (Pivnichny, Shim, and Zimmerman 1983). The data are shown in Table 1.7.

The 2-epimer is approximately $\frac{1}{100}$ as potent as avermectin B_1, whereas the Δ^2 isomer is $\frac{1}{5}$ as potent.

TABLE 1.5. Derivatives of avermectin B_{1a} and anthelmintic activity against *Trichostrongylus colubriformis* in gerbils[a].

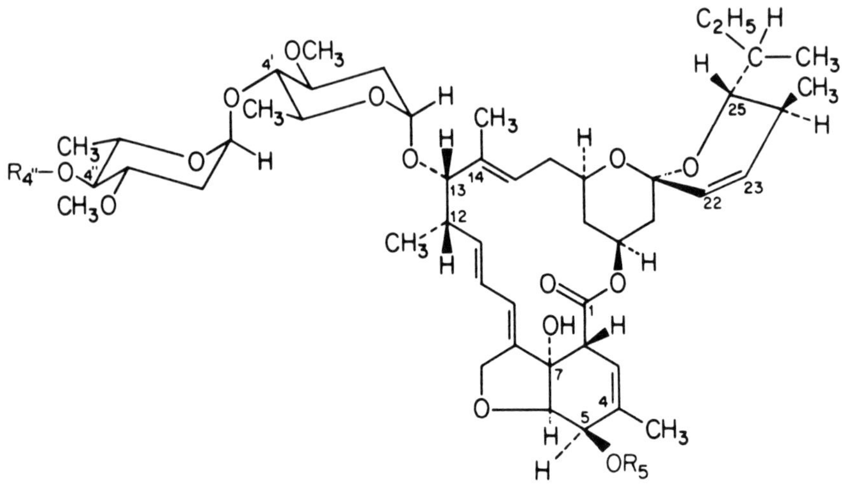

No.	R_4''	R_5	Anthelmintic act[b]
2	H	H	0.025
7	CH_3CO	H	0.031
8	H	CH_3CO	0.125
9	CH_3CO	CH_3CO	0.25
12	H	$SI(CH_3)_2C(CH_3)_3$	>2.5
13	$Si(CH_3)_2C(CH_3)_3$	$Si(CH_3)_2C(CH_3)_3$	>2.5
14	$(CH_3)_3CCO$	$Si(CH_3)_2C(CH_3)3$	
15	$(CH_3)_3CCO$	H	0.5
16	$CH_3(CH_2)_6CO$	$Si(CH_3)_2C(CH_3)_3$	
17	$CH_3(CH_2)_6CO$	H	0.125
18	$CCl_3CH_2OOCCH_2CH_2CO$	$Si(CH_3)_2C(CH_3)_3$	
19	$CCl_3CH_2OOCCH_2CH_2CO$	H	
20	$HOOCCH_2CH_2CO$	H	0.03
21	$(4\text{-}NO_2C_6H_4O)CO$	$Si(CH_3)_2C(CH_3)_3$	
22	H_2NCO	$Si(CH_3)_2C(CH_3)_3$	
23	H_2NCO	H	0.025
24	$(CH_3)_2NCO$	$Si(CH_3)_2C(CH_3)_3$	
25	$(CH_3)_2NCO$	H	0.06
26	$CH_3CONHCH_2CO$	$Si(CH_3)_2C(CH_3)_3$	
27	$CH_3CONHCH_2CO$	H	0.025

[a] From Mrozik *et al.* 1982a.

[b] Minimal doses (mg/kg needed to remove > 83% of the worm burden.

TABLE 1.6. Anthelmintic efficacy by oral administration in experimentally infected sheep[a].

See tables 4 & 5	Dose	No. of	H.c.		O.c.				C.o.		
treatment	mg/kg	sheep	EL_4	Adult	EL_4	Adult	T.a.	T.c.	EL_4	Adult	Oe.c.
none		6	(70)[b]	(442)	(1421)	(1137)	(2852)	(4110)	(193)	(1761)	(61)
1	0.1	3	3[c]	3	0	3	3	3	1	0	3
	0.05	3	2	2	0	2	2	2	1	0	2
	0.025	3	1	0	0	2	0	0	1	0	2
4	0.25	1		3		3	3	3		3	3
5	0.25	1		1		0	0	0		2	1
6	0.25	1		3		2	1	2		2	3
2	0.1	3	3	3	3	3	3	3	3	3	3
	0.05	3	3	3	3	3	3	3	3	3	3
	0.025	3	3	3	1	2	2	2	0	1	3
7	0.1	3		3	2	3	3	3	3	2	3
	0.05	3		3	0	3	3	3	2	0	3
	0.025	3		3	0	3	1	3	2	0	3
9	0.25	1		3		3	3	3		3	3
	0.15	2		3	1	3	3	3		3	3
20	0.1sc	1		3		0	2	3	3[d]	3[d]	3

[a] H.c. = *Haemonchus contortus;* O.c. = *Ostertagia circumcincta;* T.a. = *Trichostrongylus axei;* T.c. = *Trichostrongylus colubriformis;* C.o. = *Cooperia oncophora;* Oe.c. = *Oseophagostomum columbianum.*

[b] Geometric mean of the number of worms per untreated experimentally infected lamb, representative of "typical" infections encountered under standard experimental procedures.

[c] 3 = > 90% efficacy; 2 = 60–89% efficacy; 1 = 20–59% efficacy; 0 = 0–19% efficacy.

[d] *C. curticei.*

TABLE 1.7. Efficacy of avermectin isomers against *Tetranichus urticae* in a foliage assay on bean leaves.

Compound	Mortality, %					
	6.25 ppm	1.25 ppm	0.25 ppm	0.05 ppm	0.01 ppm	LC_{90} ppm
1				100	66	0.038
2	100	78	17	3		4.0
3	100	100	97	35		0.23

1: Avermectin B_1; 2: the 2-epimer, 3: the conjugatively stabilized Δ^2 isomer
Adapted from Pivnichny *et al.* 1988.

It has been reported elsewhere (Fisher 1985) that the aromatic derivative of avermectin B_1 is devoid of biological activity.

A comparison of the activities of avermectins in anthelmintic, miticidal, and insecticidal assays has been reported Mrozik 1985b). The results are shown in Table 1.8.

These data illustrate the complex structure–activity relationships among the avermectins when measured over several species. For example, while 22,23-dihydroavermectin B_1 monosaccharide is three to four-fold less active than avermectin B_1 against helminths, it is sixteen fold more active than avermectin B_1 against the southern armyworm.

TABLE 1.8. Biological activities of abamectin and ivermectin monosaccharide and aglycone derivatives.

Avermectins	In vivo anthelmintic assay ED_{90} (mg/kg)[a]	Two-spotted spider mite assay EC_{90} (ppm)[b]	Southern armyworm assay EC_{90} (ppm)[c]
B_1 (abamectin)	0.03	0.03	8.0
B_1-monosaccharide	0.1	<0.01	8.0
13-deoxy-B_1-aglycone	0.06	<0.005	—
22,23-dihydro-B_1(ivermectin)	0.03	0.05	8.0
22,23-dihydro-B_1 monosaccharide	0.1		0.5
22,23-dihydro-B_1 aglycone	0.2	>0.1	—
13-deoxy-22,23-dihydro-B_1-aglycone	0.06	0.05	0.5

Adapted from Mrozik 1985b.

REFERENCES

Albers-Schönberg G, Arison BH, Chabala JC, Douglas, AW, Eskola P, Fisher MH, Lusi A, Mrozik H, Smith JL, Tolman RL (1981) Avermectins. Structure determination. *J. Am. Chem. Soc.* 103:4216–4221

Bliard C, Escribano FC, Lukacs G, Olesker A, Sarda P (1987) Synthesis of

C-2″beta- and C-2″alfa-fluoro avermectin B_{1a}. *J. Chem. Soc., Chem. Commun.* 386–370

Bull DL, Ivie GW, MacConnell JG, Gruber VF, Ku CC, Arison BH, Stevenson JM, VandenHeuvel WJA (1984) Fate of avermectin B_1a in soil and plants. *J. Agric. Food Chem.* 32:94–102

Chabala JC, Mrozik H, Tolman RL, Eskola P, Lusi A, Peterson LH, Woods MF, Fisher MH (1980) Ivermectin, a new broad-spectrum antiparasitic agent. *J. Med. Chem.* 23:1134–1136

Chabala JC, Rosegay A, Walsh MAR (1981) Tritium labeling of avermectins B_1a and B_2a via stereoselective reduction of 5-ketoavermectins. *J. Agric. Food Chem* 29:881–884

Chiou R, Stubbs RJ, Bayne WF (1987) Determination of ivermectin in human plasma and milk by high-performance liquid chromatography with fluorescence detection. *J. Chromatogr.* 416:196–202

Chiu SHL, Buhs RP, Sestokas E, Taub R, Jacob TA (1985) Determination of ivermectin residue in animal tissue by high-performance liquid chromatography–reverse isotope dilution assay. *J. Agric. Food Chem.* 33:99–102

Danishefsky SJ, Selnick HG, Armistead DM, Wincott FE (1987) The total synthesis of avermectin Ala. New protocols for the synthesis of novel 2-deoxypyranose systems and their axial glycosides. *J. Am. Chem. Soc.* 109:8119–8120

Davies HG, Green RH (1986) Avermectins and milbemycins. Nat. Prod. Rep. 3:87–121

Els H, Celmer WD, Murai K (1958) Oleandomycin (PA-105). II. Chemical characterization (I). *J. Am. Chem. Soc.* 80:3777–3782

Fisher MH (1985) *Recent Advances in the Chemistry of Insect Control.* Janes NF (ed), Royal Soc. of Chem. Special Publication No. 53, p. 53

Fisher MH, Lusi A, Tolman RL (1980) Alkyl derivatives of C-076 compounds. U.S. Patent 4,200,581

Fisher MH, Mrozik H (1984) The avermectin family of macrolide-like antibiotics. In Omura S (ed), *Macrolide Antibiotics,* Academic Press, New York, pp 553–606

Fisher MH, Tolman RL (1979) Carbohydrate derivatives of milbemycins and processes therefor. U.S. Patent 4,134,973

Fisher MH, Tolman RL (1980) Sugar derivatives of C-076 compounds. U.S. Patent 4,203,976

Gallo VP, Kempf AJ, MacConnell J, Mrozik H, Arison B, Putter I (1983) The microbial formation of the 23-keto derivative from avermectin B_{2a} in soil. *Pestic. Sci.* 14:153–157

Hanessian S, Ugolini A, Hodges PJ, Beaulieu P, Dube D, Andre C (1987) Progress in natural product chemistry by the chiron and related approaches—synthesis of avermectin B_{1a}. *Pure & Appl. Chem.* 59:299–316

Ku CC, Hwang SC (1985) The preparation of carbon-14 labeled avermectin B1a. *J. Labelled Compd. Radiopharm.* 22:451–459

Miller TW, Chaiet L, Cole DJ, Cole LJ, Flor JE, Goegelman RT, Gullo VP, Joshua H, Kempf AJ, Krellwitz WR, Monaghan RL, Ormond RE, Wilson KE, Albers-Schönberg G, Putter I (1979) Avermectins, new family of potent antihelminthic agents: isolation and chromatographic properties. *Antimicrob. Agents Chemother.* 15:368–371

Mishima H, Kurabayashi M, Tamura C, Sato S, Kuwano H, Saito A (1975) Structures of Milbemycin betal, beta2, and beta3. *Tetrahedron Lett.* 711–714

Mrozik H (1984a) 4″-keto- and 4″-amino-4″-deoxy avermectin compounds and substituted amino derivatives thereof. U.S. Patent 4,427,663

Mrozik H (1984b) 4a-Substituted avermectin compounds. U.S. Patent 4,457,920

Mrozik H (1985a) Avermectin epoxide derivatives and method of use. U.S. Patent 4,530,921

Mrozik H, (1985b) *Chemistry and Biological Activities of Avermectin Derivatives in Biotechnology and Its Application to Agriculture.* Copping L (ed), British Crop Protection Council (BCPC) Monograph No. 32, pp. 133–143.

Mrozik H, Chabala JC, Eskola P, Matzuk A, Waksmunski F, Woods M, Fisher MH (1983) Synthesis of milbemycins from avermectins. *Tetrahedron Lett.* 24:5333–5336

Mrozik H, Eskola P, Arison BH, Albers-Schönberg G, Fisher MH (1982b) Avermectin aglycones. *J. Org. Chem.* 47:489–492

Mrozik H, Eskola P, Fisher MH (1982) Partial syntheses of avermectin B_{1a} and ivermectin from avermectin B_{2a}. *Tetrahedron Lett.* 23:2377–2378

Mrozik H, Eskola P, Fisher MH (1986) Mercuric acetate oxidation of avermectin A_{2a} as a route to the selective cleavage of the allylic C-5-methoxy group. *J. Org. Syn.* 51:3058–3059

Mrozik H, Eskola P, Fisher MH, Egerton JR, Cifelli S, Ostlind DA (1982a) Avermectin acyl derivatives with antihelminthic activity. *J. Med. Chem.* 25:658–663

Mrozik H, Eskola P, Reynolds GF, Arison BH, Smith GM, Fisher MH (1988) Photoisomers of avermectins. *J. Org. Chem.* 53:1820–1823

Mrozik H, Waksmunski FS (1985) C-8a-oxo-avermectin and milbemycin derivatives, pharmaceutical compositions and method os use. U.S. Patent 4,547,491

Nicolaou KC, Dolle RE, Papahatjis DP, Randall JL (1984) Practical synthesis of oligosaccharides. Partial synthesis of avermectin B_{1a}. *J. Am. Chem. Soc.* 106:4189–4192

Pivnichny JV, Arison BH, Preiser FA, Shim JSK, Mrozik H (1988) Base-catalyzed isomerisation of avermectins. *J. Agric. Food Chem.* 36:826–828.

Pivnichny JV, Shim JSK, Zimmerman LA (1983) Direct determination of avermectins in plasma at nanogram levels by high-performance liquid chromatography. *J. Pharm. Sci.* 72:1447–1450

Smith AB III, Thompson AS (1985) Avermectin-milbemycin studies. 2. An efficient chemical degradation of avermectin B_{1a}. *Tetrahedron Lett.* 26:4279–4282

Springer JP, Arison BH, Hirshfield JM, Hoogsteen K (1981) The absolute stereochemistry and configuration of avermectin B_{2a} aglycon and avermectin B_{1a}. *J. Am. Chem. Soc.* 103:4221–4224

Stong JD (1987) Determination of ivermectin by Fluorescence Derivatization. *Anal. Chem.* 59:266–270

Takiguchi Y, Mishima H, Okuda M, Terao M, Aoki A, Fukuda R (1980) Milbemycins, a new family of macrolide antibiotics: Fermentation, isolation and physico-chemical properties. *J. Antibiot.* 33:1120–1127

Tolan JW, Eskola P, Fink DW, Mrozik H, Zimmerman LA (1980) Determination of avermectins in plasma at nanogram levels using high-performance liquid chromatography with fluorescence detection. *J. Chromatogr.* 190:367–376

Tway PC, Downing GV, Slayback JRB, Rahn GS, Isensee RK (1984) Confirmatory assay for ivermectin in cattle tissue using chemical ionization mass spectrometry/mass spectrometry (MS/MS). *Biomed. Mass Spectrom.* 11:172–176

Tway PC, Wood JS, Downing GV (1981) Determination of ivermectin in cattle and sheep tissues using high-performance liquid chromatography with fluorescence detection. *J. Agric. Food Chem.* 29:1049–1063

Wuts PGM, Bigelow SS (1983) Total synthesis of oleandrose and the avermectin disaccharide, benzyl alfa-L-oleandrosyl-alfa-L-4-acetoxyoleandroside. *J. Org. Chem.* 48:3489–3493

CHAPTER 2

Isolation and Characterization of the Producing Organism

R.W. Burg and E.O. Stapley

Of the several thousand fermentation products that had been described through 1978, only a few were reported to have anthelmintic activity. Among these were anthelmycin, anthelvencin, the antibiotic complex S-15-1, aspiculomycin, the axenomycins, G-418, hygromycin B, the destomycins, myxin, paromomycin, and the thaimycins. Only hygromycin B has been used commercially; and, until the last decade, synthetic compounds dominated the anthelmintic market. The discovery of the avermectins changed that dramatically.

I. Source of *Streptomyces avermitilis* and Discovery of the Avermectins

The microorganism that produces the avermectins was isolated from a soil sample collected near a golf course at Kawana, Ito City, Shizuoka Prefecture, Japan. Research scientists at the Kitasato Institute in Tokyo, under the direction of Dr. Satoshi Omura, isolated this culture. This group is noted for its skill in isolating exceptional microorganisms from soil; and, as part of a joint research project between the Kitasato Institute and Merck Sharp & Dohme Research Laboratories (MSDRL), the cultures isolated at the Kitasato Institute are tested in MSDRL's screening programs. These cultures quickly gained a reputation for being a rich source of new activities, and they are used to test many new screening assays. One of the new assays being developed at MSDRL was based on the administration of test substances to mice infected with *Nematospiroides dubius*, and it was decided to test all of the Kitasato cultures in that assay.

The avermectin-producing strain was among one group of 50 Kitasato cultures grown at MSDRL and screened by the *N. dubius* assay. This strain, originally designated OS-3153, was active but quite toxic in the first assay and in a confirmatory assay. In subsequent tests, however, this culture exhibited good activity with little or no toxicity. The unknown activity received the code designation C-076, and the culture was entered into the MSDRL culture collection as MA-4680. Several accounts of the discovery of the avermectins have been published (Burg *et al.* 1979; Campbell *et al.* 1984; Stapley and Woodruff 1982; and Woodruff and Burg 1986).

II. Taxonomy of *Streptomyces avermitilis*

The taxonomy of the producing organism, MA-4680, was established using the classical method of Shirling and Gottlieb (1966) and a number of published taxonomic keys (Buchanan and Gibbons 1974; Shirling and Gottlieb 1968a, 1968b, 1969, 1972; Waksman 1961). The taxonomic description has been published (Burg *et al.* 1979) as follows:

Taxonomic studies of culture MA-4680 revealed it to be a *Streptomyces* species with sporophore forming spirals as side branches on aerial mycelia. The spirals are compact but become open as the culture ages (Figure 2.1). Spores were in chains of more than 15 and were usually spherical to oval. The spore surface was smooth as revealed by electron microscopy (Figure 2.2). Sporulation occurred on oatmeal agar, glycerol-asparagine agar, inorganic salts-starch agar, and egg albumin agar. The culture grew well at 28° and 37° C but not at 50° C. These characteristics, plus those summarized in Tables 2.1 and 2.2, were compared with those of known species in the classical references. . . . No *Streptomyces* species

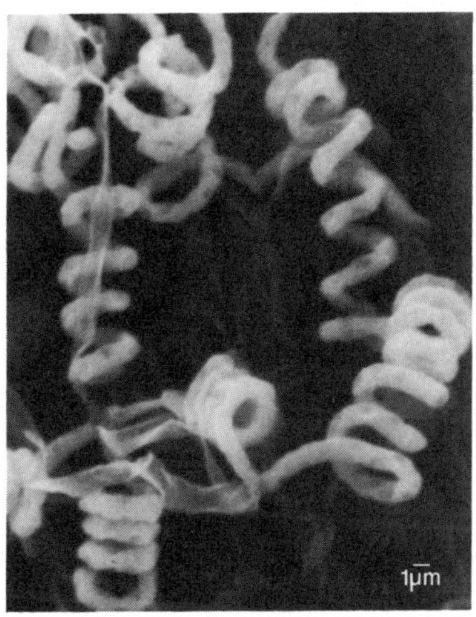

FIGURE 2.1. Scanning electron micrograph of *S. avermitilis* MA-4680 showing sporophores forming compact to open spirals.

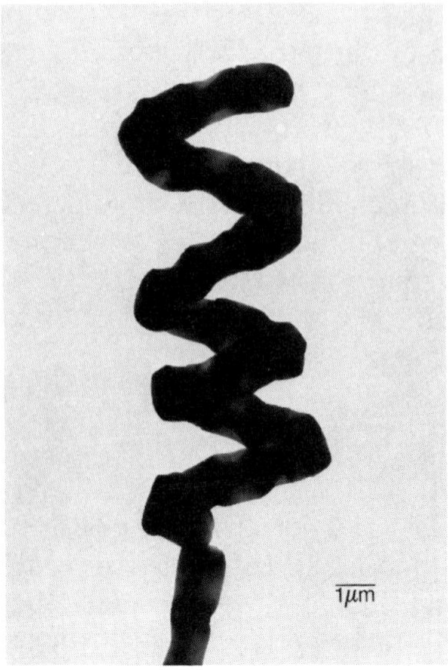

FIGURE 2.2. Transmission electron micrograph of *S. avermitilis* MA-4680 showing a sporophore with an open spiral and the smooth surface of the spherical to oval spores.

is described as having the brownish-gray spore mass color, smooth spore surface, spiral sporophore structure, production of melanoid pigments and cultural and carbon utilization patterns that together comprise the distinctive species *S. avermitilis*.

The culture was named *Streptomyces avermitilis* because of its ability to produce anthelmintic activity.

III. Isolation of the Avermectins

The avermectins were isolated by solvent extraction from the mycelia, solvent partition, and column chromatography on Sephadex LH-20 (Miller *et al.* 1979). Early work on the isolation of the avermectins proceeded slowly since it had to be guided by the mouse assay. During the isolation, the active extracts were monitored by specrophotometry; and the isolation chemists soon realized that the anthelmintic activity was correlated with a characteristic ultraviolet absorption spectrum (Miller *et al.* 1979). The examination of highly concentrated preparations by thin-layer chromatography (TLC) revealed the presence of four active components that quenched under ultraviolet light. This TLC assay guided the subsequent isolation and early work on improvement of the fermentation (Burg *et al.* 1979). Rapid progress in both areas followed the development of this physical assay. Further improvements in the assay by the use of high-performance liquid chromatography (HPLC) led to the identification and ultimate isolation of the 8 different compounds that comprise the original avermectins (Miller *et al.* 1979).

TABLE 2.1. Cultural characteristics of *S. avermitilis* MA-4680 (NRRL 8165)[a] [Burg *et al.* 1979].

Medium	Vegetative growth	Aerial mycelia	Soluble pigment
Oatmeal agar (ISP medium 3)[b]	Reverse-very dark brown	Powdery, brownish gray (41i)[c] mixed with white	Brown
Czapek-Dox agar	Poor, colorless	Scant, grayish	Light grayish tan
Egg albumin agar	Tan	Moderate, light grayish yellowish brown (3ge)[c] mixed with white	Light yellowish brown
Glycerol-asparagine agar (ISP medium 5)[b]	Reverse-yellowish brown	Powdery, brownish gray (41i)[c] mixed with white	Light yellowish brown
Inorganic salts-starch agar (ISP medium 4)[b]	Reverse-grayish-yellowish brown	Powdery, light brownish gray (4ig)[c] edged with darker brownish gray (41i)[c]	Light yellowish brown
Yeast extract–dextrose–salts agar	Reverse-dark brown	Moderate, brownish white	Brown
Yeast extract–malt extract agar (ISP medium 2)[b]	Reverse-dark brown	Moderate, brownish white	Brown
Peptone-iron–yeast extract agar	Dark brown	None	Dark brown to black
Nutrient agar	Tan	Sparse, grayish	Light brown
Nutrient starch agar	Tan	Sparse, grayish white	Light brown
Nutrient gelatin agar	Tan	Sparse, grayish white	Light brown
Gelatin stab	Brown ring	None	Greenish brown
Skim milk agar	Dark brown	None	Dark brown
Litmus milk	Dark brown growth ring	None	Dark brown
Skim milk	Dark brown growth ring	None	Dark brown
Potato plug	Tan	Brown mixed with grayish white	Grayish brown
Loeffler blood serum	Grayish tan	None	Some browning of medium
Nutrient tyrosine agar	Reverse-dark brown to black	Sparse, grayish	Dark brown

[a] All readings taken after 3 weeks at 28° C.
[b] See Shirling and Gottlieb 1966
[c] Color number designations were taken from *Color Harmony Manual,* 4th ed., Container Corp. of America, Chicago, 1958.

TABLE 2.2. Physiological properties of *S. avermitilis* MA-4680 (NRRL 8165) [Burg *et al.* 1979].

Characteristic	Observation[a]
Carbohydrate utilization[b]	Good growth: glucose, arabinose, fructose, inositol, lactose, maltose, mannitol, mannose, raffinose, rhamnose, sucrose, xylose No growth: cellulose
Melanin production[c]	Positive
H_2S production[c]	Positive
Hydrolysis of starch[d]	Good
Liquefaction of gelatin[e]	Good
Hydrolysis of casein[f]	Good
Peptonization of milk[g]	Complete, becoming alkaline (pH 8)
Liquefaction of Loeffler blood serum	None
Decomposition of tyrosine[h]	None

[a] All readings were taken after 3 weeks at 28° C.
[b] Pridham-Gottlieb basal medium plus 1% carbon source (Shirling and Gottlieb 1966)
[c] Peptone-iron–yeast extract agar (Shirling and Gottlieb 1966)
[d] Nutrient starch agar (Waksman 1961)
[e] Nutrient gelatin agar; gelatin stab (Waksman 1961)
[f] Skim milk agar (Waksman 1961)
[g] Litmus milk; skim milk (Waksman 1961)
[h] Nutrient tyrosine agar (Waksman 1961)

IV. Antibacterial and Antifungal Activity

The antibacterial spectrum of whole broth was assayed early in the study of *S. avermitilis*. The results of these first assays of the culture grown on two media (KH and JH), along with a similar assay of abamectin performed at a later date, are shown in Table 2.3 (SB Zimmerman 1975, 1984: private communication). The whole broth exhibited no detectable antibacterial activity except as a zone against *Bordetella bronchiseptica* (MB-965), an extremely sensitive bacterium. From the anthelmintic activity, the KH broth was estimated to contain at least 9 μg/ml of avermectins (Burg *et al.* 1979). The JH broth had only slight anthelmintic activity. At 500 μg/ml, abamectin gave small zones against *Bacillus* sp. 633 and *Micrococcus luteus*. At 1 mg/ml, a few other bacterial strains began to exhibit sensitivity. It is safe to conclude that the avermectins do not have significant antibacterial activity except at extremely high concentrations. Extensive studies have failed to discover any microorganism that could be used to assay for the avermectins.

The antifungal spectrum of whole broth was not determined as early in the studies of *S. avermitilis* (MA-4680), although a later isolate, *S. avermitilis* MA-5856, produced considerable activity against filamentous fungi. Table 2.4 illustrates the antifungal activity of *S. avermitilis* MA-5856 and the insignificant antifungal activity of pure abamectin (G

TABLE 2.3. Antibacterial activity of OS-3153 and abamectin.

Bacterium[a]	Zone diameter (mm)			
	OS-3153[b]		Abamectin[c]	
	KH med.	JH med.	0.5 mg/ml	1.0 mg/ml
Alcaligenes faecalis MB-10	0	0	–[d]	–
Bacillus sp. MB-633	0	0	9	0
Bacillus subtilis MB-964	0	0	0	0
Bordetella bronchiseptica MB-965	13H[e]	20	0	0
Comamonas terrrigena MB-1272	0	0	0	0
Comamonas terrigena MB-2566	0	0	0	0
Corynebacterium pseudodiphtheriticum MB-261	0	0	0	0
Enterobacter aerogenes MB-835	0	0	0	0
Erwinia carotovora subsp. *atroseptica* MB-1159	0	0	0	0
Escherichia coli MB-1418	0	0	0	0
Escherichia coli MB-1594	0	0	0	0
Escherichia coli MB-60	0	0	0	0
Klebsiella pneumoniae MB-1264	0	0	0	0
Micrococcus luteus MB-1011	0	0	10	10
Proteus mirabilis MB-3126	–	–	0	0
Proteus vulgaris MB-1012	0	0	–	0
Proteus vulgaris MB-2112	0	0	0	0
Proteus vulgaris MB-838	0	0	0	0
Pseudomonas aeruginosa MB-2824	0	0	0	0
Pseudomonas aeruginosa MB-979	0	0	0	0
Pseudomonas stutzeri MB-1231	0	0	0	0
Salmonella gallinarum MB-1287	0	0	0	0
Serratia marcescens MB-252	0	0	0	0
Staphylococcus aureus MB-1909	0	0	–	–
Staphylococcus aureus MB-2756	0	0	0	13
Staphylococcus aureus MB-108	0	0	0	12
Staphylococcus aureus MB-2949	0	0	–	–
Staphylococcus aureus MB-2983	0	0	0	13
Staphylococcus aureus MB-3032	0	0	0	12
Staphylococcus aureus MB-698	0	0	–	–
Streptococcus agalactiae MB-2875	0	0	0	0
Streptococcus faecalis MB-753	0	0	–	–
Streptococcus faecium MB-2820	0	0	0	0
Streptomyces sp. MA-4798	–	–	0	0
Xanthomonas campestris pv. *vesicatoria* MB-815	0	0	0	0

[a] All cultures were grown on nutrient agar + 0.2% yeast extract except *Streptococcus faecium* MB-2820 and *Streptococcus agalactiae* MB-2875, which were grown on brain heart infusion agar. Incubation was at 25° or 37° C.
[b] Filter paper discs (6.2 mm) were dipped into whole broth and applied to the assay plates.
[c] Filter paper discs (6.2 mm) were dipped into acetone solutions of abamectin. The disks were air dried before applying them to the assay plates.
[d] Not determined.
[e] H = hazy zone

TABLE 2.4. Antifungal activity of MA-5865 and abamectin.

Organism	Zone diameter (mm)[a]	
	MA5856[b]	Abamectin[c] 1.0 mg/ml
Filamentous fungi		
Alternaria solani MF-3550	20F	11H
Aspergillus niger MF-442	19F	0
Aspergillus niger MF-11	15F	0
Botrytis allii MF-3587	11H	0
Cephalosporium sp. MF-4641	13F	0
Ceratocystis ulmi MF-4042	19F	0
Cladosporium sp. MF-5015	0	0
Cochliobolus miyabeanus MF-4626	23F	16F
Fusarium oxysporum MF-4014	13H	0
Penicillium sp. MF-5020	10H	0
Penicillium sp. MF-5016	15F	0
Penicillium sp. MF-5014	17F	0
Phoma sp. MF-4332	20F	0
Scopulariopsis communis MF-3769	0	0
Trichoderma lignorum MF-3560	17H	0
Trichoderma sp. MF-4064	18F	0
Ustilago maydis MF-1996	14	0
Verticillium serrae MF-3794	0	0
Yeasts		
Brettanomyces bruxellensis MY-315	–	0
Candida albicans MY-992	15H	0
Candida albicans MY-1099	–	0
Candida albicans MY-1028	–	9V
Candida guilliermondi MY-1019	–	0
Candida pseudotropicalis MY-1100	–	0
Candida rugosa MY-1022	–	0
Candida tropicalis MY-1012	–	0
Cryptococcus albidus MY-1070	–	0
Cryptococcus laurentii MY-1073	–	0
Cryptococcus laurentii MY-1077	–	0
Cryptococcus laurentii MY-1074	–	8V
Kluyvermyces fragilis MY-1113	–	0
Saccharomyces cerevisiae MY-34	–	0
Saccharomyces cerevisiae MY-410	–	0
Torulopsis glabrata MY-1062	–	0
Torulaspora hansenii MY-321	–	0

[a] F = Fuzzy edge, S = Slightly hazy, H = Hazy, V = Very hazy, – = Not determined.

[b] Whole broth was applied to 6.2 mm filter paper discs.

[c] Abamectin in 25% aqueous DMSO was applied to 6.2 mm filter paper discs (25 ul/disc) and air dried before applying to the seeded assay plates.

Garrity 1988: private communication). A report that avermectin had antifungal activity (Calcott and Fatig 1984) proved erroneous, probably due to the authors' use of a crude avermectin preparation. In refuting this work, Onishi and Miller (1985) reported that pure avermectin B_{1a} lacks any detectable antifungal activity at 400 μg/ml and that *S. avermitilis* produces both a polyene and oligomycin. In fact, the first paper on the avermectins (Figure 2 in Burg *et al.* 1979) described a "Peak D" on a densitometer tracing of a thin-layer chromatogram of a mycelial extract of *S. avermitilis* MA-4680 as "a fermentation product unrelated to the avermectins." This product had already been identified as oligomycin (T Miller 1976: personal communication).

References

Buchanan RE, Gibbons NE (eds) (1974) *Bergey's Manual of Determinative Bacteriology,* 8th ed, The Williams & Wilkins Co., Baltimore

Burg RW, Miller BM, Baker EE, Birnbaum J, Currie SA, Hartman R, Kong Y-L, Monaghan RL, Olson G, Putter I, Tunac JB, Wallick H, Stapley EO, Oiwa R, Omura S (1979) Avermectins, new family of potent anthelmintic agents: producing organism and fermentation. *Antimicrob. Agents Chemother.* 15:361–367

Calcott PH, Fatig RO III (1984) Inhibition of chitin metabolism by avermectin in susceptible organisms. *J. Antibiot.* 37:253–259

Campbell WC, Burg RW, Fisher MH, Dybas RA (1984) The discovery of ivermectin and other avermectins. In Magee PS, Kohn GK, Menn JJ (eds), *Pesticide Synthesis through Rational Approaches,* American Chemical Society, Washington, DC, pp 5–20

Miller TW, Chaiet L, Cole DJ, Cole LJ, Flor JE, Goegelman RT, Gullo VP, Joshua H, Kempf AJ, Krellwitz WR, Monaghan RL, Ormaond RE, Wilson KE, Albers-Schönberg G, Putter I (1979) Avermectins, new family of potent anthelmintic agents: isolation and chromatographic properties. *Antimicrob. Agents Chemother.* 15:368–371

Onishi JC, Miller TW (1985) The lack of antifungal activity by avermectin B_{1a}. *J. Antibiotics* 38:1568–1572

Shirling EB, Gottlieb D (1966) Methods for characterization of *Streptomyces* species. *Int. J. Syst. Bacteriol.* 16:313–340

Shirling EB, Gottlieb D (1968a) Cooperative description of type cultures of *Streptomyces* II. Species descriptions from first study. *Int. J. Syst. Bacteriol.* 18:69–189

Shirling EB, Gottlieb D (1968b) Cooperative description of type cultures of *Streptomyces* III. Additional descriptions from first and second studies. *Int. J. Syst. Bacteriol.* 18:279–392

Shirling EB, Gottlieb D (1969) Cooperative description of type cultures of *Streptomyces* IV. Additional descriptions from second, third and fourth studies. *Int. J. Syst. Bacteriol.* 19:391–512

Shirling EB, Gottlieb D (1972) Cooperative description of type cultures of *Streptomyces* V. Additional descriptions. *Int. J. Syst. Bacteriol.* 22:265–394

Stapley EO, Woodruff HB (1982) Avermectins, antiparasitic lactones produced by *Streptomyces avermitilis* isolated from a soil in Japan. In Umezawa H, Demain AL, Hata T, Hutchinson CR (eds), *Trends in Antibiotic Research,* Japan Antibiotics Research Association, Tokyo, pp 154–170

Waksman SA (1961) *The Actinomycetes,* Vol 2, The Williams & Wilkins Co., Baltimore

Woodruff HB, Burg RW (1986) The antibiotic explosion. In Parnham MJ, Bruinvels J (eds), *Discoveries in Pharmacology, Vol 3: Pharmacological Methods, Receptors & Chemotherapy,* Elsevier Science Publishers, Amsterdam, pp 303–351

CHAPTER 3

Fermentation Development and Process Improvement

Mary Nallin Omstead, Louis Kaplan, and Barry C. Buckland

I. Introduction

Streptomyces avermitilis was originally isolated from soil as described in Chapter 2. The first fermentations of the culture used a standard screening approach: a loopful of slant growth was inoculated into a seed flask which was incubated and then transferred into two types of production flasks. Seed cultures were grown for 48 to 72 hours in baffled flasks containing 50 ml seed medium I (Burg *et al.* 1979). Production flasks were inoculated by transferring 2.0 ml of seed growth into 40 ml production medium A (Burg *et al.* 1979) and incubated for 4 days. The production cultures were then harvested and assayed for activity as indicated in Chapter 2.

This chapter describes the development of an optimized process for the large-scale fermentation of *Streptomyces avermitilis,* beginning with the original strain. Improvements in the process involved multiple parameters—including strain improvement, seed and production media development, and modification of physical fermentation parameters (such as aeration, temperature, pH, and length of incubation). Furthermore, scaling up the avermectin process to large fermentation tanks demanded the optimization of yet another set of parameters—such as oxygen transfer and media sterilization.

II. Process Improvement—Shake Flask Scale

A. Culture Development

After the discovery that the avermectins possess anthelmintic activity—and the intense interest that fact elicited—it became an obvious goal to develop and improve the avermectin fermentation process. Process improvement can and usually does proceed along several different avenues of investigation. In the case of the avermectins, various fermentation parameters were studied simultaneously. These parameters included developing the *S. avermitilis* strain itself, modifying and/or altering the composition of the seed and production media constituents, and determining the nutritional and physiological requirements of the organism. To perform the latter studies, one must develop either an adequate synthetic medium or a resting cell system. In either case, the system must be capable of supporting a basal level of product formation against which gains or losses can be measured.

To develop the *S. avermitilis* strain, several mutational procedures were examined and adapted to obtain a number of different mutant cultures. As a rule, these procedures were performed on spores suspended in 0.1M HEPES buffer, pH 7.4. However, several of the methods also were used to treat washed vegetative mycelia suspended in various media. Suspensions of treated cultures were plated on complex media to guarantee optimal recovery of survivors. Survival curves were determined for all mutations. The frequency of mutation was determined by calculating the degree of morphological variation induced by the mutation, the frequency of induced auxotrophy, or the resistance to growth inhibitory levels of various compounds.

The first method used to induce mutations involved irradiating spores with ultraviolet (UV) light, varying exposure times (Clarke and Hopwood 1976). The irradiated suspensions were plated and grown in the dark to prevent possible photoreactivation. The resulting decrease in viability was directly related to the exposure time. Irradiation also induced obvious mutations in some of the survivors, as evidenced by their altered morphologies (Table 3.1). These morphological changes proved to be stable through several reisolation (generational) events.

The second type of mutation involved the use of various alkylating agents—including nitrosoguanidine (NTG) (Awerbuch and Stark 1979; Godfrey 1974; Kirkpatrick and Godfrey 1973), nitrosomethylurethane (NMU) (Awerbuch and Stark 1979), and ethylmethane sulfonate (EMS) (Awerbuch and Stark 1979; Sega 1984). Suspensions of these mutagens were prepared as follows: the NMU and EMS were dissolved in the same buffer as that in which the spores were suspended, 0.1M HEPES buffer, pH 7.4; initially, the NTG was dissolved in 0.05 or 0.1M Tris-maleate buffer, pH 6.0. After it was discovered that the Tris itself was adversely affecting the culture, subsequent experiments used HEPES-buffered NTG solutions. As with the irradiation method, exposure times for NTG and NMU were varied. EMS exposure times had to be prolonged because of the apparent resistance of the *S. avermitilis* to this mutagen as

TABLE 3.1. Types of *Streptomyces avermitilis* mutants.

Types of mutants	Relative avermectin production titers[a]
A. Morphological variants	
1 altered spore pigmentation	I, R, NP
2 absence of aerial mycelia (''balds'')	NP
3 loss of melanin production	NP
B. Nonproducing mutants	NP
C. Auxotrophs (various nutritional requirements)	R, NP
D. Modified avermectin-producing mutants	
1 des-methyl macrolide ring	I, R
2 des-methyl oleandrose	R
3 open furan ring	R
4 aglycone	R
5 altered ratio of components	I, R

[a] : Titers obtained from mutant strains compared to the titers of their specific parental strain
I: improved, increased
R: reduced
NP: nonproducer

demonstrated by the low level of kill and the low frequency of morphological variants. EMS is also a less effective mutagen for other organisms (Sega 1984). In all procedures using alkylating agents the mutagen either was removed from the suspension by centrifugation or was inactivated by adding 10% sodium thiosulfate to the reaction mixture.

Treating *S. avermitilis* with these alkylating agents resulted in various types of mutants. Morphological variants were easily detected. These survivors consisted of the following types: nonsporulating (i.e., "bald") colonies, sporulating colonies which displayed altered spore pigmentation, colonies which failed to produce the melanin pigment typical of the *S. avermitilis* parent, and colonies which displayed various combinations of these characteristics. Mutants categorized within each type of variant class exhibited a range in the ability to produce avermectin: many exhibited lowered production as compared to the parental type, while some had become complete nonproducers. Auxotrophic strains were also detected and purified. They, too, varied in the amount of avermectin produced, although generally their titers were significantly reduced. Other mutants produced structurally modified avermectin components, including the aglycone or monosaccharide avermectins (Ikeda, Kotaki, and Omura 1987; Schulman *et al.* 1985); components which no longer contained completely closed furan ring structures (Goegelman, Gullo, and Kaplan 1983); and des-methyl avermectins (either on the macrolide ring or on the oleandrose units) (Schulman *et al.* 1985; Schulman *et al.* 1986). Once again, these mutants produced reduced total avermectin components. In addition, other mutants were isolated which synthesized all the avermectin components (a total of 8 structural types) (Miller *et al.* 1979) but produced them in different ratios than the original parental strain.

Treating various parental strains by the procedures described resulted in the accumulation of many mutants of each type. They were subsequently tested as to whether any of them were capable of cross-feeding each other. These tests were done either by cofermenting the mutant strains in a mixed fermentation or by feeding to one fermentation an extract prepared from another fermentation broth. The cofermentations were generally difficult to interpret, although they were adequate in evaluating whether strains that had independently lost the ability to produce melanin could regain that function if cocultured. Experiments that involved feeding one strain with an extract from another strain proved to be more useful. This type of feeding study enabled us to categorize our nonproducing mutants into several classes based on their ability to convert a given substrate (e.g., an aglycone avermectin) into an easily distinguishable product (in the example cited, a standard avermectin). In this fashion, it was possible to differentiate nonproducing mutants even further.

There remains one final type of mutant, that which is most important to any strain improvement program: a strain that produces significantly more total avermectin (and more of the active B_1 components) than its parent. Table 3.2 depicts the partial genealogy of improved avermectin producers, both in terms of $B_{1(a+b)}$ components and in relation to the total avermectin produced. Several features of this table warrant further attention. Culture 1 is the original soil isolate, the first to manifest avermectin activity (Burg *et al.* 1979). There was a clear gain in activity between this and the next culture (2): a twenty-onefold increase in B_1 titer and a twenty-fivefold improvement in total avermectin produced. The levels cited in Table 3.2 represent accumulated gains in titer achieved through strain improvement, media development, and fermentation condition changes. Prior to discussing subsequent cultures, it should be emphasized that *S. avermitilis* was first described as having a brownish-gray spore mass color (Burg *et al.* 1979). Culture 4, and all cultures obtained subsequently, displayed altered spore pigmentation: isolates were blue-green. Moreover, this change in morphological appearance was correlated with an increase in avermectin production. Through culture 7 all improved producers showed a coupled response between improved B_1 titer and improved total avermectin production. Cultures 8b and 12, however, exhibited improved B_1 titers but a concomitant reduction in the other components, resulting in a smaller increase in total avermectin levels (103X vs 91X and 108X vs 92X, respectively). Culture 12 was particularly important because it demonstrated that one could continue to enhance B_1 production while maintaining the other components at reduced levels.

B. Seed Media Development

Along with developing improved avermectin-producing strains, we were studying and modifying the fermentation process itself. A particular set of conditions had been defined for the original parental strain (Burg *et al.*

TABLE 3.2. *Streptomyces avermitilis* genealogy.

Culture	Fold improvements[a] B1[b]	Total	Comments
1	(1.0)	(1.0)	Original soil isolate; brownish-gray spore coloration
2	21X	25X	brownish-gray spore coloration
4	34X	38X	spore pigmentation mutant (blue-green coloration)
7	56X	69X	blue-green spore coloration
8b	103X	91X	blue-green spore coloration; reduced "A" components
12	108X	92X	blue-green spore coloration; reduced "A" components

[a]: As shown in this table, the fold improvement includes increases in titer due to the following factors: strain improvement, seed and production media modifications, and changes in physical fermentation parameters

[b]: B_1 refers to the combined titers for $B_{1a} + B_{1b}$

1979). This set specified a seed medium (II) grown for 24 to 48 hrs, with subsequent transfer to production medium (B) which fermented at 28° C for 5 to 6 days. As the *S. avermitilis* strain was being developed, we wanted to be sure that the fermentation conditions (including media composition, temperature, aeration, and length of fermentation) would not become limiting to the new, improved strains. To start, we examined the initial seed medium. As reported (Burg *et al.* 1979), seed medium II contained distiller's solubles (a particulate raw material), lactose, and Ardamine PH. Our first manipulation of this medium involved testing the effect of various carbon sources. Of those, cerelose is optimal for *S. avermitilis* in this medium. Seed medium II is one in which cerelose was the primary source of carbon. As shown in Table 3.3, this single seed medium change, combined with superior mutants (note culture improvement in Table 3.3), resulted in five- to elevenfold improvement in avermectin production. The original seed medium (II) demonstrated about the same degree of improvement (six to tenfold) based on improved cultures alone. However, simultaneously modifying the seed and the production media produced even better results. Seed medium III, combined with production medium C, resulted in sixteen- to twenty-onefold improved avermectin production, whereas seed medium II with production medium C netted only thirteen- to fourteenfold improvement. Therefore, the combined effects of culture improvement and modification

TABLE 3.3. Seed medium development.

		Production media[a]			
Seed medium	Culture	B	C	D	E
II	1	(1.0)	ND[b]	ND	ND
	3	6X	14X	ND	ND
	4	10X	13X	ND	ND
	5	8X	ND	ND	ND
III	3	7X	18X	ND	ND
	4	5X	16X	ND	ND
	5	11X	21X	23X	ND
IV	3	1X	12X	ND	ND
	4	1X	18X	ND	ND
	5	2X	24X	37X	40X
	7	ND	ND	ND	56X
	8	ND	ND	ND	66X
V	5	ND	22X	ND	ND
VI	5	ND	ND	29X	ND
VII	5	ND	ND	ND	32X
	7	ND	ND	ND	44X
	8	ND	ND	ND	54X

[a]: Values shown are total fold improvements in $B_{1(a+b)}$ titers, including increases due to the following factors: strain improvement, seed and production media modifications, and changes in the physical fermentation parameters
[b]: Not determined

of both the seed and production media resulted in an optimal improvement in avermectin formation of twenty-onefold. The degree of improvement cited in Table 3.3 is relative to the avermectin titer produced by the original strain grown in seed medium II and fermented in production medium B.

Despite these impressive yield improvements, a problem occurred concomitant with the change made in the seed medium. Cultures which had been superior avermectin producers in the original fermentation process were no longer so. Culture 4 was no longer producing higher titers than culture 3 in production medium C, whether it was grown in seed medium II or III (13X vs 14X from seed II, and 16X vs 18X from seed III). Interestingly, culture 5 demonstrated superiority only when grown in seed III. Similarly, culture 4 displayed superior production when seed II was fermented in production medium B but not when fermented in production medium C (10X vs 6X for culture 3, compared to 13X vs 14X, respectively). Apparently, the ability to detect superior mutants with higher avermectin titers was strongly dependent on the specific fermentation conditions (seed medium, production medium combinations) being used.

Clearly, this situation demanded a seed medium that would be neither specific to a given culture nor so strongly dependent on the subsequent production medium. To formulate a reasonable mixture of ingredients, we compared the formulations used in several published *Streptomycete* fermentations (Aharonowitz and Demain 1977; Godfrey 1973; Hirsch and Ensign 1976; Kirkpatrick and Godfrey 1973; Stark, Hoehn, and Knox 1967). As a consequence, we developed medium IV, and coupled this formulation to the specific nutritional requirements of *S. avermitilis*. Results from the original tests of this medium did not meet expectations. Cultures 3, 4, and 5—grown in seed IV and transferred to production medium B—produced quite poorly (1X or 2X levels). However, when these same cultures (grown in seed IV) were transferred into production C, quite impressive results were obtained. Not only had avermectin production increased twenty-fourfold, but the mutant cultures maintained the superiority they had originally shown. Seed medium IV had an additional benefit: unlike its predecessors, it was completely soluble and essentially defined.

Seed medium development continued with the acquisition of new mutant strains but was constantly checked against seed medium IV (the best at that time). Three additional seed media were devised and tested: V, VI, and VII. As shown in Table 3.3, cells grown in seed medium V failed to synthesize as much avermectin from production medium C as they had when grown in seed IV (22X vs 24X, respectively). Using culture 5, seed medium VI transferred into production medium D resulted in the production of more avermectin (29X) than when seed medium III was used (23X). Changing to seed medium IV and keeping the other parameters (culture and production medium) the same, avermectin production was improved to thirty-sevenfold. Once again, seed medium IV proved to be the most flexible in terms of demonstrating culture superiority and in relation to use of the various production media. Seed medium VII, which was developed later, was tested only in production medium E. Seed medium VII clearly demonstrated the superiority of improved mutants (32X, 44X, and 54X for cultures 5, 7, and 8, respectively) fermented in production medium E. However, when cultures 5, 7, or 8 were grown in seed medium IV rather than seed medium VII, avermectin production was higher still: 40X versus 32X for culture 5, 56X versus 44X for culture 7, and 66X versus 54X for culture 8. A total evaluation of the data contained in Table 3.3 indicates that maximum avermectin production was obtained from superior cultures when they had been grown in seed medium IV and were fermented in production medium E. Overall, the accumulated results demonstrate that it is essential to monitor the fermentation process continually to guarantee optimal product formation.

C. Production Media Development

As the seed medium was being developed, so too was the production medium. Early studies involved classical titration experiments: the concentration of a given component of production medium B (Burg *et al.* 1979) was varied while the remaining ingredients were held constant. In this approach, one looks for the occurrence of maxima (in this case, highest avermectin titers) as they are collected from tests of each ingredient assessed independently (Box, Hunter, and Hunter 1978). It was exactly this approach that led to the development of production medium C from production medium B (Table 3.3). Individual ingredients of production medium B were titrated while the remaining ingredients were maintained at constant levels. Concentrations of each individual component that resulted in maximum avermectin production were then simply combined to yield the composition of production medium C. As seen in Table 3.3, combining any of the seed media and any of the cultures fermented in production medium C increased the avermectin titer compared to that obtained under the identical conditions in production medium B. Focusing on culture 5 (Table 3.4), avermectin titers improved by a factor of 24 when fermented in production medium C. Obviously, this approach does have merit; its use can have a definite positive impact on process development.

We then pursued a somewhat different but equally "classical" approach to medium development. These tests substituted various nitrogen sources for the peptonized milk ingredient in medium C. Protein sources such as soy, pork, cottonseed, and fish, as well as soybean and cottonseed meals, were substituted based on their nitrogen equivalence. The best avermectin titer obtained from any of these substituted media was only 42% of that obtained from the control medium. The avermectin

TABLE 3.4. Production medium development.

Culture	Seed medium	Production media[a]						
		B	C	D	E	F	G	J
1	II	(1.0)	ND[b]	ND	ND	ND	ND	ND
5	IV	2X	24X	37X	40X	ND	ND	ND
7	IV	ND	ND	ND	56X	ND	41X	36X
8b	IV	ND	ND	ND	ND	87X	103X	117X
12	IV	ND	ND	ND	ND	ND	108X	128X

[a]: Values shown are total fold improvements in $B_{1(a+b)}$ titers including increases due to the following factors: strain improvement, seed and production media modifications, and changes in the physical fermentation parameters
[b]: Not determined

production levels in the other media ranged from 0 to 25% of control values. When the yeast ingredient was varied, production values varied within only 3% to 4%. Therefore, of the various media ingredients we tested, none improved avermectin production relative to those ingredients currently in the production medium.

In summary, we used the classical approach to medium development to devise production medium C. Substituting the nitrogen source and yeast component in medium C did not improve avermectin titers. There are, however, other approaches to medium/process development that could be pursued (Box, Hunter, and Hunter 1978; Greasham and Inamine 1986). Despite the improvement in avermectin synthesis, it should be recognized that the classical approach has an inherent weakness. It fails to consider the possibility that individual ingredients may interact with one another in some way, altering their role in the overall medium composition. In addition, factors other than medium formulation also influence the fermentation's outcome—factors such as culture, temperature, aeration, and pH. Although experiments can be devised to consider all these parameters, they would be extremely laborious and time-consuming. Alternatively, it is possible to use various statistical methods that allow testing of multiple variables concurrently (Box, Hunter, and Hunter 1978; Greasham and Inamine 1986).

Frequently the development of production media follows a sequential path, beginning with Plackett-Burman studies designed to identify independent variables (e.g., media ingredients) of interest (Greasham and Inamine 1986). Once the variables that impact product accumulation have been determined, the next step is to optimize the level of each identified variable. Generally, this optimization procedure uses response surface methodology (Box, Hunter, and Hunter 1978), which allows estimation of up to 5-variable interactions. Response surface methodology involves generating contour curves (Box, Hunter, and Hunter 1978; Greasham and Inamine 1986). It is precisely along these curves where the optima occur. To adequately (mathematically) identify each maximum point, a variable must be tested at 3 levels. A 5-variable interaction study therefore requires 247 trials to identify the optimum for each of the 5 variables. Obviously, this many trials become unwieldy and impractical to perform. As a consequence, partial factorial designs have been constructed (Greasham and Inamine 1986). Partial factorials consist of selected points extracted from a full factorial design; those points are used to obtain an estimated response. A partial factorial result may only indicate where an optimum may be, and a second set of trials may be needed to confirm that optimum. As a general rule, the use of partial factorials followed by independent experiments to confirm identification of optima results in better and ultimately faster process improvement than alternative approaches.

Tables 3.3 and 3.4 demonstrate the consequences of using response surface methodology to develop production media. As previously stated, production medium C was composed using the classical approach. Production medium D, however, was developed using partial factorial experiments, followed by secondary trials to confirm acquisition and location of optimum values. As shown in both Tables 3.3 and 3.4, culture 5 fermented in production medium D produced thirty-sevenfold more avermectin than the original strain. Furthermore, it produced higher avermectin titers in D than in C (37X vs 24X, respectively). Medium modification as a consequence of observations made on statically growing cultures (and applied to those in liquid media) resulted in the formulation of production medium E. Culture 5, fermented in production medium E, yielded fortyfold improved avermectin production compared to that in medium D. Clearly, culture 5 demonstrated improved avermectin synthesis as it progressed through the various production media (Table 3.4). The compositions of production media E and F are identical. The differences in titer obtained from these media demonstrate the importance of examining modifications in physical fermentation parameters (such as aeration, pH, and length of incubation) as the media are developed and as newly acquired strains are obtained. Production media G and J were derived once again as a consequence of partial factorial experiments with subsequent confirmation trials. As Table 3.4 indicates, improved cultures (7, 8b, and 12) demonstrated improved ability to synthesize avermectin in the new production media: 56X in production E, 87X in production F, and 108X in production G, respectively. Furthermore, both cultures 8b and 12 showed improvement in avermectin production based only on the developed production media. For culture 8b, titers improved from 87X to 103X to 117X as the production changed from medium F to G to J. Similarly, culture 12 displayed improvement to 128X in medium J compared to 108X in medium G. Interestingly, the data in Table 3.4 also indicate that not all cultures will overproduce product in all media. For example, culture 7 produced significantly less avermectin in medium J (36X) and in medium

G (41X) than in medium E (56X). Obviously, media G and J had not been optimized for use with this culture. In general, these data definitely prove that production medium development, coupled with culture improvement and modifications in the physical fermentation parameters, can and does result in improved processes for the fermentation of secondary metabolites.

Figure 3.1 illustrates the shake flask fermentation of culture 8 in production medium J. Avermectin production began sometime between the second and third day of the fermentation, after logarithmic growth had ceased. Although avermectin production has been reported to be catabolite repressible (Ikeda, Kotaki, and Omura 1987; McCann-McCormick *et al.* 1981), using the cultures and conditions described herein avermectin production was unaffected by glucose. Neither ammonia nor pH levels rose until relatively late in the fermentation cycle, indicating that the culture had not lysed. Now that we had developed superior cultures and

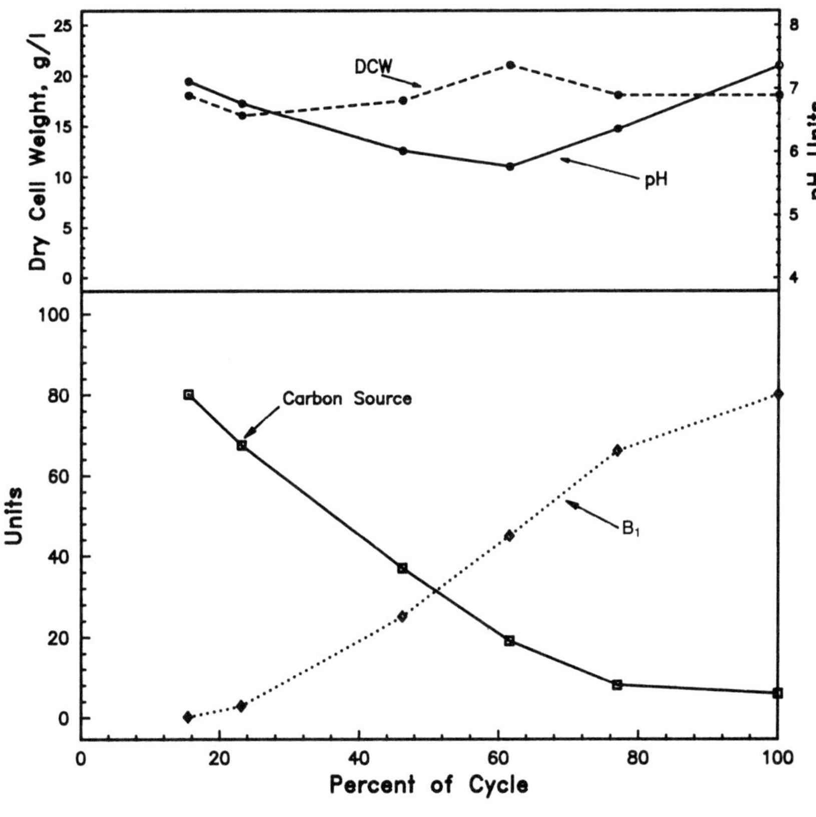

FIGURE 3.1. Avermectin formation and growth of *Streptomyces avermitilis* in shake flasks.

optimized the media and fermentation parameters in shake flasks, it remained to transfer and translate the whole system to larger vessels.

III. Process Scale-Up

The objective was to scale up a process developed in shake flasks (20 ml in a 250 ml flask) to production-scale fermentors (50,000L operating volume), i.e., a scale-up factor of 2.5 million. In practice, the scale-up was accomplished in two steps, first by developing a stirred-tank process at the 500L scale (pilot plant), followed by a hundredfold scale-up to the factory.

A. Fermentation Kinetics: Stirred Tanks

In a typical avermectin fermentation in stirred tanks, rapid cell growth is followed by a prolonged period of product synthesis with no evidence of further cell mass accumulation. Under the range of conditions investigated within our pilot plant, the formation of avermectin occurs only when cell growth is extremely low, perhaps zero. A typical fermentation profile is shown in Figure 3.2. This is similar to that obtained in shake flasks (Figure 3.1) and also to that previously described by Burg *et al.* (1979).

The relative mixture of different avermectin components produced in

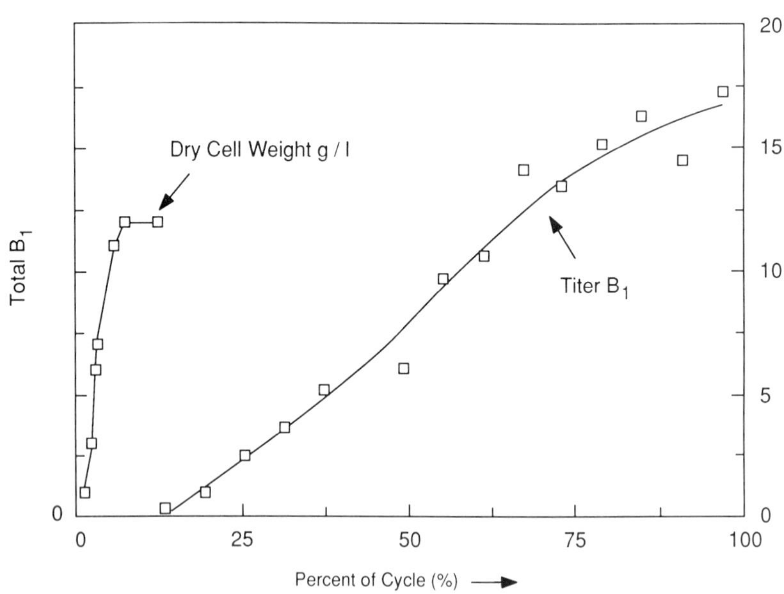

FIGURE 3.2. Avermectin formation and growth of *Streptomyces avermitilis* in stirred tank formentor.

stirred tanks is similar to that obtained in the shake flask process. This presents a special challenge for downstream extraction; the desired B_{1a} and B1b components must be separated during the purification process. An additional challenge to the purification is that *S. avermitilis* also synthesizes lipids in large amounts. These consist primarily of a mixture of triglycerides (Metz *et al.* 1988) possessing C14-C17 free fatty acids.

B. Prediction of Cell Mass On-Line

Using a combination of mass spectrometry, mass flow meters, and minicomputer (Buckland *et al.* 1985), it is possible to obtain a very accurate on-line measurement of oxygen consumption rates (expressed as mmoles of oxygen consumed per liter of fermentation broth per hour) for any of our stirred tank fermentations. For *S. avermitilis* in a variety of different media, there was an excellent correlation between total oxygen consumed—obtained on-line by integrating the sum of the oxygen uptake rates—and cell mass accumulation during the active growth phase of the fermentation (Figure 3.3) according to Equation 1. This correlation cannot be used after the period of rapid growth.

$$X = Y\ o/x \sum_{t=0}^{t} OUR \cdot \Delta t$$

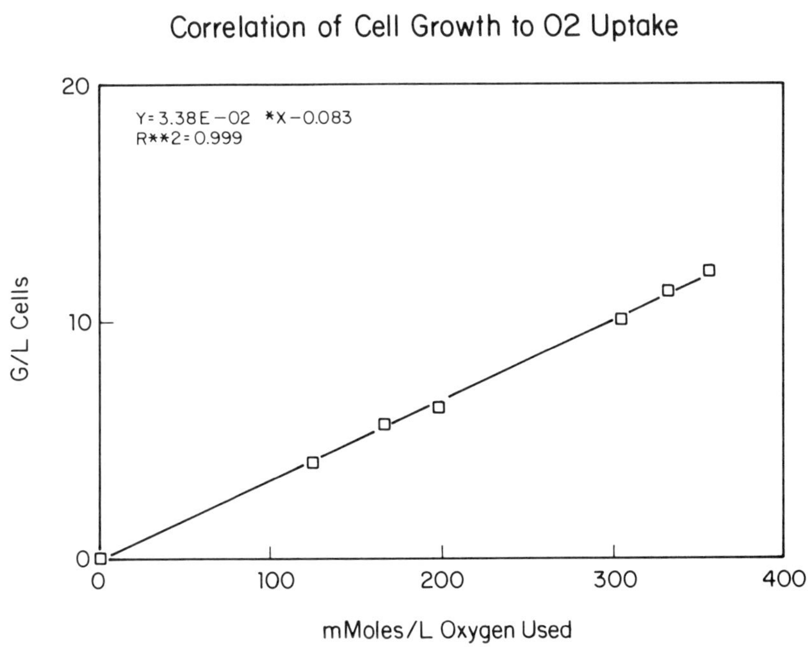

FIGURE 3.3. Correlation between cell growth and oxygen uptake (from Buckland et al. 1985).

Where t = time
OUR = oxygen uptake rate (mmoles/l/h)
$Y\,o/x$ = ratio of total oxygen consumed to cell concentration
X = cell concentration (g dry cell weight/l)

Therefore the function OUR · Δ t denotes the total oxygen consumed, easily calculated by on-line computer summation of the oxygen uptake rate with respect to time.

Assuming that there is a constant yield coefficient between cell mass and total oxygen consumed during this time period, it is possible to extend this model further by dividing the oxygen uptake rate by the total oxygen consumed; this provides an estimation of the specific growth rate of the culture (gram increase in cell mass/ total cell mass in grams/hour). Using the power of the minicomputer, this estimation can be done on-line.

$$\mu = \frac{1}{x}\frac{dx}{dt} = \frac{OUR}{\sum_{t=0}^{t} OUR \cdot \Delta t}$$

Where μ = specific growth rate, reciprocal hours
x = cell concentration [g (dry cell weight)/l]

The on-line estimation of both cell mass and cell growth rate (Figure 3.4) (Buckland *et al.* 1985) has proven to be accurate, reliable, and a very

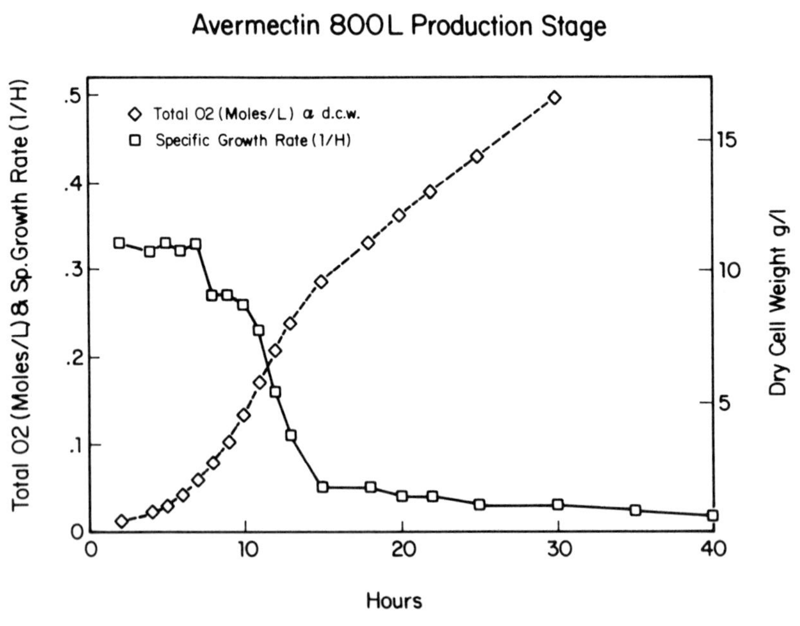

FIGURE 3.4. On-line estimation of cell concentration and specific growth rate (from Buckland *et al.* 1985).

powerful tool for process development. An example is given [Figure 3.5 (Brix, Drew, and Buckland 1988)] in which two fermentations were run at different temperatures, one 4° C higher than the other. The resulting difference in specific growth rate is very pronounced.

C. Oxygen Transfer

As the cell mass increases, the cells' mycelia begin to tangle, making the broth viscous (Figure 3.6). This increase in viscosity adversely affects oxygen transfer. It has been determined experimentally (Buckland *et al.* 1988) that the oxygen transfer coefficient is approximately proportional to the reciprocal of the square root of the viscosity. This effect limits the maximum achievable cell concentration and therefore the reactor's volumetric productivity. Consequently, the study of oxygen transfer efficiency was especially important for this process.

Computer-controlled, highly instrumented fermentors can calculate on-line a number of different parameters for a single fermentation batch. In one series of experiments (Buckland *et al.* 1988), the performance of a large-diameter axial flow hydrofoil impeller was compared to that of a conventional Rushton radial flow impeller. Two fermentations were run side by side and the oxygen uptake rate profiles for the 2 different agitator

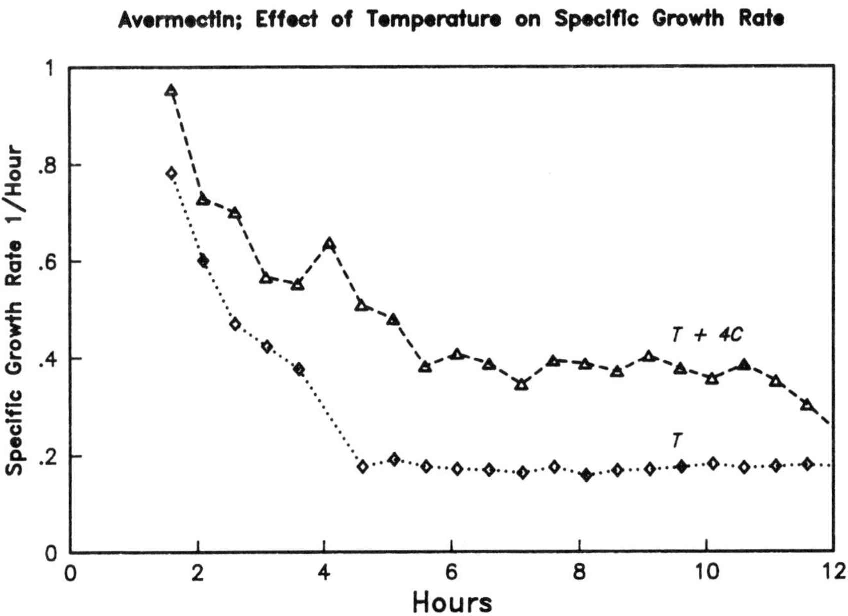

FIGURE 3.5. Specific growth rate (estimated on-line) for two fermentations at different temperatures. Standard temperature (T) and standard temperature plus 4° C (T + 4C) (from Brix, Drew, and Buckland 1988).

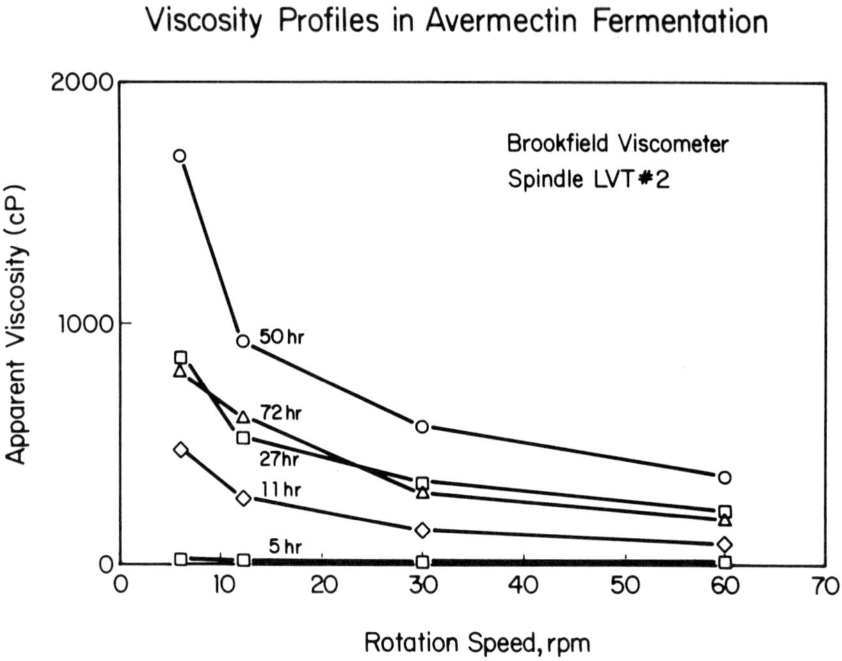

FIGURE 3.6. Viscosity profile for the avermectin fermentation. 400mL samples of broth, taken at different fermentation ages, were measured on Brookfield Viscometer. The rotation speed of the spindle LVT #2 was varied from 6, 12, 30, and 60 rpm to determine torque deflection. The % torque deflection was converted to apparent viscosity (cP) units using calibration charts provided by Brookfield instruments.

types are compared (Figure 3.7). The dissolved oxygen profiles are also similar (Figure 3.8). The on-line calculation of the oxygen transfer coefficient (KLa) is made using the data from Figures 3.7 and 3.8; not surprisingly, the profiles are also similar (Figure 3.9). The most striking difference is in the relative power consumption of the 2 different agitator types (Figure 3.10). The results of this study (and others) demonstrated that—for a viscous mycelial fermentation of this type—a large-diameter axial flow impeller is much more efficient at oxygen transfer than the more conventional Rushton radial flow impeller.

D. STRATEGY USED FOR SUCCESSFUL SCALE-UP

There were a number of key issues related to successful scale-up from 250 ml shake flasks to 50,000L production fermentors. These include the following:

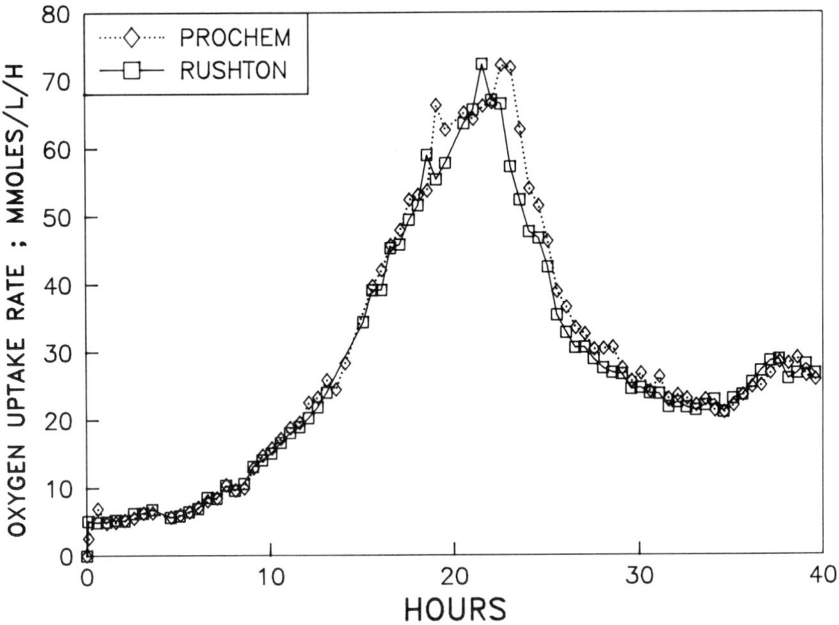

FIGURE 3.7. Oxygen uptake rate profiles for two avermectin fermentations: one using Rushton impellers and the other using Prochem impellers (from Buckland *et al.* 1988).

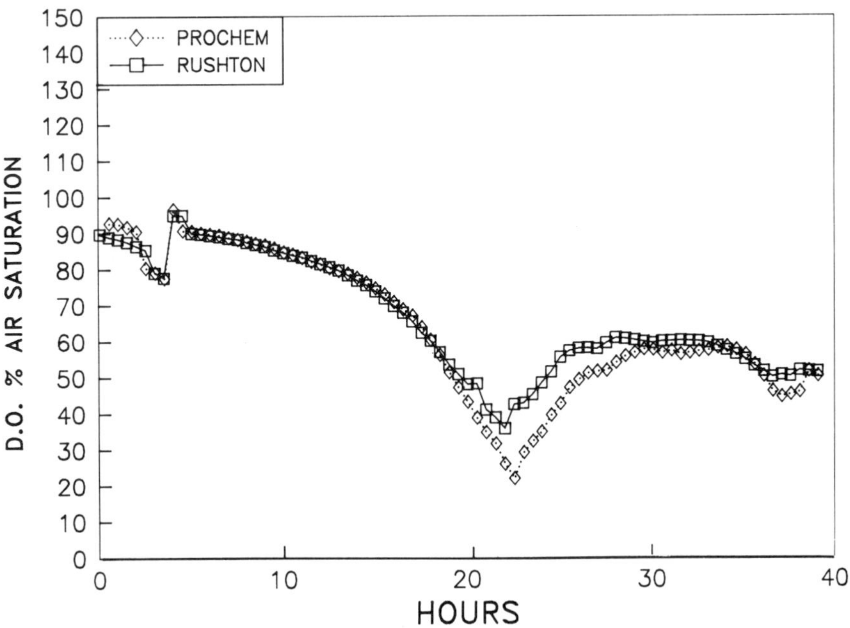

FIGURE 3.8. Dissolved oxygen profiles for same two fermentation described in Figure 3.7 (from Buckland *et al.* 1988).

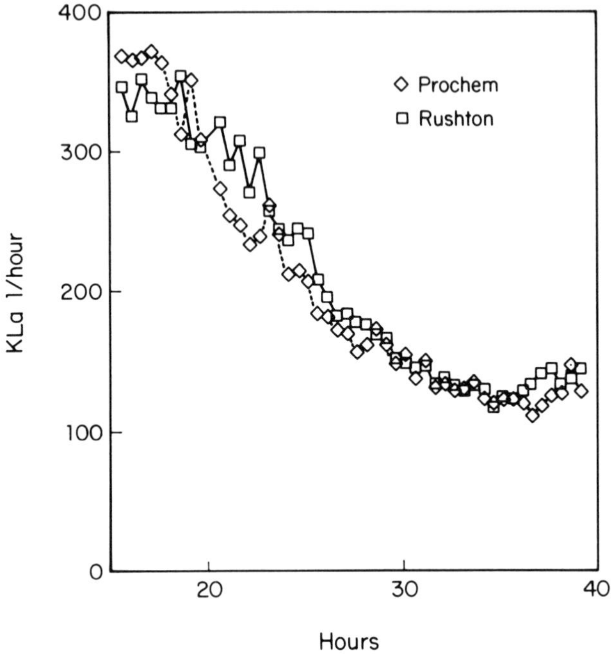

FIGURE 3.9. On-line calculation of the oxygen transfer coefficient for the same two avermectin fermentations described in 3.7 (from Buckland *et al.* 1988).

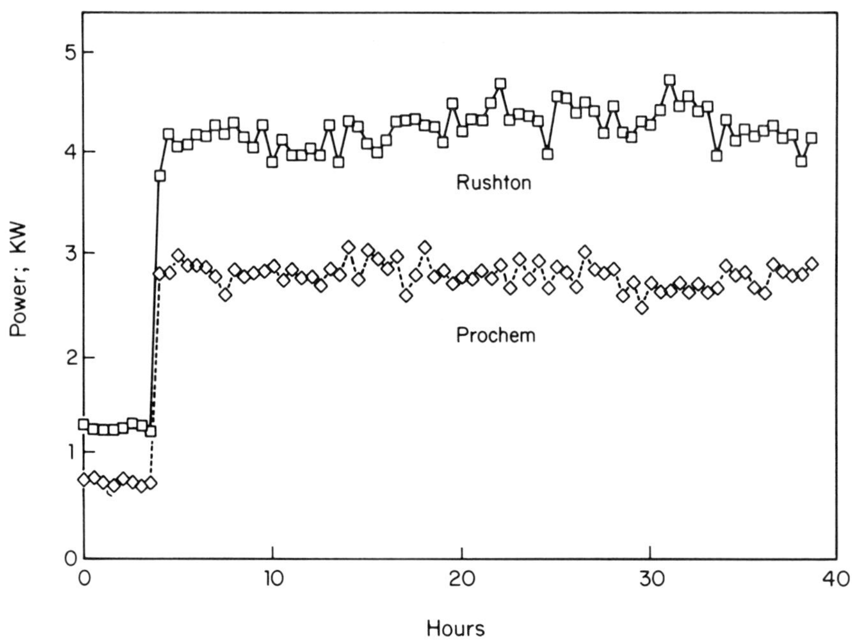

FIGURE 3.10. Agitator power draw for the same two avermectin fermentations described in Figure 3.7 (from Buckland *et al.* 1988).

Environmental Containment

Streptomyces avermitilis is not known to be unusually harmful; nevertheless, it was necessary to maintain a high level of containment because the product—avermectin—is very potent and could have a potential environmental impact on aquatic life forms. Containment concerns extended to both the fermentation operations and to the downstream purification facility. These considerations were incorporated into the factory design from the beginning and were resolved successfully: all possible exit streams from the process are captured and the avermectin therein degraded chemically.

Media Sterilization

As with many processes of this type, media sterilization is an important variable (Jain and Buckland 1988) for both the seed tank stages and the production stage. By necessity, more stringent conditions are required as scale is increased to achieve the same assurance of complete sterilization (Buckland 1985). With a batch procedure, this is normally accomplished by increasing time at sterilization temperature; with a continuous sterilizer either the time or the temperature can be easily increased. Superimposed on the requirement for sterility is the fact that a number of chemical changes occur in the medium during sterilization, some of which can have a great impact on culture productivity. This therefore becomes an important area for optimization and, if possible, chemical analysis.

Oxygen Transfer

Because of the viscous characteristics of the broth, the ability to transfer sufficient oxygen to the individual microbial cell ultimately limits the cell mass and hence productivity of the fermentation, assuming that the other critical physical and chemical parameters that influence metabolism have been chosen correctly to achieve high levels of product expression. When evaluating a proposed process change in the pilot plant, it is necessary to be sure that the oxygen requirements of the new process can be met adequately in the larger-scale equipment. One simple method for doing this is to run the pilot-scale fermentor in a way that mimics the limitations of the factory equipment. An example is given in Figure 3.11, in which a new medium formulation was evaluated in the pilot plant (medium 2). It was immediately apparent that the oxygen demand of the new process was in fact less than that for the standard process; given that the broth viscosities were similar, introducing this process into the factory would not result in starving the cells for oxygen.

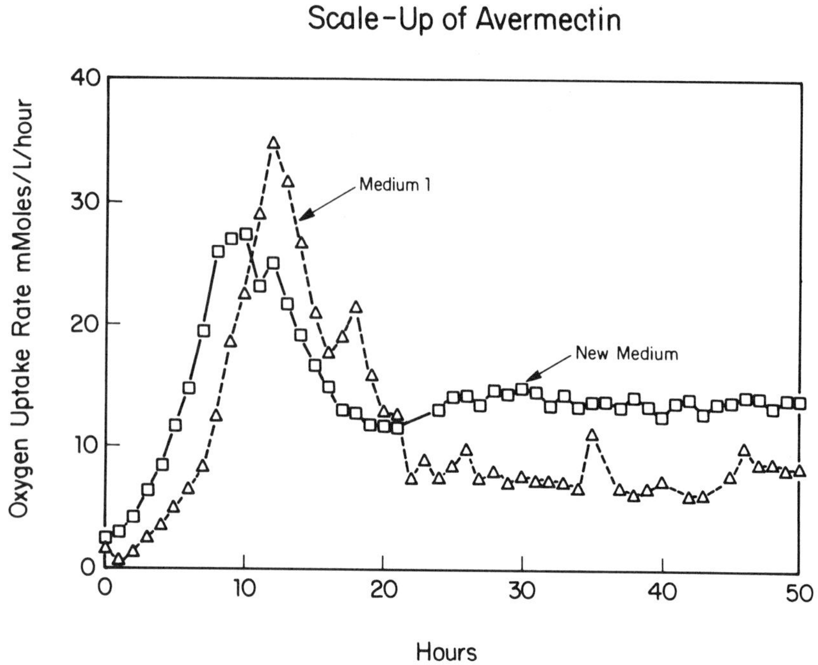

FIGURE 3.11. Scale-up information for new avermectin process (from Buckland 1985).

IV. Downstream Extraction

The challenge to develop an economic process for the purification of the desired B_1 component of avermectin from this fermentation broth was formidable. The harvested fermentation broth contains the following components:

- various unused substrates from a complex fermentation medium
- other closely related avermectin compounds (A_{1a}, A_{1b}, B_{2a}, B_{2b}; see Chapter 1)
- a mixture of triglycerides possessing C14–C17 acyl groups (Metz *et al.* 1988), made by the culture
- low levels of C15–C17 free fatty acids, squalene and diglycerides (Metz *et al.* 1988), made by the culture
- significant amounts of chemical defoamer added to the medium
- other unidentified metabolites produced by the culture

An early process scheme for achieving this purification was described by Miller *et al.* (1979). It is interesting to contrast this very elaborate procedure with an improved version described in a recent patent by Bagner and Wildman (1983). In the revised process, the fermentation broth is first acidified and then mixed with an extractant such as toluene at high temperature. The extractant is then decanted away from the aqueous phase and, after just a few more processing steps, transferred to the final crystallization tank.

References

Aharonowitz Y, Demain AL (1977) Influence of inorganic phosphate and organic buffers on cephalosporin production by *Streptomyces clavuligerus*. *Arch. Microb.* 115:169–173

Awerbuch TE, Stark AA (1979) Plate diffusion assay as a rapid method for dosimetry of mutagens. *Appl. & Envir. Microb.* 38:1127–1131

Bagner C, Wildman AS (1983) Process for the whole broth extraction of avermectin. U.S. Patent #4,423,211

Box GE, Hunter WG, Hunter JS (1978) Response surface methods. *Statistics for Experimenters,* John Wiley & Sons, Inc., New York, pp 510–539

Brix T, Drew SW, Buckland BC (1988) Fermentation process development within a computer controlled pilot plant. In Bushell ME (ed), *Progress in Industrial Microbiology,* Vol 25, Elsevier, New York, pp 151–193

Buckland BC (1985) The translation of scale in fermentation processes: the impact of computer process control. *Bio/Technology* 2:875–883

Buckland BC, Brix T, Fastert H, Gbewonyo K, Hunt G, and Jain D (1985) Fermentation exhaust gas analysis using mass spectrometry. *Bio/Technology* 3:982–988

Buckland BC, Gbewonyo K, DiMasi D, Hunt G, Westerfield E, Nienow AW (1988) Improved performance in viscous mycelial fermentations by agitator retrofitting. *Biotech. & Bioeng.* 31:737–742

Burg RW, Miller BM, Baker EE, Birnbaum J, Currie SA, Hartman R, Kong YL, Monaghan RL, Olson G, Putter I, Tunac JB, Wallick H, Stapley EO, Oiwa R, Omura S (1979) Avermectins, new family of potent anthelmintic agents: producing organism and fermentation. *Antimicrob. Agents Chemother.* 15:361–367

Clarke CH, Hopwood DA (1976) Ultraviolet mutagenesis in *Streptomyces coelicolor:* induction of reversions in a polyauxotrophic strain. *Mutat. Res.* 41:201–208

Godfrey OW (1973) Isolation of regulatory mutants of the aspartic and pyruvic acid families and their effect on antibiotic production in *Streptomyces lipmanii.* Antimicrob. Agents Chemother. 4:73–79

Godfrey OW (1974) Directed mutation in *Streptomyces lipmanii.* Canad. J. Microb. 20:1479–1485

Goegelman RT, Gullo VP, Kaplan L (1983) Novel C-076 compounds. U.S. Patent #4,378,353

Greasham R, Inamine E (1986) Nutritional improvement of processes. In Demain AL, Solomon NA (eds), *Manual of Industrial Microbiology and Biotechnology,* American Society For Microbiology, Washington DC, pp 41–48

Hirsch CF, Ensign JC (1976) Nutritionally defined conditions for germination of *Streptomyces viridochromogenes* spores. *J. Bacter.* 126:13–23

Ikeda H, Kotaki H, Omura S (1987) Genetic studies of avermectin biosynthesis in *Streptomyces avermitilis*. *J. Bacter.* 169:5615–5621

Ikeda H, Kotaki H, Tanaka H, Omura S (1988) Involvement of glucose catabolism in avermectin production by *Streptomyces avermitilis*. *Antimicrob. Agents Chemother.* 32:282–284

Jain D, Buckland BC (1988) Scale-up of the efrotomycin fermentation using a computer controlled pilot plant. *Bioproc. Eng.* 3:31–36

Kirkpatrick JR, Godfrey OW (1973) The isolation and characterization of auxotrophs of the aspartic acid family from *Streptomyces lipmanii*. *Folia Microb.* 18:90–101

McCann-McCormick PA, Monaghan RL, Baker EE, Goegelman RT, Stapley EO (1981) Studies on the avermectin fermentation. In Moo-Young M, Robinson CW, Vezina C (eds), *Advances in Biotechnology,*Pergamon Press, New York, pp 69–74

Metz P, Omstead DR, Kaplan L, Liesch JM, Stearns RA, VandenHeuvel WJA (1988) Characterization of a lipid-rich fraction synthesized by *Streptomyces avermitilis*. J. Chromatog. 441:31–44

Miller TW, Chaiet L, Cole DJ, Cole LJ, Flor JE, Goegelman RT, Gullo VP, Joshua H, Kempf AJ, Krellwitz WR, Monaghan RL, Ormond RE, Wilson KE, Albers-Schonberg G, Putter I (1979) Avermectins, new family of potent anthelmintic agents: isolation and chromatographic properties. *Antimicrob. Agents Chemother.* 15:368–371

Schulman MD, Valentino D, Hensens OD, Zink D, Nallin M, Kaplan L, Ostlind DA (1985) Demethylavermectins: biosynthesis, isolation and characterization. *J. Antibiot.* 38:1494–1498

Schulman MD, Valentino D, Nallin M, Kaplan L (1986) Avermectin B2 O-methyltransferase activity in *Streptomyces avermitilis* mutants that produce increased amounts of the avermectins. *Antimicrob. Agents Chemother.* 29:620–624

Sega GA (1984) A review of the genetic effects of ethyl methanesulfonate. Mutat. Res. 134:113–142

Stark WM, Hoehn MM, Knox NG (1967) Mebramycin, a new broad-spectrum antibiotic complex. I. Detection and biosynthesis. *Antimicrob. Agents Chemother.* pp 314–323

Stark WM, Knox NG, Wilgus R, DuBus R (1976) The nebramycin fermentation: culture and fermentation development. In *Developments in Industrial Microbiology,* American Society for Microbiology, Washington DC, pp 61–77

CHAPTER 4

Biosynthesis

S. T. Chen, O. D. Hensens, and M. D. Schulman

I. Introduction

The avermectins are a family of oleandrose disaccharide derivatives of pentacyclic lactones. Figure 4.1 presents a generalized structure of the avermectins produced by *Streptomyces avermitilis*. In addition, a number of key intermediates in the biosynthesis of the avermectins have been identified. These structures are as follows: aglycones lack the oleandrose disaccharide and possess a hydroxyl at C13; demethylavermectins lack one or more methoxyls on the oleandrose disaccharide and possess a hydroxyl at either or both the C3″ and C3′; desfurano avermectins lack the oxygen at C8a and C6 and possess a CH_3 at C8a and an H at C6; and 5-keto avermectins lack the hydroxyl (or methoxyl) at C5 and possess a keto group at C5.

Presently, the pathway for avermectin biosynthesis is not completely understood. The pathway proposed in this chapter is based on evidence obtained from four types of studies: the incorporation of labeled precursors into the avermectins; the conversion of proposed intermediates into avermectins by producing strains and blocked mutants; the *in vitro* measurement of enzymes involved in the biosynthesis of the avermectins; and the production of incomplete avermectins by administration of specific enzyme inhibitors.

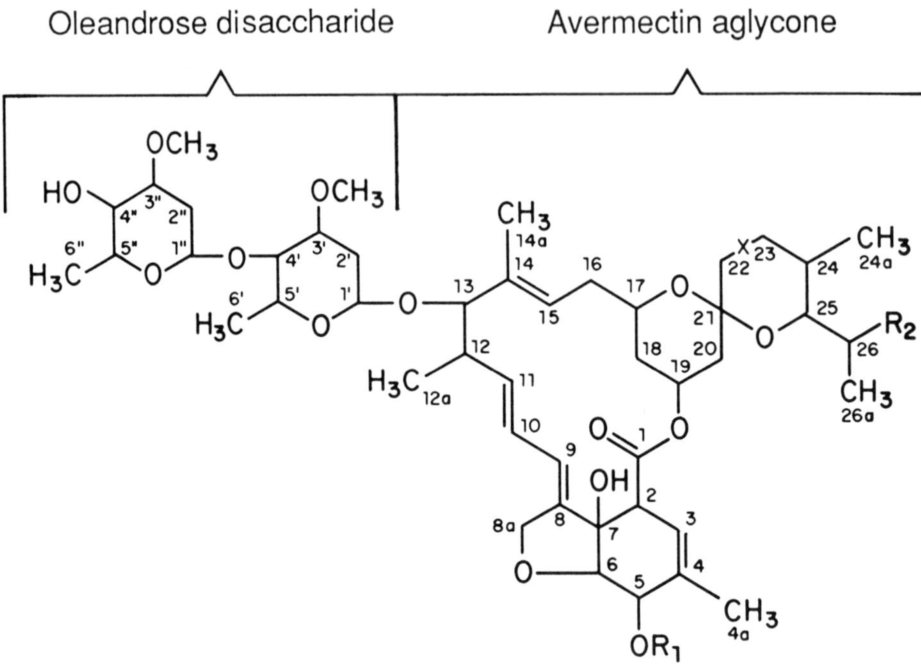

FIGURE 4.1. Avermectin terminology is as follows: X = CH = CH for "1" components; X = CH_2CHOH for "2" components; R_1 = H for "B" components, R_1 = CH_3 for "A" components; R_2 = CH_2CH_3 for "a" components; R_2 = CH_3 for "b" components (from Schulman, Ruby 1987).

II. Incorporation of Labelled Precursors

Figure 4.2 summarizes results obtained from incorporation studies with [1-^{13}C] acetate, [1-^{13}C] propionate (Cane *et al.* 1983); [2-^{13}C] acetate, [1,2-^{13}C] acetate, [3-^{13}C] propionate, [2,3-^{13}C] propionate, [1-^{13}C] 2-methylbutyrate, [1-^{13}C] isobutyrate (Chen *et al.* in press); [U-^{14}C] valine, [U-^{14}C] isoleucine (G. Albers-Schonberg, A.W. Douglas, R.T. Goegelman, L. Kaplan, A. Kempf, and J.B. Tanac, unpublished observations); [1-^{14}C] acetate, [2-^{14}C] acetate, [1-^{14}C] propionate, [2-^{14}C] propionate, [methyl ^{14}C] methionine, and [methyl ^{13}C] methionine (Schulman, Valentino, and Hensens 1986). Tables 4.1 through 4.4 present incorporation data from the most important of these studies. The data show that the aglycone is derived from a head to tail condensation of seven acetates and five propionates. The 2-methylbutyryl group (C25–C28) of the "a" components and the isobutyl group (C25–C27) of the "b" components were not labeled by either precursor; instead, they were derived from isoleucine and valine, respectively. This is supported by the efficient incorporation of [^{14}C] isoleucine into the "a" components and

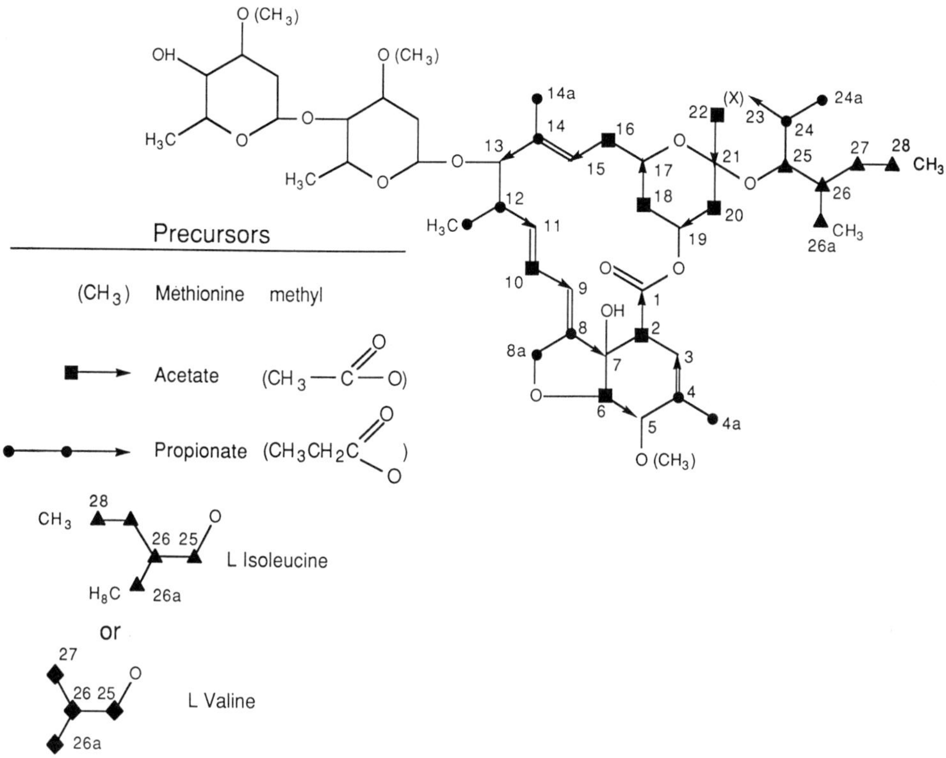

FIGURE 4.2. Incorporation of labeled precursors in the avermectins. (CH3) = S-CH_3 of methionine; ■⟶ = acetate unit; ●-●⟶ = propionate unit; ▲ = carbons derived from isoleucine found in "a" components; ♦ = carbons derived from valine found in "b" components.

[^{14}C] valine into the "b" components (Table 4.2). In addition, there was high enrichment (twenty-fivefold) at C25 of avermectin B_{1a} by [1-^{13}C] 2-methylbutyrate (Table 4.1) and of avermectin B_{1b} [1-^{13}C] by isobutyrate. The metabolism of [1-^{13}C] 2-methylbutyrate to [1-^{13}C] propionate accounts for the enrichment at C3, C7, C11, C13, C23 of B_{1a}.

The methoxyl substituents at C5 of the macrolide moiety and C3′ and C3″ of the oleandrose disaccharide are derived from the methyl of methionine. It was shown using both ^{14}C and ^{13}C-methyl methionine and [2-^{14}C] methionine that the S-methyl and not the carbon backbone is incorporated into avermectin (Tables 2.3, 2.4, and 2.5). The methyl is incorporated equally into all 3 methoxyl groups.

The origin of the oxygen atoms in the macrolide moiety was investigated by measuring the incorporation of [1-^{13}C, 1-^{18}O] acetate and [1-^{13}C, 1-^{18}O] propionate (Cane *et al.* 1983). The oxygens at C1, C5, C7, C13, C17, C19, and C23 (for the "2" components) retained their isotope

TABLE 4.1. Incorporation of [^{13}C] precursors in avermectins by *S. avermitilis*.

Carbon No.	Relative ^{13}C abundance in avermectin B_{1a} biosynthesized from			^{J}CC in avermectin B_{1a} from	
	[2-^{13}] acetate	[3-^{13}C]propionate	[1-^{13}C]2-methylbutyrate	[1,2-$^{13}C_2$]acetate	[2,3-$^{13}C_2$]propionate
C-1	1.4	1.0	1.1	59.3Hz	N.D.[2]
C-2	3.2	1.2	0.9	59.3Hz	N.D.
C-3	1.8	1.4	6.7	N.D.[a]	N.D.
C-4	3.0	1.2	1.3	N.D.	43.4 Hz
C-4a	2.2	5.8	1.2	N.D.	43.4 Hz
C-5	1.0	1.3	0.8	40.7 Hz	N.D.
C-6	3.8	1.2	1.0	40.7 Hz	N.D.
C-7	1.6	1.4	7.7	N.D.	43.2 Hz
C-8	2.8	1.3	1.2	N.D.	43.2 Hz
C-8a	2.4	6.2	1.0	N.D.	N.D.
C-9	1.1	1.0	1.2	55.9 Hz	N.D.
C-10	3.2	1.3	0.9	55.9 Hz	N.D.
C-11	1.8	1.5	6.4	N.D.	N.D.
C-12	2.6	1.5	1.0	N.D.	35.5 Hz
C-12a	2.4	6.8	1.1	N.D.	35.5 Hz
C-13	1.2	1.4	5.9	N.D.	N.D.
C-14	2.9	0.9	0.9	N.D.	44.0 Hz
C-14a	2.3	6.6	1.1	N.D.	44.0 Hz
C-15	1.1	1.2	1.0	43.7 Hz	N.D.
C-16	3.0	1.1	1.1	43.7 Hz	N.D.
C-17	1.2	1.1	1.3	36.3 Hz	N.D.
C-18	4.4	1.3	1.0	36.5 Hz	N.D.

C-19	1.2	1.1	1.3	36.3 Hz	N.D.
C-20	3.8	1.3	0.9	36.3 Hz	N.D.
C-21	1.3	0.9	1.2	54.9 Hz	N.D.
C-22	3.7	1.3	1.0	54.9 Hz	N.D.
C-23	1.8	1.5	5.6	N.D.	N.D.
C-24	2.7	1.7	0.9	N.D.	35.2 Hz
C-24a	2.8	6.7	1.2	N.D.	35.2 Hz
C-25	2.2	1.0	24.5	N.D.	N.D.
C-26	1.3	1.1	0.8	N.D.	N.D.
C-26a	1.3	1.0	0.9	N.D.	N.D.
C-27	1.4	1.0	1.1	N.D.	N.D.
C-28	1.3	1.0	0.9	N.D.	N.D.
C-1′	1.2	1.0	0.9		
C-1″	1.1	1.0	1.0		
C-2′	1.3	1.0	1.0		
C-2″	1.2	1.0	1.0		
C-3′	1.2	1.0	1.0		
C-3″	1.1	1.1	1.1		
C-4′	1.1	1.1	1.1		
C-4″	1.1	1.1	1.0		
C-5′	1.1	1.3	0.8		
C-5″	1.0	1.1	1.0		
C-6′	1.0	1.1	1.0		
C-6″	1.0	1.1	1.0		
3′,3″O-CH_3	1.7	1.2	1.3		

[a]: Not determined.

TABLE 4.2. The incorporation of [U-^{14}C] valine, isoleucine, and sodium isobutyrate into the C-25 sidechain of avermectin B_{1a} and B_{1b}.

			Labeled avermectin			
			Spec. radioact. (μCi/mmole)		Spec. incorporation into C25 sidechain (%)	
Substrate	Conc (uM)	Spec. radioact. (μCi/mmole)	B_{1a}	B_{1b}	B_{1a}	B_{1b}
Valine	4.1	5.85	0.54	1.57	12.3	21.3
Isoleucine	7.3	3.28	2.32	0.40	70.4	14.7
Isobutyrate	1.1	11.00	0.17	0.57	1.5	5.0
	2.2	6.36	0.14	0.69	6.4	10.9
	3.3	3.62	0.71	0.82	4.7	22.7
	4.4	2.58	0.27	0.77	10.5	29.8

TABLE 4.3. [^{14}C]Methionine incorporation into avermectins (from Schulman, Valentino, and Hensens 1986).

	^{14}C in avermectins				
Precursor	Incorporation (%)	Specific activity of A components (dpm/μmol)	Specific activity of B components (dpm/μmol)	Ratio A/B	^{14}C in cell constituents (%)
[methyl-^{14}C]methionine	60–63	179,155	107,521	1.67	23–27
[2-^{14}C]methionine	0	0	0	0	16–20

TABLE 4.4. [Methyl-^{14}C]methionine incorporation in avermectin aglycones (from Schulman, Valentino, and Hensens 1986).

Avermectin component	Specific activity[a] (dpm/μmol)	Original specific activity (%)
A_{1a}	30,075	100
Deglycosylated A_{1a}	11,910	40
A_{2a}	45,409	100
Deglycosylated A_{2a}	17,787	39

[a]: Determined following isolation of the pure component.

TABLE 4.5. Incorporation of [methyl-^{13}C]methionine into avermectins (from Schulman, Valentino, and Hensens 1986).

	Isotopic enrichment[a]		
Avermectin component	C3′ methoxyl	C3″ methoxyl	C5 methoxyl
A_{2a}	5.5	6.5	4.2
A_{1a}	4.3	4.2	6.2
B_{1a}	2.9	2.5	—

[a]: The assignments of the C3′ and C3″ methoxyl carbons are not unequivocal. The C3′ methoxyl carbon is arbitrarily chosen as the high field resonance.

TABLE 4.6. Incorporation of [1-$^{18}O_2$, 1-^{13}C]acetate and [1-$^{18}O_2$, 1-^{13}C]propionate into avermectins (from Cane et al. 1983).

C	4	^{13}C shift, ppm[a]	[1-$^{18}O_2$, ^{13}C]Ac	[1-$^{18}O_2$, ^{13}C]Pr	$^{16}O : ^{18}O$
1	A_1	173.96	0.035	N.D.[c]	50 : 40 : 10[a]
	A_2	173.76	0.035	N.D.	60 : 35 : 5[a]
	B_1	173.69	0.035	N.D.	65 : 35
	B_2	173.54	0.035	N.D.	70 : 30
5	A_1	77.03	0.023	N.D.	60 : 40
	A_2	77.03	0.017	N.D.	60 : 40
	B_1	67.76	0.023	N.D.	70 : 30
	B_2	67.72	0.023	N.D.	70 : 30
7	A_1	80.64	N.D.	0.023	60 : 40
	A_2	80.66	N.D.	0.023	60 : 40
	B_1	80.44	N.D.	0.023	60 : 40
	B_2	80.52	N.D.	0.023	70 : 30
13	A_1	82.06	N.D.	0.023	55 : 45
	A_2	81.82	N.D.	0.023	60 : 40
	B_1	81.99	N.D.	0.023	60 : 40
	B_2	81.77	N.D.	0.023	60 : 40
17	A_1	68.49	b	N.D.	b
	A_2	68.42	0.029	N.D.	60 : 40
	B_1	68.42	0.029	N.D.	60 : 40
	B_2	68.37	0.029	N.D.	60 : 40
19	A_1	68.44	0.023	N.D.	60 : 40
	A_2	67.72	0.035	N.D.	60 : 40
	B_1	68.32	b	N.D.	b
	B_2	67.61	b	N.D.	b
21	A_1	95.84	0.0	N.D.	100 : 0
	A_2	99.73	0.0	N.D.	100 : 0
	B_1	95.83	0.0	N.D.	100 : 0
	B_2	99.70	0.0	N.D.	100 : 0
23	A_2	69.93	N.D.	0.017	60 : 40
	B_2	69.93	N.D.	0.023	60 : 40

[a]: C^{13} O^{18} peak due to excess intramolecular multiple labeling by 90% acetate precursor.

[b]: Signal obscured by overlap with other peaks.

[c]: Not determined.

TABLE 4.7. Incorporation of specifically labeled glucose into avermectin A_{2a} and methyl oleandrose.

Position of label in glucose fed	$^3H^{14}C$ of glucose	Avermectin A_{2a} $^3H/^{14}C$	Avermectin A_{2a} ^3H retention %	Methyl oleandrose $^3H/^{14}C$	Methyl oleandrose ^3H retention
6-^{14}C, 1-^3H	0.91	0.14	15.4	0.67	74
6-^{14}C, 6-^3H	0.46	0.10	21.7	0.46	100

content (Table 4.6). Several conclusions were drawn from these results: (1) the avermectin "1" components which contain a double bond at C22-23 arise from the "2" components by dehydration of the hydroxyl at C23; (2) the oxygen at C21 is probably derived from the 2-methylbutyryl or isobutyryl sidechain (C25); (3) the avermectins are not derived from a milbemycin type intermediate by late-stage oxidation at C13 (Ono *et al.* 1983).

To investigate the origin of the oleandrose backbone, studies with $^3H/^{14}C$ and ^{13}C labeled glucose were conducted. Comparison of the $^3H/^{14}C$ ratio in the labeled avermectin and the methyl oleandrose obtained by methanolysis (Table 4.7) indicated a direct conversion of glucose to oleandrose (Chen *et al.* in press). This was confirmed by studies with [1-^{13}C] glucose and [U-^{13}C] glucose which showed high enrichment of the oleandrose units (Schulman, Valentino, and Hensens 1986).

Studies with labeled glucose provided some insight into the metabolic origin of the avermectin precursors (Schulman, Valentino, and Hensens 1986). Equal incorporation of [1-^{14}C], [2-^{14}C] and [6-^{14}C] glucose into the avermectin aglycone provided strong evidence for the symmetrical cleavage of glucose via the Embden-Myerhoff pathway. A parallel study with [U-^{13}C] glucose demonstrated that the entire avermectin molecule is synthesized from glucose (Figure 4.3). The oleandrose units derived directly from glucose had the highest incorporation rate. The methoxyls of the oleandrose units which are derived from the methyl of methionine were also enriched. Methyl-labeled methionine can be synthesized from glucose via a known microbial pathway that involves serine and serine transhydroxymethylase. The carbons derived from acetate were enriched 3.3-fold over those derived from propionate. This is due to a dilution of acetate by the passage through the tricarboxylic acid cycle to yield propionate (via succinate). The asymmetric labeling of the 2-methylbutyrate-derived sidechain is explained by assuming isoleucine is formed from oxalacetate via the known pathway in the presence of threonine aldolase.

III. Bioconversion of Intermediates

To study the biosynthetic interrelationships among the avermectin "a" components, ^{14}C-labeled A_{1a}, A_{2a}, B_{1a}, B_{2a} were individually fed to cultures of *S. avermitilis* for 5.5 days (Chen *et al.* in press). The "a"

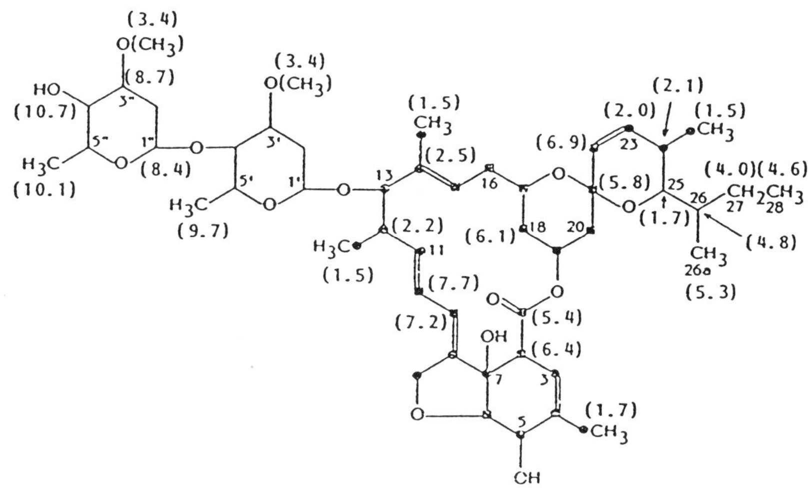

FIGURE 4.3. Incorporation of [U[13]C] glucose into avermectin B_{1a}. CH_3●-●-● = propionate carbons; ■ = acetate carbons; (CH_3) = S-methyl of methionine. Numbers in parentheses are % ^{13}C incorporated (from Schulman, Valentino, and Hensens 1986).

components were then isolated and the distribution of radioactivity was determined. The results, summarized in Table 4.8, show that 30% of the B_{2a} was converted to A_{2a} and 3% of the B_{1a} was converted to A_{1a}. Neither A_{1a} nor A_{2a} was converted into any other avermectin, suggesting that they are the end products of the pathway. Further feeding studies with ^{14}C-labeled B_{2a} aglycone and B_{2a} monosaccharide indicate the biosynthetic reaction sequence B_{2a} aglycone → B_{2a} monosaccharide → B_{2a} → A_{2a}.

Avermectins A_{1a} and B_{1a} were not labeled by B_{2a} aglycone and B_{2a} monosaccharide, indicating that neither compound is the precursor of the "1" components. Avermectin A_{2a} aglycone was converted to A_{2a} by a nonproducing blocked mutant of *S. avermitilis*. Feeding of desfurano avermectins (Figure 4.4) to this blocked mutant revealed that 6,8a-seco-6,8a-deoxy-5 keto$_{1a}$ avermectin aglycone (Figure 4.4, I) was converted exclusively to avermectins A_{1a} and B_{1a}; 6,8a-seco-6,8a-deoxy-5 keto$_{2a}$ avermectin aglycone (Figure 4.4, II) was converted exclusively to A_{2a} and B_{2a}. These results demonstrate that the 5-keto desfurano "2" components are not precursors of the "1" series avermectins and indicate that dehydration at C22-23 must occur before formation of the desfurano avermectins. 6,8a-seco-6,8a-deoxy B_{1a} aglycone (Figure 4.4, III) and 6,8a-seco-6,8a-deoxy A_{2a} aglycone (Figure 4.4, IV) were not bioconverted into complete avermectins; instead they were converted to their respective desfurano mono- and disaccharides. This suggested that formation of the furan ring cannot occur in the presence of a C5 hydroxy or methoxyl and requires a keto group at C5. Avermectin 5-keto aglycone in the 2 series was bioconverted into B_{2a} and A_{2a} in agreement with the

TABLE 4.8. Radioactivity distribution in the avermectins after feeding ^{14}C-labeled avermectins A_{1a}, A_{2a}, B_{1a}, B_{2a}, B_{2a} monosaccharide ($B_{2a}MS$) and B_{2a} aglycone ($B_{2a}AG$) to *S. avermitilis*.

Compounds fed	Radioactivity fed, dpm	Incubation time hr	Total radioactivity recovered in avermectins, dpm					
			$B_{2a}AG$	$B_{2a}MS$	A_{1a}	A_{2a}	B_{1a}	B_{2a}
A_{1a}	3.99×10^5	156	ND[b]	ND	4.02×10^5 (100)[a]	ND	ND	ND
A_{2a}	1.92×10^5	156	ND	ND	ND	1.78×10^5 (93)	ND	ND
B_{1a}	8.3×10^5	156	ND	ND	0.22×10^5 (2.7)	ND	7.77×10^5 (93.6)	ND
B_{2a}	5.59×10^5	156	ND	ND	ND	1.66×10^5 (29.7)	ND	3.82×10^5 (68.3)
$B_{2a}AG$	5.4×10^5	144	2.50×10^5 (46.3)	0.3×10^5 (5.6)	ND	0.5×10^5 (9.3)	ND	1.72×10^5 (31.6)
$B_{2a}MS$	4.16×10^5	144	ND	1.34×10^5 (32.2)	ND	0.78×10^5 (18.6)	ND	1.88×10^5 (45.2)

[a]: Values in parenthesis are given in percent.
[b]: Not detected.

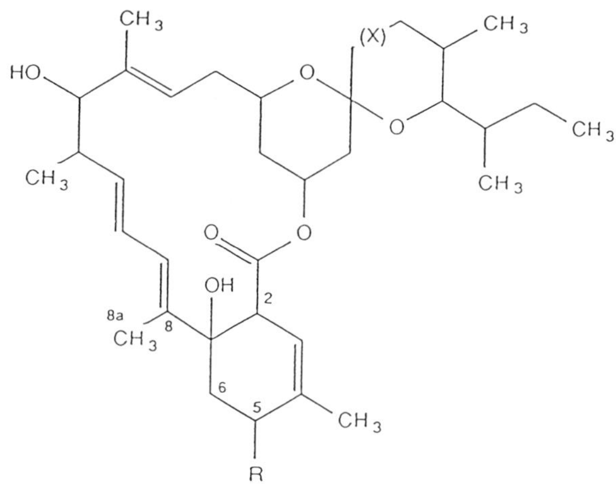

	R	X
I. 6,8a-seco-6,8a-deoxy-5-keto 1a aglycone	=O	—CH=CH—
II. 6,8a-seco-6,8a-dexoy-5-keto 2a aglycone	=O	—CH_2—CHOH—
III. 6,8a-seco-6,8a-deoxy B_{1a} aglycone	—OH	—CH=CH—
IV. 6,8a-seco-6,8a-deoxy A_{2a} aglycone	—OCH_3	—CH_2—CHOH—

FIGURE 4.4. Structure of 6,8a-seco-6,8a-deoxy-5-keto avermectin aglycone.

hypothesis that reduction of the C5 keto occurs after the formation of the furan ring.

Glycosylation to the mono- and disaccharide was observed with a variety of intermediates, indicating that the glycosyltransferases lacked specificity. When [5-methoxyl-^{14}C] A_{2a} bisdemethylavermectin and unlabeled methionine were fed to wild-type *S. avermitilis,* the unaltered substrate was the only radioactive compound recovered (Schulman and Ruby 1987). Its specific radioactivity was virtually identical to that added. This demonstrates that methylation of the oleandrose units is not a terminal step in avermectin biosynthesis and that it occurs before attachment of the sugars to the macrolide ring. The addition of 6,8a-deoxy-5,13,23-triketo avermectin to a nonproducing blocked mutant did not yield any natural avermectin compound, indicating this compound is not a biosynthetic intermediate.

IV. Enzyme Studies

Avermectin B O-methyltransferase

Avermectin B O-methyltransferase catalyzes the conversion of avermectin "A" components to "B" components by transferring the methyl of S-adenosylmethionine to the C5 hydroxyl of the "B" component, yielding the "A" component and S-adenosylhomocysteine (Figure 4.5). This enzyme has been purified and characterized (Schulman, Valentino, and Ruby 1985). It has a molecular weight of 70,000 and is composed of two identical subunits. The enzyme's substrate specificity for the avermectins, in order of decreasing activity, is as follows: B_{2a} aglycone> B_{2a} monosaccharide> B_{1a} aglycone> B_{1a} monosaccharide> B_{2a}> B_{1a}. Avermectin "2" components react faster than "1" components; within each group the order of activity is aglycones> monosaccharides> disaccharides. There was virtually no activity detected with B1a as substrate.

The time course of avermectin B O-methyltransferase activity and avermectin production was measured in several high-producing mutants of *S. avermitilis* (Schulman *et al.* 1986). Table 4.9 presents the average specific activity of the avermectin B O-methyltransferase, the maximum observed specific activity of the O-methyltransferase, and the avermectin titers of 4 mutant strains. Both average specific activity and the maximum observed specific activity increased in direct proportion to the quantity of avermectin formed. These data support the hypothesis that genes coding for enzymes involved in the secondary metabolism biosynthesis may be coordinately expressed.

Avermectin 5-ketoreductase

Avermectin 5-ketoreductase catalyzes the NADPH specific reduction of 5-keto avermectins to B components as shown in Figure 4.6. The time course of enzyme activity and avermectin production was determined in a number of high-producing strains of *S. avermitilis* (M.D. Schulman, unpublished observations). The maximal specific activity of 5-ketoreductase was proportional to avermectin production in these strains, as shown in Figure 4.7. These data further support the hypothesis that genes coding for enzymes involved in secondary metabolism is coordinately regulated.

Avermectin Aglycone Glycosyltransferase

Avermectin aglycone glycosyltransferase, which catalyzes the stepwise addition of oleandrose units from the nucleotide sugar thymidine diphosphate oleandrose to the avermectin aglycone (Figure 4.8), has been demonstrated in cell-free extracts of *S. avermitilis* (M.D. Schulman, D. Valentino, S. Acton, S., and B.H. Arison, unpublished observations).

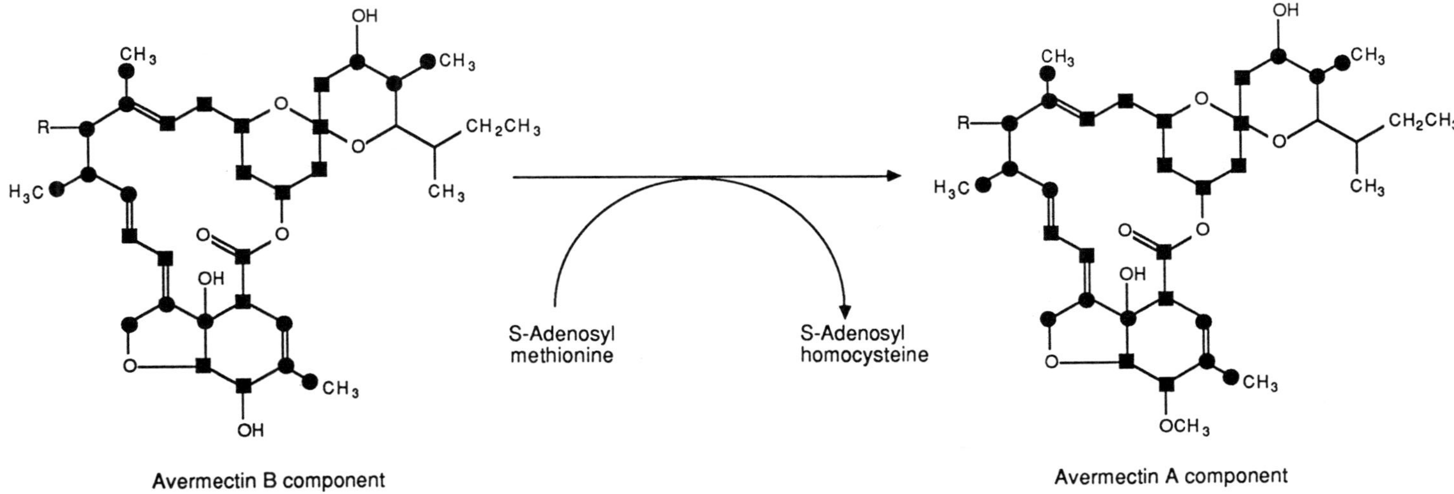

FIGURE 4.5. Reaction of avermectin B O-methyltransferase. R = oleandrose disaccharide.

TABLE 4.9. Avermectin B O-methyltransferase activity and avermectin production in strains A, B, C, and D (From Schulman *et al.* 1986).

Strain	Sp. act. of O-methyltransferase (nmol/h per mg of protein)		Total avermectin at 144 h (relative units)	Fold increase in:		
				Sp. act. of O-methyltransferase		
	Maximum observed	Avg (48 to 144 h)		Maximum	Avg	Avermectin
A	0.37	0.26	0.85	1	1	1
B	0.86	0.54	2.10	2.3	2.1	2.5
C	1.06	0.63	2.4	2.9	2.5	2.8
D	1.35	0.85	3.0	3.6	3.3	3.5

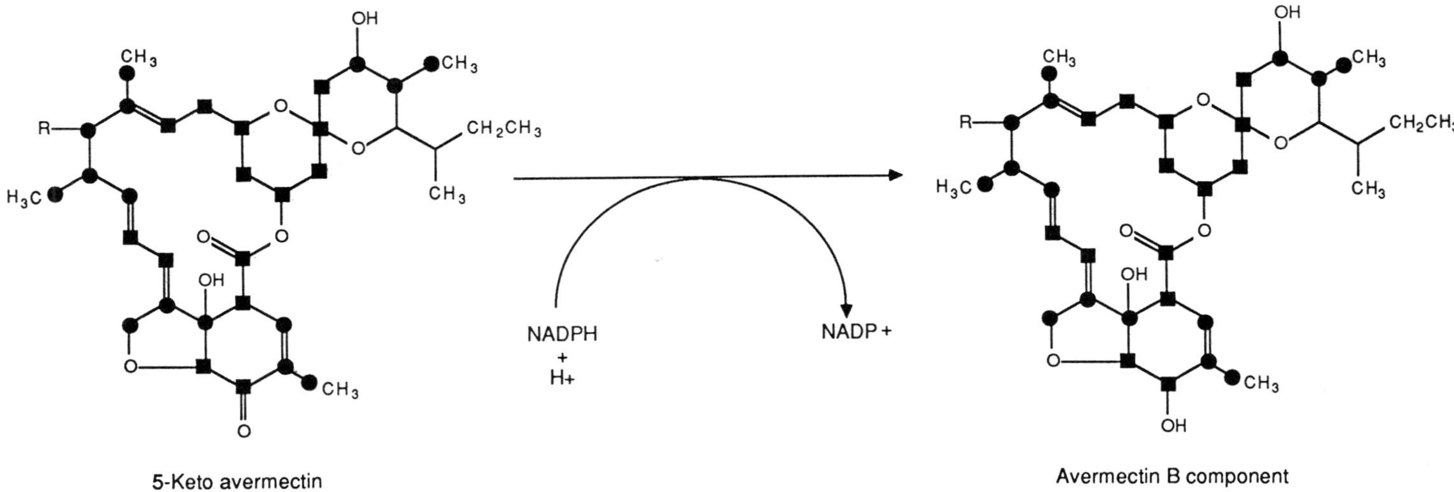

FIGURE 4.6. Reaction of avermectin 5-ketoreductase. R = oleandrose disaccharide.

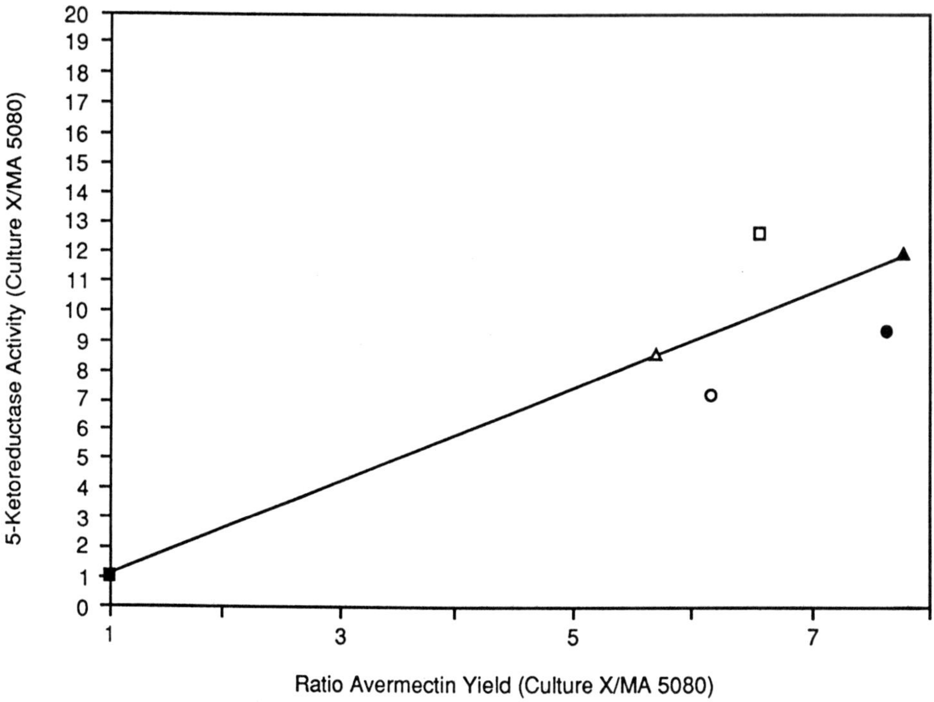

FIGURE 4.7. Avermectin production versus avermectin 5-ketoreductase activity in high-producing strains of *S. avermitilis*. ■ MA5080, ▲ MA5502, ● MA5508, □ MA5856, ○ MA6016, △ MA6233. Line represents a linear regression.

It has not yet been determined if both sugars are transferred by a single enzyme or if two enzymes are required. It is clear, however, that the sugars are transferred sequentially.

V. Effect of Specific Inhibitors

Sinefungin, an analogue of S-adenosylmethionine, is a potent inhibitor of methyltransferases and has been shown to inhibit avermectin B O-methyltransferase *in vitro* (Schulman, Valentino, and Ruby 1985). When fed to a culture that produces virtually only avermectin aglycone "A" components (91%–99%), sinefungin inhibited the formation of "A" components and caused a concomitant accumulation of "B" components (Schulman *et al.* 1985). Sinefungin thus inhibited the conversion of "B" components to "A" components *in vivo*. When sinefungin was added to wild-type *S. avermitilis,* new avermectin components lacking methoxyl groups on the C-3′ and C-3″ of the oleandrose accumulated (Schulman *et al.* 1985b). In this case, sinefungin inhibited methylation of the oleandrose

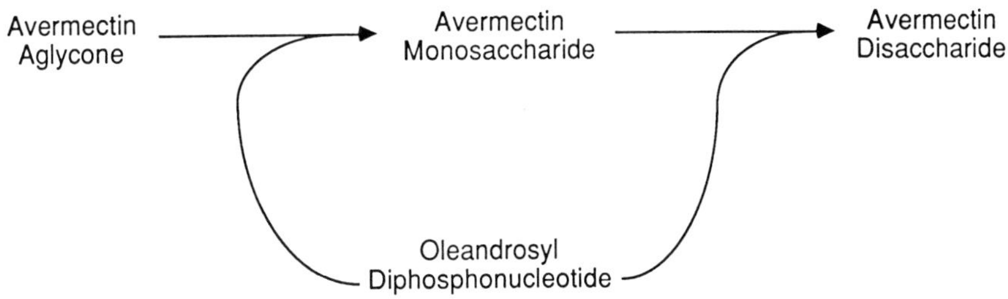

FIGURE 4.8. Reaction of avermectin aglycone glycosyltransferase.

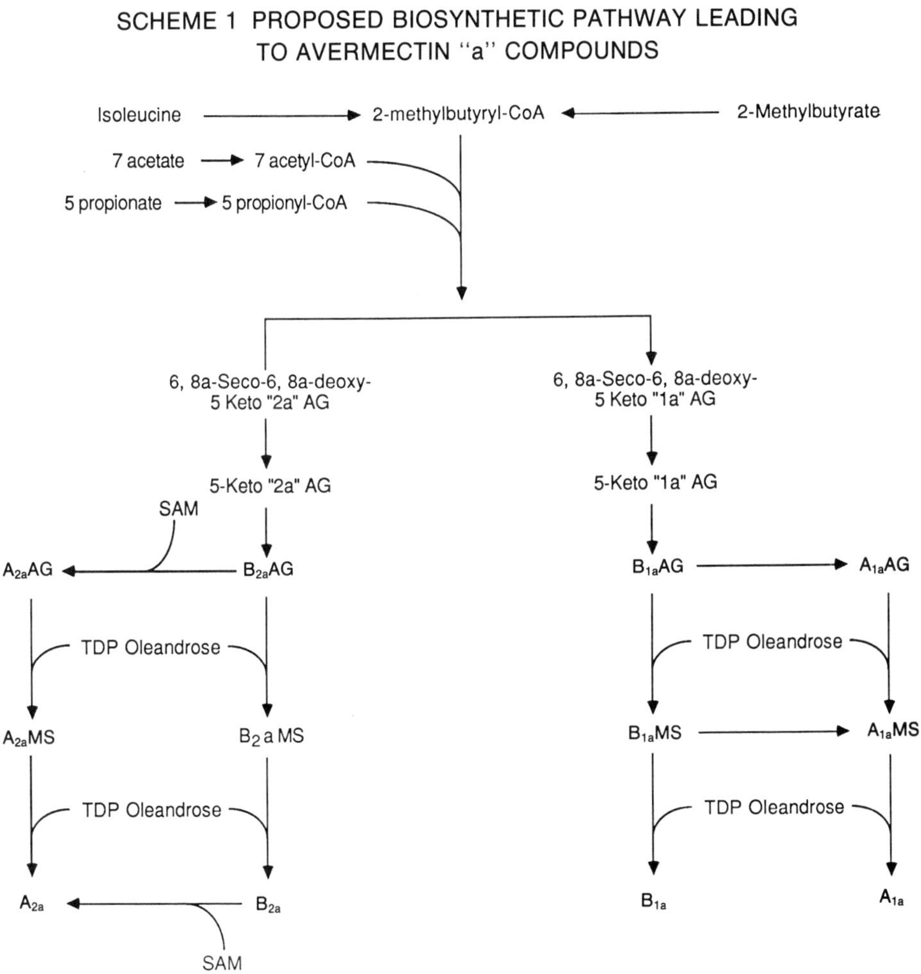

SCHEME 1. Proposed pathway for biosynthesis of the avermectins in *S. avermitilis*.

units, indicating that an S-adenosylmethionine-dependent methyltransferase is involved.

VI. Conclusions

The proposed pathway for biosynthesis of the avermectin "a" components is presented in Figure 4.9. An exactly analagous pathway is envisioned for the "b" components, with valine, isobutyrate, and isobutyryl-CoA replacing isoleucine, 2-methylbutyrate, and 2-methylbutyryl-CoA. Isoleucine undergoes transamination and decarboxylation to yield 2-methylbutyryl-CoA, which serves as the primer for chain elongation. 2-methylbutyryl-CoA can also arise from fed 2-methylbutyrate by activation via a thiokinase. Chain elongation proceeds by addition of acetate and propionate via their CoA esters in a fashion analagous to fatty acid synthesis. At some point during the process, a precursor of the "2" components is dehydrated at C22-23 to yield a precursor of the "1" compounds. From this point on, biosyntheses of the "1" and "2" components proceed in parallel to produce the respective aglycones. Because the methyltransferase and the glycosyltransferase display little specificity, the aglycones are either methylated or glycosylated to produce "A" and "B" disaccharides. At the disaccharide level, B_{2a} can be methylated to A_{2a} but B_{1a} cannot be methylated to A_{1a}.

References

Cane DE, Liang T-C, Kaplan LK, Nallin MK, Schulman MD, Hensens OD, Douglas AW, Albers-Schonberg G (1983) Biosynthetic origin of the carbon skeleton and oxygen atoms of the avermectins. *J. Am. Chem. Soc.* 105:4110–4112

Chen TS, Arison BH, Gullo VP, Inamine ES (in press) Further studies on the biosynthesis of the avermectins. *J. Indust. Microbiol.*

Chen TS, Inamine ES (in press) Studies on the biosynthesis of avermectins. *Arch. Biochem. & Biophys.*

Ono M, Mishima M, Takiguchi Y, Teroa M (1983) Milbemycins, a new family of macrolide antibiotics. Studies on the biosynthesis of milbemycins $\alpha 2$, $\alpha 4$ and D using 13C labelled precursors. *J. Antibiot.* 36:991–1000

Schulman MD, Ruby C (1987) Methylation of demethylavermectins. *Antimicrob. Agents Chemther.* 31:964–965

Schulman MD, Valentino D, Hensens OD (1986) Biosynthesis of the avermectins by *Streptomyces avermitilis*. *J. Antibiot.* 39:541–549

Schulman MD, Valentino D, Hensens OD, Zink D, Nallin MK, Kaplan LK, Ostlind DA (1985) Demethylavermectins. Biosynthesis, isolation and characterization. *J. Antibiot.* 38:1494–1498

Schulman MD, Valentino D, Nallin MK, Kaplan LK (1986) Avermectin B_2 O-methyltransferase activity in *Streptomyces avermitilis* mutants that produce increased amounts of the avermectins. *Antimicrob. Agents Chemother.* 29:620–624

Schulman MD, Valentino D, Ruby C (1985) Avermectin B O-methyltransferase of *Streptomyces avermitilis*. *Fed. Proc.* 44:931

CHAPTER 5

Mode of Action of Ivermectin

M.J. Turner and J.M. Schaeffer

I. Introduction

The anthelmintic activity of the avermectins was first described in 1979 (Burg *et al.* 1979; Egerton *et al.* 1979; Miller *et al.* 1979). The mode of action of these compounds, however, has remained elusive. Identifying the mode of action is all the more difficult because the avermectins have been studied in so many different model systems with an array of experimental protocols. For example, direct injection of avermectin (AVM) into *Ascaris suum* results in a rapid paralysis that is neither flaccid nor rigid; incubation of the free living nematode, *Caenorhabditis elegans,* with AVM results in slow-onset rigid paralysis; and incubation of *Haemonchous contortus ex vivo* with AVM has no observable effect. Exactly why AVM affects these 3 AVM-sensitive nematodes differently is unknown, but it may reflect in part the drug's ability to reach its site of action. The problems in identifying the mechanism(s) by which the avermectins work have been further confounded by several additional factors: the drug acts at multiple sites; various target species have different sensitivities to the drug; and avermectins have poor solubility in aqueous solutions.

The actions of avermectins on vertebrate and invertebrate systems are distinct and will be dealt with separately. Although the most parsimonious explanation for how avermectins work is that they specifically increase membrane chloride ion permeability, there are clearly other sites of action at which avermectins affect either the host or target organism.

It is likely that the entire series of avermectins share a common mode of action; therefore, we will refer to all of the avermectins with the generic abbreviation, AVM. In actuality, nearly all of the studies discussed in this review used either avermectin B_{1a} or 22,23-dihydroavermectin B_{1a} (ivermectin, IVM).

II. Invertebrates

A. Electrophysiological Studies

The earliest studies designed to elucidate the mode of action of AVM were reported by Fritz, Wang, and Gorio (1979). They demonstrated that when lobster stretcher muscle is perfused with $10^{-5}-10^{-6}$M AVM, the inhibitory postsynaptic potentials are rapidly eliminated, followed by a more gradual reduction in the amplitude of excitatory postsynaptic potentials. In these preparations, AVM reduces the input resistance of the muscle fiber by increasing its permeability to chloride (Cl^-) ions. These effects were not reversed by washing. The reduction of both excitatory potentials and input resistance, however, was reversed by picrotoxin (a GABA antagonist active at the chloride channel). It was hypothesized that these responses to AVM were caused by an increase of membrane permeability to chloride ions, perhaps due to its interaction with GABA binding sites or by regulating the release of endogenous GABA. These findings have subsequently been confirmed (Mellin, Busch, and Wang 1983; Albert *et al.* 1986).

The motor nervous system of *Ascaris lumbricoides* is an excellent experimental system to study avermectin's mode of action. An elegant description of the nervous system is available (Stretton *et al.* 1978) which outlines the connections and electrical characteristics of the neurons. The neurons, moreover, are large enough to be penetrated with microelectrodes. Using this model system, Kass and his collaborators (1980, 1984) demonstrated that AVM ($\simeq 5 \times 10^{-6}$M) inhibits transmission between interneurons and excitatory motoneurons in the ventral nerve cord (Figure 5.1), as well as inhibiting transmission between inhibitory motoneurons and muscle; it has little effect, however, on excitatory neuromuscular transmission. Picrotoxin can reverse the AVM-induced block of interneuron-excitatory motoneuron transmission but has no effect on the inhibitory motoneuronal synapse in either the presence or absence of AVM. These findings suggest that AVM can function either as a GABA agonist or as a stimulator of GABA release from presynaptic inhibitory terminals.

Duce and Scott (1983, 1985) demonstrated that within the extensor tibiae muscle of the locust (*Schistocerca gregaria*), specific muscle bundles are sensitive to GABA, whereas a separate population of muscle bundles, which receive only excitatory innervation, are GABA-insensitive. This specificity within a single preparation of muscle fibers was exploited to investigate the interaction of AVM with the GABA receptor-ionophore complex in insect muscle. The muscle bundle that is sensitive to GABA receives inhibitory innervation and exhibits both reversible and irreversible responses to AVM. There is a reversible dose-dependent increase in Cl^- permeability in response to very low doses of AVM ($\simeq 10^{-10}$M); these effects appear to be due to an interaction of AVM with the GABA receptor-Cl^- ion channel complex. Higher AVM concentrations ($\simeq 10^{-8}$M) evoke an irreversible increase in Cl^- conductance that continues to rise after removal of AVM. GABA-insensitive neurons with no inhibitory innervation were also examined; in this case

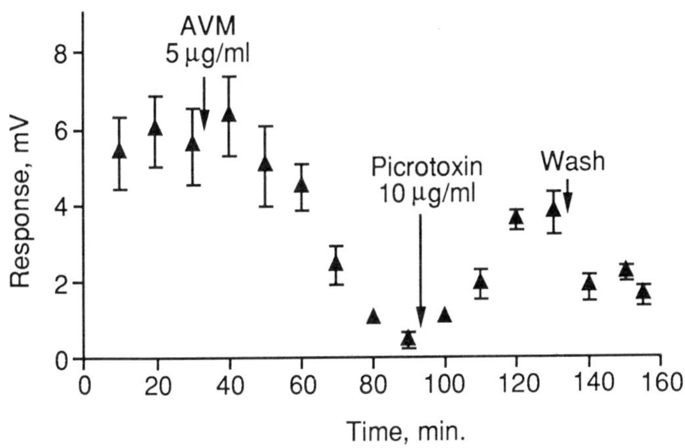

FIGURE 5.1. Responses to indirect stimulation of DE1. Each point represents the mean of five responses. All recordings are from the same dorsal muscle cell. Drugs were added at arrows. (From *Kass et al.* 1980).

AVM ($\simeq 10^{-10}$M) induces only irreversible increases in Cl^- conductance. These important results clearly demonstrate a site of action for AVM distinct from the GABA receptor chloride channel complex. Mellin, Busch, and Wang (1983) studied the effect of AVM on the extensor tibialis muscle from cockroach (*Periplaneta americanus*) walking leg. This preparation consists of numerous fibers which lack an inhibitory GABA innervation. AVM had no effect on the "fast" axon excitatory electrical responses (glutamatergic synapses). The reason for the contradictory effect of AVM on the non-GABA neurons in locust and cockroach has not been resolved.

Recently, single Cl^- channels have been studied by patch-clamping techniques. Martin and Pennington (1988) examined the effect of AVM on single channels in *Ascaris suum* muscle membranes. A progressive stepwise opening of chloride ion channels at AVM concentrations of 2×10^{-12}M and above was observed, with a concentration-dependent delay in onset. The amplitude of the channel was about 1 pA, with a conductance of 12 pS. The duration of opening was very long (>1 second) and was irreversible. This chloride channel is not voltage dependent, it is not GABA-gated, and it is not sensitive to any other neurotransmitters examined. Using the same preparation, GABA-gated channels were also studied. GABA produced a 35-msec opening of a 22-pS conductance channel. Effects of AVM on this channel could be seen only at concentrations of $>10^{-8}$M, at which levels antagonism of the GABA effect was observed.

6. Biochemical Studies

1. IVM Binding Sites

Specific AVM binding sites have been identified in membranes prepared from the nonparasitic nematode, *Caenorhabditis elegans* (Schaeffer and Haines, in press). Specific binding is saturable with an apparent dissociation constant of 2.6×10^{-10}M (Figure 5.2). Kinetic analysis of the binding showed that the reaction proceeds by a 2-step mechanism. Initially, a rapidly reversible complex is formed; after additional incubation this complex is transformed to a much more slowly reversible complex (see Equation 5.1).

$$\mathrm{IVM} + \mathrm{R} \underset{k_{-1}}{\overset{k_{+1}}{\rightleftharpoons}} \mathrm{IVM} \cdot \mathrm{R} \underset{k_{-2}}{\overset{k_{+2}}{\rightleftharpoons}} \mathrm{IVM} \cdot \mathrm{R}^*$$

Stereospecificity of AVM binding was demonstrated by competition with a series of avermectin derivatives. As shown in Figure 5.3, the AVM analogs that are the most potent anthelmintics are also the analogs with the highest affinity for the AVM binding site. Several neurotransmitters, including GABA, were found to have no effect on AVM binding. Specific

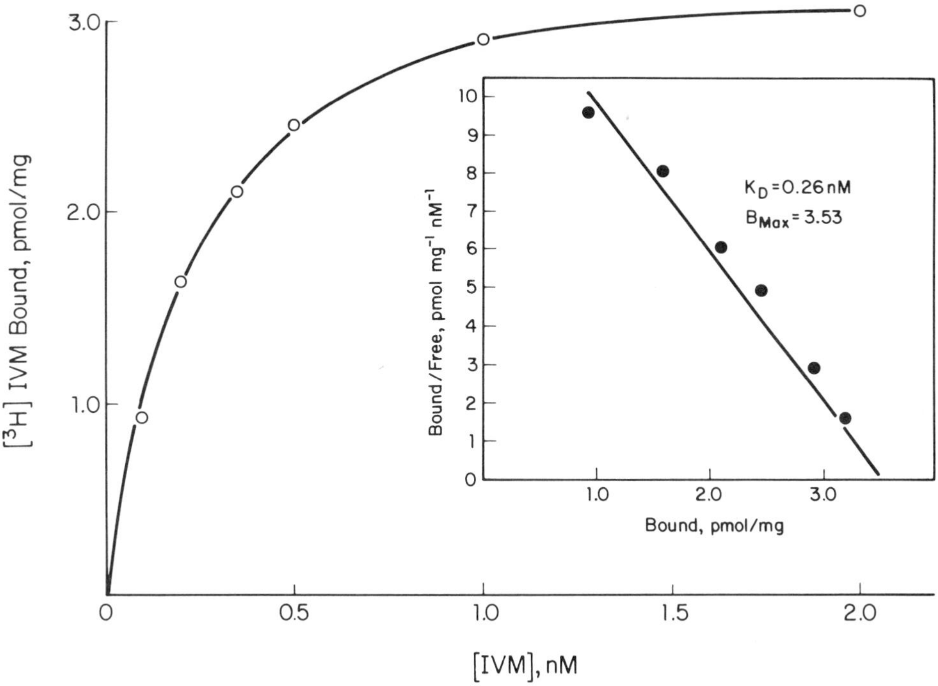

FIGURE 5.2. Equilibrium binding of [^{3}H] IVM to *C. elegans* membranes. Increasing concentrations of [^{3}H] IVM were incubated with *C. elegans* membranes and specific binding was determined as described in the text. Each point is the average of 4 determinations. Replicate experiments gave similar results. A scatchard analysis (inset) of the saturation data is shown. (From Schaeffer and Haines, in press).

AVM binding sites identified in rat brain have an approximately one hundredfold lower affinity than that observed in *C. elegans,* and the stereospecificity is also different (see below).

Specific, high-affinity GABA binding sites ($K_D = 3.7 \times 10^{-8}$M) were also identified in *C. elegans,* and AVM (10^{-10} to 10^{-6}M) had no effect on [^{3}H]-GABA binding (Schaeffer and Bergstrom, 1988). However, in other invertebrate systems AVM-sensitive GABA binding sites have been observed. Lummis and Sattelle (1985) identified a GABA binding site in nerve cord extracts from the cockroach, *Periplaneta americana,* with a K_D value of 3.84×10^{-7}M. AVM enhances the amount of binding of [^{3}H]-GABA over a narrow range concentration ($0.5–5.0 \times 10^{-6}$M). No effects of AVM were seen at lower or higher concentrations. Unfortunately, this study does not report whether AVM alters the affinity of GABA for its binding site. Abalis and Eldefrawi (1986) have reported that AVM acts as a partial agonist at the GABA binding site and competes with [^{3}H] muscimol for specific binding to membranes prepared from honey bees.

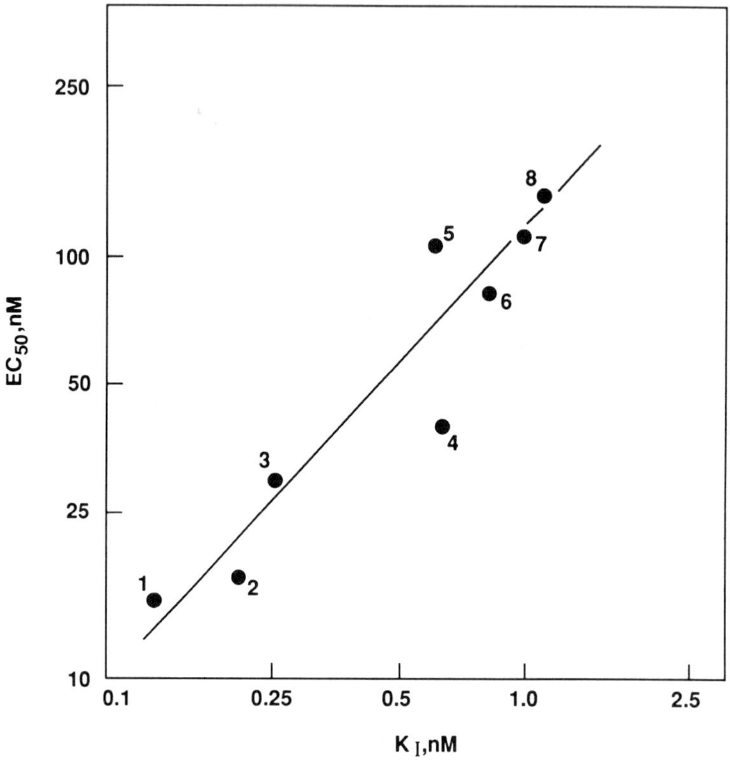

FIGURE 5.3. Correlation between binding affinities of AVM analogs and their biological potencies of *C. elegans* motility *in vivo*. ED_{50} is the concentration of AVM needed to produce immotility in 50% of the worms. The results are the mean values from 2 to 10 experiments (SEM less than 15%). A correlation coefficient (r) of 0.975 was calculated by linear regression analysis. For the log-log plot, r = 0.923. The compounds tested were (1) IVM; (2) AVM B_{2a}; (3) AVM B_{1a} 4′-0-phosphate; (4) 22,23-dihydro-AVM B_{1a} aglycone; (5) 22,23-dihydro-AVM B_1 monosaccharide; (6) AVM B_1 monosaccharide; (7) 2-dehydro-4-hydro-α-2,3-AVM B_1; and (8) AVM B_{1a}-5-ketone. (From Schaeffer and Haines, in press).

2. Chloride Uptake

The action of AVM on chloride uptake was studied on the perfused leg muscle of the American cockroach, *Periplaneta americana* (Tanaka and Matsumura 1985). AVM stimulated chloride uptake at concentrations as low as 10^{-8}M. The AVM-stimulated chloride uptake is antagonized by picrotoxin and to a lesser extent by bicuculline methiodide. At 10^{-7}M AVM the leg muscles fail to respond to external stimuli. This inhibition was postulated to be due to an increase of chloride uptake by the leg muscle. These results suggest that AVM is opening the chloride channel on the plasma membrane. Since AVM had no stimulatory effect on [^{3}H] muscimol or [^{3}H] dihydropicrotoxinin binding to the muscle membranes, the authors suggest that AVM is not active at the GABA binding site but directly at the site of the chloride ion channel. It should be pointed out that the quantitative determination of chloride flux using $^{35}Cl^-$ is very difficult because of the high background in these experiments, and the results presented in this paper are equivocal. The basal rate of chloride uptake (100.00 ± 5.42%) does not seem to be significantly different from the maximal AVM-stimulated chloride uptake (114.56 ± 6.07%).

3. Acetylcholine Release

Nicholson and colleagues (1988) measured AVM-induced presynaptic acetylcholine release in a cockroach CNS synaptosomal preparation. The synaptosomes were preloaded with [^{3}H]choline and perfused under various conditions. AVM causes a release of radioactivity presumed to be acetylcholine (this was not verified). The threshold AVM concentration for acetylcholine release was 10^{-10}M, the ED_{50} value was 10^{-8}M, and maximum stimulation required 10^{-6}M. The effect was chloride dependent and could be antagonized by picrotoxin, trioxabicyclooctaines, and hexachlorocyclohexane. In contrast, the β-isomer of hexachlorocyclohexane potentiated the AVM effect. The authors conclude that in the insect CNS, AVM induces the opening of a presynaptic chloride ion channel (not GABA-activated), leading to efflux of chloride ions, depolarization of the nerve terminal, and hence, to neurotransmitter release.

4. Interaction with Retinol Binding Proteins

A novel mode of action for the AVMs was suggested by Sani and Vaid (1988), who demonstrated that AVM specifically binds to retinol-binding protein isolated from parasitic worms of the family *Filarioidea*. Interestingly, AVM has no affinity toward retinol-binding proteins isolated from the host organism, and AVM has no affinity for retinoic acid–binding proteins from either parasite or host tissues. Binding studies using radiolabeled AVM and retinol reveal that AVM has a higher affinity than retinol for the parasite retinol-binding protein. In addition, a correlation exists between the binding affinities of AVM analogs and their antiparasitic activities. These experiments suggest a binding protein–mediated interrelationship may exist between the actions of retinol and AVM in the parasites, but not in the host. This hypothesis will require further experimentation.

5. Inhibition of Chitin Synthesis

AVM was reported to inhibit fungal growth by interfering with chitin metabolism (Calcott and Fatig 1984a). The evidence for this conclusion was based on data obtained with a methanol extract of a *Streptomyces avermitilis* culture. The sample inhibited N-acetylglucoseamine incorporation into chitin, reduced chitin turnover in brine shrimp, and inhibited purified chitinase. These results could not be confirmed using purified AVM (Onishi and Miller 1985), and it was subsequently reported that the antifungal activity was due to oligomycin and a polyene in the extract (Gordnier, Brezner, and Tanenbaum 1987).

III. Vertebrates

Avermectins have been tremendously successful anthelmintic agents because of their ability to kill parasites without affecting the host organism. Many of the reports describing AVM effects in vertebrates require concentrations of AVM far in excess of those that will ever be attained outside of the laboratory. For this reason, the effects of AVM on nontarget vertebrate species cannot necessarily be related to the mode of action against invertebrate target species.

A. AVM Stimulated Neurotransmitter Release

AVM stimulates the release of endogenous GABA from rat cerebral cortex synaptosomes with an EC_{50} of approximately 2×10^{-6}M (Pong, Wang, and Fritz 1980). This response appears relatively specific because endogenous glutamate was not released. Using rat brain slices from the region of the caudate nucleus, Ishiko, Inagake, and Takaon (1985) perfused the tissue with AVM (10^{-3} to 10^{-2}M) and demonstrated an inhibitory effect of calcium-dependent, potassium-stimulated dopamine release. The inhibitory effect of AVM was completely antagonized by 10^{-5}M picrotoxin and 10^{-4}M bicuculline. The superpharmacological concentrations of AVM required to elicit these responses suggests that they may not be of importance in understanding the mode of action of AVM in target species.

B. AVM Binding Sites

At least 4 different laboratories have investigated the specific binding of [^{3}H]AVM to membranes prepared from dog or rat brains. Pong and Wang (1982) used synaptosomes prepared from dog brain and identified specific AVM binding with an apparent dissociation constant, K_D of 1.2×10^{-9}M. This high-affinity binding was saturable, and the density of binding sites was estimated to be 1.54 pmol/mg protein. Results from competition experiments suggest that the binding is stereospecific and the affinity to the binding sites correlates well with anthelmintic activity. The binding sites are unevenly distributed in the dog brain; the highest density is in the cerebellum (this is also the region of the brain with the highest concentration of GABA binding sites). Similar binding sites were observed in rat brain tissue. Significantly, these authors did not observe any effect of GABA on AVM binding sites. Drexler and Sieghart (1984a, 1984b, 1984c) confirmed the existence of specific AVM binding sites in rat brain membrane preparations. They also report an affinity of approximately 2×10^{-9}M. In contrast to Pong and Wang (1982), however, these investigators observed partial inhibition of AVM binding in the presence of GABA (approximately 40% inhibition of specific AVM binding in the presence of 3×10^{-4}M GABA). Other GABA agonists had similar effects, and this could be blocked by GABA antagonists and also by chloride ions. The presence of chloride ions in the incubation solution may explain why Pong and Wang (1982) observed no effect of GABA on [^{3}H]AVM binding. Specific high-affinity binding of [^{3}H]AVM was also stimulated by the convulsant picrotoxin and inhibited by the anticonvulsant pentobarbital and the anxiolytic etazolate. These results support an interaction between the AVM binding site and the GABA-benzodiazepine receptor chloride channel complex. Two other laboratories have examined [^{3}H]AVM binding to rat brain membranes and report K_D values in the range of 20 nM (Schaeffer and Haines, in press; Huang and Burg 1986). The reason for the discrepancy in the binding affinity is not clear but may be explained by differences in nonspecific binding: in the more recent reports (Huang and Burg 1986; Schaeffer and Haines, in press) the glass fiber filters used in the binding assay were pretreated with polyethyimine and Triton X-100, resulting in a 90% decrease of nonspecific binding.

C. AVM Effect on [^{3}H]GABA Binding

Because the data obtained in invertebrate systems suggest a link between the action of AVM and GABA binding sites, the effect of AVM on [^{3}H]GABA binding has been extensively investigated in rat brain tissue. Pong and Wang (1982) reported that AVM stimulates [^{3}H]GABA binding to washed rat brain membranes (Figure 5.4). Scatchard analysis demonstrated that AVM does not alter the affinity of GABA for its binding site but, rather, increases the number of binding sites by approximately 60%. The AVM effect on GABA binding was antagonized by both bicuculline and picrotoxin and is chloride-dependent. Similar experiments were reported by Olsen and Snowman (1985). However, they report that AVM (10^{-7}M) decreases GABA binding to rat brain membranes (approximately 50% inhibition) and increases the binding of the GABA antagonist [^{3}H]bicuculline, an effect that was potentiated by picrotoxin. These results are a direct contradiction to those of Pong and Wang (1982), and the explanation for this discrepancy is not known. Calcott and Fatig (1984b) also report that AVM increases [^{3}H]GABA binding to rat brain membranes. The maximal stimulation was approximately 50% in the

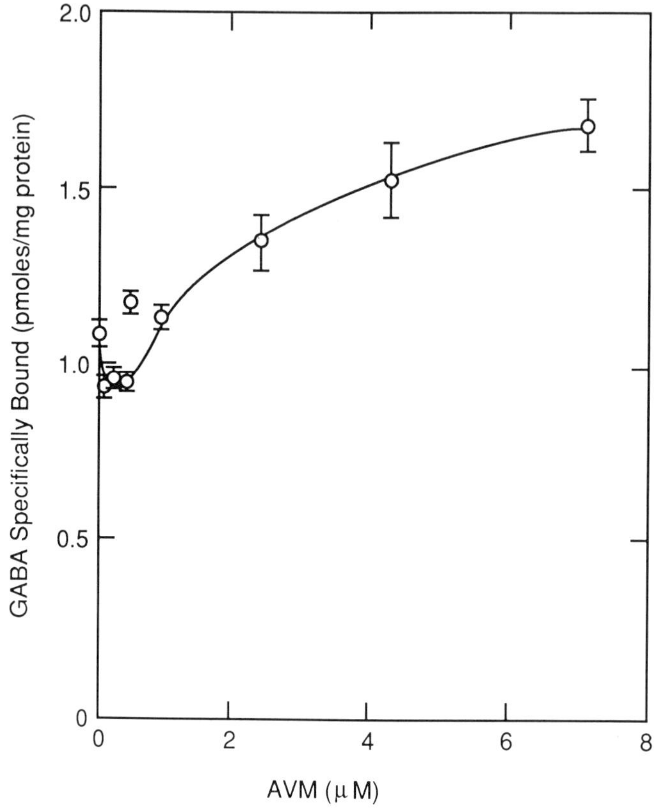

FIGURE 5.4. Dose-response enhancement of Na^+-independent [^{3}H] GABA binding by AVM in washed rat brain membrane preparations. The concentration of [^{3}H] GABA was 10 nM. Each point is the mean ± S.D. of 3 experiments performed in triplicate (from Pong and Wang 1982).

presence of 4×10^{-7}M AVM. At higher and lower concentrations of AVM, the stimulatory effect was less pronounced.

D. AVM Effect on Benzodiazepine Binding Sites

It is well documented that benzodiazepine agonists increase the affinity of $GABA_A$ recognition sites associated with the GABA receptor/chloride ion channel complex (Guidotti, Tottano, and Costa 1978; Meiners and Salama 1982). Several laboratories have reported that AVM potentiates benzodiazepine receptor binding in rat, mouse, and human brain membrane preparations (Figure 5.5; Williams and Yarbrough 1979; Paul, Skolnick, and Zatz 1980; Pong, DeHaven, and Wang 1981; Supavilai and Karobath 1981; Williams and Risley 1984; Sieghart *et al.* 1985). These studies clearly demonstrate that AVM causes a concentration-dependent

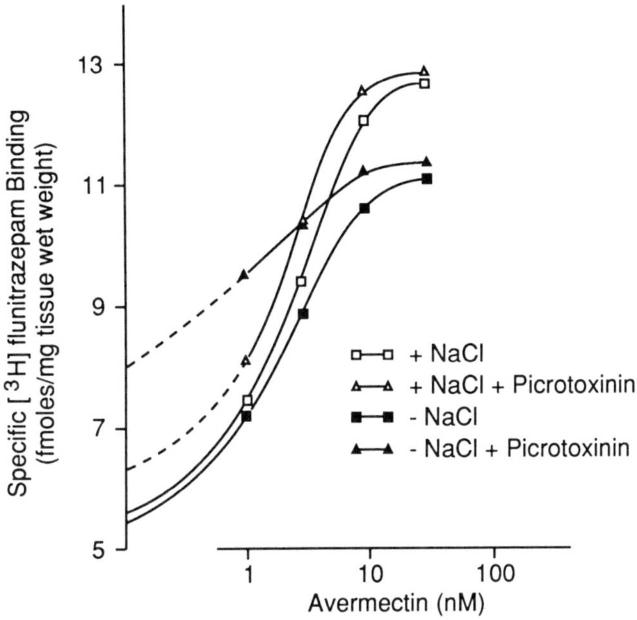

FIGURE 5.5. Effect of AVM on [^{3}H]flunitrazepam binding and modulating of AVM-stimulated [^{3}H]flunitrazepam binding by chloride ions and picrotoxinin. Membranes from rat cerebellum were incubated with 1 nM [^{3}H]flunitrazepam and various concentrations of AVM in the absence or presence of μM diazepam in a solution containing 50 mM Tris-citrate, pH 7.3, in the absence or presence of 150 mM NaCl and/or 30 μM picrotoxinin. Incubations were performed at 23°C for 30 minutes, and membranes were then filtered through Whatman GF/B filters and washed as described in Materials and Methods. Results are from a typical experiment which was repeated three times with identical results (from Williams and Yarbrough 1979).

increase in the *in vitro* binding of [^{3}H]benzodiazepine to rat brain membranes. AVM elicits both an increase in the affinity and number of binding sites for [^{3}H]benzodiazepine. The concentration of AVM required to increase the benzodiazepine binding varies in these reports from EC_{50} values of 40 to 250 $\times$ 10^{-9}M. In addition, the magnitude of the increase in binding varies from 15% to 100% of the control.

AVM does not inhibit the binding of the benzodiapine receptor inverse agonist [^{3}H]β-carboline-carboxylate methyl ester, and it enhances the binding of the cage convulsant [^{35}S]t-butyl cyclophosphorothionate to picrotoxin receptor sites. Interestingly, Williams and Risley (1982) examined a similar system and report that AVM does enhance [^{3}H]β-carboline carboxylate binding to rat brain membranes. The increase in binding reflects an increase in the B_{max} with no change in the K_D value. This change is bicuculline insensitive.

[^{35}S]tert-butylbicyclophophorothionate (TBPT, a potent convulsant that is thought to bind to the chloride channel associated with the GABA benzodiazepine receptor complex) binding is stimulated by AVM in rat brain membrane preparations (Drexler and Sieghart 1984c). Conversely, TBPT either weakly stimulates or does not significantly influence the specific high-affinity binding of [^{3}H]AVM to the same membranes in the absence or presence of chloride ions. These results indicate that AVM and TBPT bind to different but closely associated binding sites.

E. Chloride Uptake

Neurosynaptosomal preparations provide a model system for the study of chloride influx into neuronal tissue (Harris and Allen 1985; Schwartz *et al.* 1986). It has been clearly established that GABA stimulates Cl^- influx into neuronal tissues. Soderlund and colleagues (1987) reported that in rat neurosynaptosomes AVM is a weak activator of chloride uptake in the absence of GABA as well as an inhibitor of GABA-stimulated chloride uptake. Conversely, when these authors used mouse brain tissue, AVM acted only as a noncompetitive antagonist of GABA-stimulated uptake. The authors conclude that AVM binds with high affinity to a site associated with, but not identical to, the GABA receptor. It is unclear why mice and rats would have such different responses to AVM. In addition, these results are difficult to reconcile with the fact that, in other systems, AVM increases membrane permeability to chloride ions and is acting as a GABA agonist, not a GABA antagonist. Our laboratory (Schaeffer and Bergstrom, in press) recently demonstrated that GABA increases Cl^- uptake into rat cerebral cortex neurosynaptosomes 125% with an EC_{50} value of 3×10^{-4}M. AVM has no effect on chloride influx; it does, however, potentiate the GABA-stimulated chloride influx, without increasing the maximal response to GABA (the EC_{50} value is shifted to 9×10^{-5}M). The reasons for the difference between these results and those presented in earlier reports (Soderlund *et al.* 1987) are not understood. However, the suggestion that AVM stimulates chloride uptake into neurosynaptosomes correlates very well with the results reported by Sigel and Baur (1987). They injected chick brain mRNA into Xenopus oocytes and demonstrated the expression of functional GABA receptors. The oocyte was voltage clamped and the effects of various compounds on the GABA-induced chloride current were monitored. AVM strongly enhanced the GABA-induced chloride current in a dose-dependent manner (Figure 5.6). The half-maximal dose of AVM was 10^{-7}M, which may be physiologically significant in the mammalian system (however, not in invertebrate systems). Interestingly, AVM did not affect the reversal potential of the current or the maximal response elicited by GABA, nor did it alter membrane permeability in the absence of GABA. The major effects of AVM were a shift of the K_a for GABA from 21 to 2×10^{-6}M, and a decrease of the apparent Hill coefficient for GABA from 1.7 to 1.1.

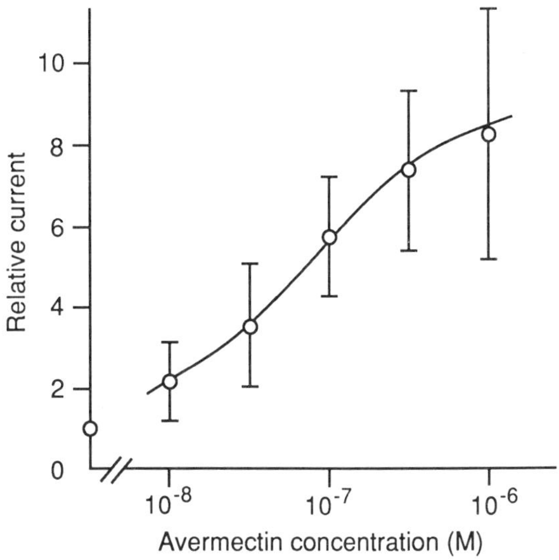

FIGURE 5.6. Concentration dependence of the stimulatory effect by avermectin B_{1a}. The measurements were standardized by assigning the value of 1 to the current amplitude elicited by a control application of 5 μM GABA. Different concentrations of avermectin B_{1a} were applied for 3 minutes alone and then in combination with 5 μM GABA. For each point the Mean $\pm$ standard deviation is given for at least three determinations performed on different oocytes (from Sigel and Baur 1987).

F. Other Actions of AVM

Graham, Pfeiffer, and Betz (1982) identified and characterized glycine binding sites associated with membranes isolated from rat spinal cord. They report that AVM inhibits the binding of the glycine antagonist, strychnine, with a K_I value of 1.3×10^{-6}M. The high concentration of AVM required for this action suggests that this may not be of physiological significance.

There has been at least one report that AVM is a specific inhibitor of protein kinase C activity isolated from rat brain (Ellis *et al.* 1987); in these experiments, however, 10^{-6}M AVM was required to inhibit 50% of the enzyme activity. Once again, this high dose may not be physiologically significant.

IV. Conclusions

It is not possible to assign a single mechanism of action for AVM in the various systems that have been studied. In target organisms, the effect of AVM is mediated via a specific, high-affinity ($\simeq 10^{-10}$M) binding site. The physiological response to AVM binding is an increase in membrane permeability to chloride ions, which is independent of GABA-mediated chloride ion channels. GABA-gated chloride ions may also interact with AVM, but at significantly greater AVM concentrations ($\approx 10^{-7}$M). In addition to their interaction with chloride channels, several other actions of the AVMs have been proposed; the importance of these remains to be resolved.

References

Abalis IM, Eldefrawi AT (1986) [^{3}H]Muscimol binding to a putative GABA receptor in honey bee brain and its interaction with avermectin B_{1a}. *Pestic. Biochem. Physiol.* 25:279–287

Albert J, Lingle DH, Marder E, O'Neil MB (1986) A GABA-activated chloride-conductance not blocked by picrotoxin on spiny lobster neuromuscular preparations. *Brit. J. Pharmacol.* 87:771–779

Burg RW, Miller BM, Baker EE, Birnbaum J, Currie JA, Harman R, Kong VL, Monaghan RL, Olson G, Putter I, Tunac JP, Wallick H, Stapley EO, Oiwa R, Omura S (1979) The action of avermectin on identified central neurons from *Helix* and its interaction with acetylcholine and gamma-aminobutyric acid responses. *Antimicrob. Agents Chemother.* 15:361–367

Calcott PH, Fatig RO (1984a) Inhibition of chitin metabolism by avermectin in susceptible organisms. *J. Antibiot.* 37:253–259

Calcott PH, Fatig RO (1984b) Avermectin modulation of gamma-aminobutyric acid binding to membranes of rat brain, brine shrimp and a fungus, *mucor miehei*. *J. Antibiot.* 37:797–801

Drexler G, Sieghart W (1984a) Properties of high affinity binding site for tritium-labeled avermectin B_{1a}. *Eur. J. Pharmacol.* 99:269–277

Drexler G. Sieghart W (1984b) Evidence for association of a high affinity avermectin binding site with benzodiazepine receptor. *Eur. J. Pharmacol.* 101:201–207

Drexler G. Sieghart W (1984c) Sulfur-35-labeled tert-butyl-bicyclophosphorothionate and avermectin bind to different sites associated with the gamma-aminobutyric acid-benzodiazepine receptor complex. *Neurosci. Let.* 50: 273–277

Duce IR, Scott RH (1983) GABA sensitivity in the distal bundles of the locust extensor tibiae muscle. *J. Physiol.* 343:32P

Duce IR, Scott RH (1985) Actions of dihydroavermectin B_{1a} on insect muscle. *Brit. J. Pharmacol.* 85:395–401

Egerton JR, Ostlind DA, Blair LS, Eary DH, Suhayda D, Cifelli S, Riek RF, Campbell WC (1979) Avermectins, new family of potent anthelmintic agents: efficacy of the B_{1a} component. *Antimicrob. Agents Chemother.* 15:372–378

Ellis C, Nathwani B, Morrice N, Parker P, Evans FJ, Aitken A (1987) Ivermectin: an inhibitor of protein kinase C−: A potential target enzyme for onchocerciases chemotherapy. *Brit. J. Pharmacol.* 91:22P

Fritz LC, Wang CC, Gorio A (1979) Avermectin B_{1a} irreversibly blocks presynaptic potentials at the lobster neuromuscular junction by reducing muscle membrane resistance. *Proc. Natl. Acad. Sci. USA* 76:2062–2066

Gordnier PM, Brezner J, Tanenbaum, SW (1987) Chitin metabolism: not a target of avermectin/milbemycin activity in insects. *J. Antibiot.* 40:110–112

Graham D, Pfeiffer F, Betz H (1982) Avermectin B_{1a} inhibits the binding of strychnine to the glycine receptor of rat spinal cord. *Neurosci. Let.* 29:173–176

Guidotti A, Tottano G, Costa, E (1978) An endogenous protein modulates the affinity of GABA and benzodiazepine receptors in rat brain. *Nature* 275:553–555

Harris RA, Allen AM (1985) Functional coupling of GABA receptors to chloride channels in brain membranes. *Science* 228:1108–1110.

Huang L, Burg R (1986) The avermectin receptor of the American cockroach. *Soc. Neurosci. Abstr.* #9.9

Ishiko J, Inagake C, Takaori S (1985) Effects of avermectin B_{1a} and picrotoxin on striatal release of dopamine with reference to replacement of extracellular chloride with nitrate. *Neuropharm.* 24:1147–1154

Kass IS, Stretton AOW, Wand CC (1984) The effects of avermectin and drugs related to acetylcholine and 4-aminobutyric acid on neurotransmission in *Ascaris suum. Molec. & Biochem. Parasit.* 13:213–225

Kass IS, Wang CC, Walrond JP, Stretton AOW (1980) Avermectin B_{1a}, a paralyzing anthelmintic that affects interneurons and inhibitory motoneurons in *Ascaris. Proc. Natl. Acad. Sci. USA* 77:6211–6215

Lummis CR, Sattelle DB (1985) GABA and benzodiazepine binding sites in insect CNS. *Pestic. Sci.* 16:61–65.

Martin R, Pennington AJ (1988) Effect of dihydroavermectin B_{1a} on Cl single-channel currents in *Ascaris* muscle. *Neurotox. '88 Abstr.* 141

Meiners BA, Salama AI (1982) Enhancement of benzodiazepine and GABA binding by the novel anxiolytic, tracazolate. *Euro. J. Pharmacol. 78:315–322*

Mellin TN, Busch RD, Wang CC (1983) Postsynaptic inhibition of invertebrate neuromuscular transmission by avermectin B_{1a}. *Neuropharm.* 22:89–96

Miller TW, Chaiet L, Cole DJ, Flor JE, Goegelman RT, Gullo VP, Joshua H, Kempf AJ, Krellwitz WR, Monaghan RL, Ormond RE, Wilson KE, Albers-Schonberg G, Putter I (1979) Avermectins, a new family of potent anthelmintic agents: isolation and chromatographic properties. *Antimicrob. Agents Chemother.* 15:368–371

Nicholson R, Robinson PS, Palmer PJ, Casida JE (1988) Ivermectin-stimulated release of neurotransmitter in the insect central nervous system: modulation by external chloride and inhibition by a novel trioxabicyclooctane and two polychlorocyloalkane insecticides. *Neurotox '88 Abstr.* #96

Olsen RW, Snowman AM (1985) Avermectin B_{1a} modulation of gamma-aminobutyric acid-benzodiazepine receptor binding in mammalian brain. *J. Neurochem.* 44:1074–1082

Onishi JC, Miller TW (1985) The lack of antifungal activity by avermectin B_{1a}. *J. Antibiot.* 38:1568–1572

Paul SM, Skolnick P, Zatz M (1980) Avermectin B_{1a}: an irreversible activator of the gamma-aminobutyric acid-benzodiazepine-chloride-ionophore receptor complex. *Biochem. Biophys. Res. Commun.* 96:632–638

Pong S-S, DeHaven R, Wang CC (1981) Stimulation of benzodiazepine binding to rat brain membranes and solubized receptor complex by avermectin B_{1a} and GABA. *Biochem. Biophys. Acta* 646:143–149

Pong S-S, Wang CC (1982) Avermectin B_{1a} modulation of gamma-aminobutyric acid receptors in rat brain membranes. *J. Neurochem.* 38:375–379

Pong S-S, Wang CC, Fritz LC (1980) Studies on the mechanism of action of avermectin B_{1a}: stimulation of release of gamma-aminobutyric acid from brain synaptosomes. *J. Neurochem.* 34:351–358

Sani BP, Vaid A (1988) Specific interaction of ivermectin with retinol-binding protein from filarial parasites. *Biochem. J.* 249:929–932

Schaeffer JM, Bergstrom AR (1988) Identification of gamma-aminobutyric acid binding sites in *Caenorhabditis elegans*. *Life Sci.* 43:1701–1706

Schaeffer JM, Bergstrom AR (in press) The effect of ivermectin on chloride uptake by rat brain synaptosomes. *Biochem. Biophys. Res. Comm.*

Schaeffer JM, Haines H (in press) Avermectin binding in *Caenorhabditis elegans:* a two-state model for the avermectin binding site. *Biochem. Pharm.*

Schwartz RD, Sudak PD, Paul SM (1986) GABA- and barbituate-mediated chloride uptake in rat brain synaptoneurosomes: Evidence for a rapid desensitization of the GABA receptor-coupled chloride ion channel. *Molec. Pharm.* 30:419–426

Sieghart W, Eichinger A, Riederer P, Jellinger K (1985) Comparison of benzodiazepine receptor binding in membranes from human or rat brain. *Neuropharm.* 24:751–760

Sigel E, Baur R (1987) Effect of avermectin B_{1a} on chick neuronal gamma-aminobutyric acid receptor channels expressed in *Xenopus* oocytes. *Molec. Pharm.* 32:749–752

Soderlaud DM, Adams PM, Bloomquist JR (1987) Differences in the action of avermectin B_{1a} on the $GABA_A$ receptor complex of mouse and rat. *Biochem. Biophys. Res. Commun.* 146:692–698

Stretton AOW, Fishpool RM, Southgate E, Donmoyer JE, Walrond JP, Moses JER, Kass IS (1978) Structure and physiological activity of the motorneurons of the nematode *Ascaris*. *Proc. Natl. Acad. Sci. USA* 75:3493–3497

Supavilai P, Karobath M (1981) *In vitro* modulation by avermectin B_{1a} of the GABA/benzodiazepine receptor complex or fat cerebellum. *J. Neurochem.* 36:798–805

Tanaka K, Matsumura F (1985) Action of avermectin B_{1a} on the leg muscles and nervous system of the American cockroach. *Pest. Biochem. Physiol.* 24:124–135

Williams M, Risley EA (1982) Interaction of avermectins with $[^3H]\beta$-carboline-3 carboxylate ethyl ester and $[^3H]$ diazepam binding sites in rat brain cortical membranes. *Eur. J. Pharmacol.* 77:307–312

Williams M, Risley EA (1984) Ivermectin interactions with benzodiazepine receptors in rat cortex and cerebellum *in vitro*. *J. Neurochem.* 42:745–753

Williams M, Yarbrough GG (1979) Enhancement of *in vitro* binding and some of the pharmacological properties of diazepam by a novel anthelmintic agent, avermectin B_{1a}. *Eur. J. Pharmacol.* 56:1273–276

CHAPTER 6

Toxicology

George R. Lankas and Lea R. Gordon

I. Introduction

Abamectin (MK-0936) is a natural fermentation product of *Streptomyces avermitilis*. Ivermectin (MK-0933) is a synthetic derivative of abamectin. The chemical structure of abamectin differs from ivermectin only in the bond between carbons 22 and 23; abamectin has a double bond where ivermectin has a single bond and additional hydrogens on C-22 and C-23 (Figure 6.1). Both compounds are a mixture of homologous products with B_{1a} and B_{1b} components. The B_{1b} component differs chemically from the B_{1a} component by only 1 methylene (CH2) unit at the 26-carbon position: the ethyl group (C2H5) is a methyl group (CH3) in the B_{1b} form. Abamectin and ivermectin are defined as containing a minimum of 80% B_{1a} and a maximum of 20% B_{1b} components. Studies in our laboratories have clearly demonstrated that the individual components have very similar biological and toxicological properties and, for all practical purposes, can be considered equivalent.

GABA receptors. Abamectin and ivermectin increase calcium perme-

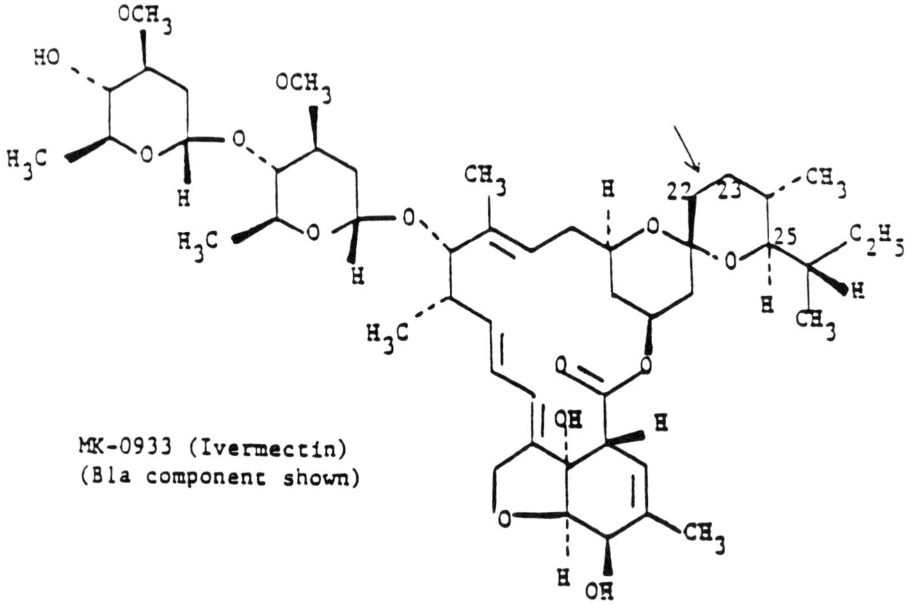

MK-0933 (Ivermectin)
(Bla component shown)

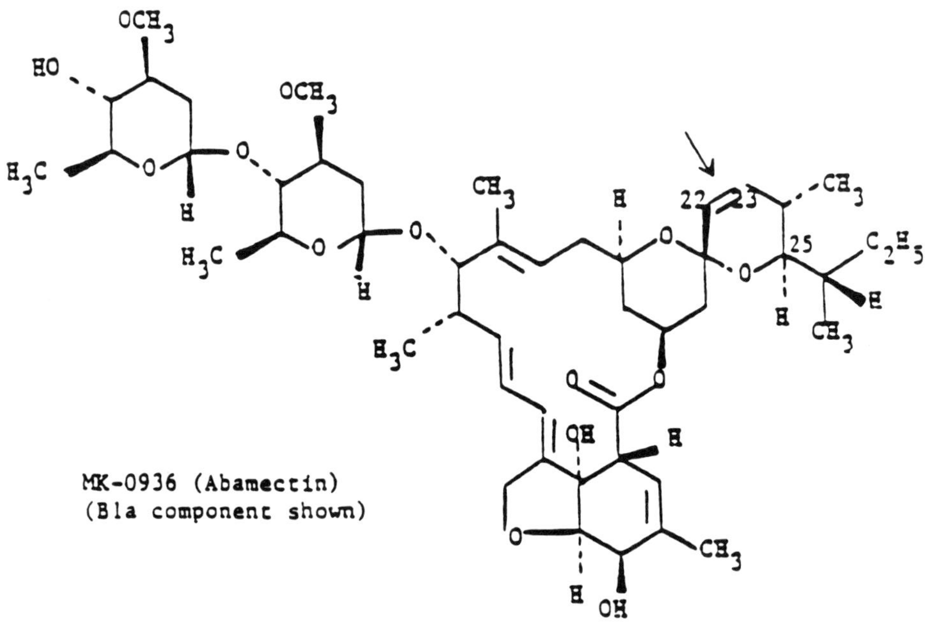

MK-0936 (Abamectin)
(Bla component shown)

FIGURE 6.1. The chemical structures of ivermectin B_{1a} (above) and abamectin B_{1a}.

ability by their interaction with GABA-gated chloride channels but it is now thought that this is not the primary basis of their anthelmintic action (see Chapter 5). The compounds' mechanism of toxicity in mammals is unknown but GABA is a mammalian central nervous system neurotransmitter and effects on GABA may be relevant to their safety in mammals. The fact that much higher concentrations of these compounds are needed in mammals as compared to nematodes to affect neurological function may be due to the lack of a specific, high affinity site associated with neuronal function or to the relatively poor penetration of these large molecular weight compounds into the CNS.

In general ivermectin is slightly less toxic than abamectin in laboratory animals. Clinical signs of toxicity for abamectin and ivermectin in laboratory animals are identical, depending on the species: mydriasis (pupillary dilatation) in dogs, emesis in monkeys, and convulsions and/or tremors and coma at higher doses in most species.

II. Toxicity Studies Conducted with Ivermectin (MK-0933)

A. Genotoxicity Studies

Ivermectin has been tested for genotoxic activity in a series of *in vitro* bacterial and mammalian cell assays. In bacteria ivermectin was studied for mutagenic activity by assessing its ability to revert *Salmonella typhimurium* (strains TA1535, TA1537, TA98, and TA100) from histidine prototrophy to auxotrophy as described by Ames (Ames, McCann, and Yamasaki 1975). Each component of ivermectin was tested separately in a similar fashion, and all tests were done with and without metabolic activation systems prepared from rat liver. None of the agents studied produced significant increases in reversion to histidine prototrophy under any of the test conditions, at concentrations up to 2000 ug/plate.

Ivermectin was studied in the mouse lymphoma assay (Clive *et al.* 1972; Clive and Spector 1975) to evaluate the compound's potential to produce a forward mutation at the thymidine kinase (TK) locus of Fischer L5178Y mouse lymphoma cells. The cytotoxicity dose range-finding studies revealed that ivermectin apparently is detoxified in the presence of S-9 rat liver homogenate, a microsomal activation system. Therefore, higher doses of the test compound could be used with L5178Y cells in the presence of S-9 than in its absence. The drug, dissolved in DMSO, was added to cell cultures with and without S-9. Final concentrations of ivermectin were 5 to 20 ug/ml in the absence of the S-9 system and 20 to 60 ug/ml in the presence of S-9. The cells were treated for 4 hours, and then washed, fed, and cultured in growth medium for 3 days. At the end of this expression period, $TK^{-/-}$ mutants were detected by cloning the cells in selection medium containing bromodeoxyuridine for 10 to 14 days. The surviving cell population was determined by plating diluted aliquots in nonselective growth medium.

The results showed that ivermectin at concentrations up to 60 ug/ml did not produce any significant increase in mutation frequency (with or without an S-9 metabolic activation system) when compared with appropriate negative controls.

Unscheduled DNA synthesis (UDS) occurs after cellular DNA is damaged by agents that induce either base, short-patch, or long-patch excision repair (Wilkins and Hart 1973; Setlow and Carrier 1964). The damaged bases are enzymatically excised from their DNA strand, creating a gap; new bases are inserted and polymerized to fill the gap, using the intact opposite strand as template. Since many carcinogenic and mutagenic agents have been demonstrated to induce UDS, the assay is considered to be a measure of genotoxicity (Williams, Laspia, and Dunkel 1982).

Ivermectin was assayed for its ability to induce UDS in an *in vitro* assay using a normal human embryonic lung fibroblast cell strain, IMR-90, at concentrations of 10 to 1000 ug/ml. The compound was tested with and without the addition of a rat liver S-9 metabolic activation system. Ivermectin did not induce UDS in human cells at any dose level.

In conclusion, ivermectin was tested *in vitro* for genotoxic activity in microbial and mammalian cell mutagenesis assays and in human fibroblasts for DNA damage as measured by unscheduled DNA synthesis. In all instances, ivermectin had no genotoxic activity.

B. Acute Toxicity of Ivermectin

As discussed in Chapter 5, ivermectin interacts with GABA receptors, resulting in enhanced release and binding of GABA to its receptors. In contrast to lower organisms, GABA is found only in the brain and spinal cord of mammals, with no detectable levels in the peripheral nervous system (Cooper 1982). Therefore, it was expected that the acute toxicity of ivermectin would be due to its effects in the CNS. This hypothesis has proved correct in acute toxicity studies conducted in a variety of laboratory animal species, although the exact mechanism of neurotoxicity remains unknown.

Table 6.1 shows the acute LD_{50} values for ivermectin in a variety of species using several different routes of administration. Rodents are significantly more sensitive to ivermectin toxicity than are other species. In mice the LD_{50} values after oral and intraperitoneal administration were approximately 25 and 30 mg/kg, respectively. The acute oral LD_{50} values in mice of the individual ivermectin components (ivermectin B_{1a} and B_{1b}) were comparable to each other and to ivermectin.

TABLE 6.1. Acute toxicity of ivermectin.

Species	Route of administration	LD50 (mg/kg)
Mouse	Oral	25
Mouse	Intraperitoneal	30
Rat	Oral	50
Rat	Intraperitoneal	55
Rat (infant)	Oral	2 to 3
Rat	Inhalation	—[a]
Rat	Dermal	>660
Rabbit	Dermal	406
Dog	Oral	~ 80
Rhesus monkey	Oral	> 24

[a] Maximum attainable concentration of 5.11 mg/litter produced transient irritation of mucous membranes but no deaths or other evidence of toxicity after 1 hour exposure.

The drug's effects in mice were similar after either oral or intraperitoneal administration: they consisted of ataxia (uncoordinated movement), bradypnea (abnormally slow respiration rate), and tremors at all dosage levels within approximately 1 hour of treatment. Death, preceded by loss of righting, occurred from 75 minutes to 6 days after dosing, with most occurring within 24 hours. There were no significant sex-related differences in acute toxicity in mice after either route of administration.

In rats treatment-related physical signs consisted of ataxia, ptosis (drooping upper eyelids), and decreased activity; the symptoms appeared from about 4 to 24 hours after oral or intraperitoneal administration. Death, generally preceded by loss of righting, occurred overnight to the second day. Body weight gains during the 2-week observation period appeared unaffected by drug administration. There were no significant sex-related differences.

Ivermectin was more toxic in infant rats (1–2 days old) than in young adult rats. As discussed in more detail in Section D, this enhanced sensitivity is believed due to postnatal development of the blood-brain barrier in rats (Betz and Goldstein 1981) (in humans this structure is formed prenatally; Bohr and Mollgard 1974). This conclusion is supported by significantly higher brain/plasma drug concentration ratios in neonatal rats compared to adults.

In rats and rabbits acute dermal LD_{50} values for ivermectin after 24 hours of occluded exposure were >660 and 406 mg/kg, respectively. These values are significantly greater than those discussed previously for oral exposure in rats and mice, suggesting that ivermectin is poorly absorbed percutaneously. The poor dermal absorption of abamectin has been confirmed in rhesus monkey (*Macaca mulatta*) studies, demonstrating that 0.5% or less of a dermally applied dose is absorbed (see section III A below).

The acute oral toxicity of ivermectin in dogs was assessed by administration of the drug dissolved in sesame oil at dosage levels of 5, 10, 20, 40, or 80 mg/kg to groups of 2 males and 2 females each. Mydriasis was the most sensitive indicator of toxicity in dogs, occurring at all dosage levels. The incidence and duration of mydriasis were dose-related, with the effect lasting up to several days in some dogs. More severe signs of CNS intoxication, including ataxia and tremors, occurred at doses of 10 mg/kg and above. Two animals in the 80 mg/kg group died between 12 and 24 hours posttreatment, while 1 dog in the 40 mg/kg group died 4 days after treatment. These deaths were preceded by a comatoselike state. On the basis of this data, the oral LD_{50} in dogs is approximately 80 mg/kg.

In view of the increased sensitivity of rodents, particularly mice, to the acute toxicity of ivermectin compared to other species, including humans, a comparative acute oral toxicity study in rhesus monkeys was conducted with ivermectin and abamectin to determine the sensitivity of nonhuman primates to these compounds. In this study single oral doses of either ivermectin or abamectin dissolved in sesame oil were administered to groups of 2 males and 2 females. The doses for each compound ranged from 0.2 to 24 mg/kg, with intervals of 2 to 3 weeks between administration of the next higher dose to the same group of monkeys. Plasma concentrations of both compounds were measured at frequent intervals after treatment, with doses of 2, 8, and 24 mg/kg. After each treatment, all animals were carefully examined for clinical signs of drug effect.

No drug-related physical signs were found with either drug at doses of 0.2, 0.5, or 1.0 mg/kg. As shown in Table 6.2, the most sensitive indicator of toxicity was emesis, which occurred in 1 of 4 monkeys with both compounds at 2.0 mg/kg. Therefore, the no-observable-effect level in rhesus monkeys with each compound is 1.0 mg/kg. At doses up to 12.0 mg/kg the only consistent effect was an increase in the incidence and a decrease in the time of onset of emesis from about 8 to 4 hours after treatment. At 24.0 mg/kg, the highest dose tested, marked mydriasis occurred, as well as slight sedation and emesis. Recovery from these effects was complete by 48 hours for both ivermectin and abamectin. No tremors or convulsions were observed in any monkeys, and all survived the highest dose tested of 24.0 mg/kg.

The minimum toxic dose (MTD) in rhesus monkeys is 2.0 mg/kg, about tenfold higher than the human therapeutic dose for onchocerciasis therapy (Greene *et al.* 1985). The peak plasma concentrations following the MTD are shown in Table 6.2. The 110 ng/ml plasma level for ivermectin at this dose is approximately 5.5-fold the mean peak plasma level of 20 ng/ml in humans administered the 0.2 mg/kg therapeutic dose of ivermectin (M. Dobrinska, personal communication; see Chapter 20).

Despite the approximately proportional increases in plasma levels with increasing dose, the severity of clinical signs did not worsen appreciably. Even at 24 mg/kg of ivermectin, a dose producing plasma levels about thirty-fourfold above the human therapeutic level, all monkeys survived. Therefore, the relatively steep dose-response curve in rodents for toxicity

TABLE 6.2. Acute toxicity and plasma concentrations of ivermectin and abamectin in rhesus monkeys and humans.

	Monkeys		Humans
	Ivermectin	Abamectin	Ivermectin
Therapeutic dose			0.2 mg/kg
Peak-plasma levels	—	—	20 ng/ml
Minimum effect level	2 mg/kg	2 mg/kg	—[a]
Peak-plasma levels	110 ng/ml	76 ng/ml	
Signs	emesis	emesis	
Toxic effect level	8 mg/kg	8 mg/kg	6.6–8.6 mg/kg
Peak-plasma levels	270 ng/ml	150 ng/ml	unknown
Signs	emesis	emesis	emesis, mydriasis, sedation
Toxic effect level	24 mg/kg	24 mg/kg	—[a]
Peak-plasma levels	680 ng/ml	390 ng/ml	
Signs	emesis, mydriasis, sedation		
Fatalities	no deaths		no deaths

[a] —Not determined

with the avermectins is not reproduced in monkeys, indicating that in primates clinical evidence of toxicity may occur well in advance of serious or life-threatening toxicity. This view is further supported by the case of a child who survived a dose of ivermectin of about 7 to 8 mg/kg (Table 6.2) with comparable signs of toxicity as observed in rhesus monkey at similar dosage levels (R.J. Nessel, personal communication).

Monkeys can tolerate doses of ivermectin that produce more severe forms of toxicity or death in other species, most notably the mouse but also the dog and the rat. For example, acute oral doses of ivermectin at or slightly above the 0.2 mg/kg therapeutic dose have produced toxicity and even death in some mice. At this dose no adverse effects are produced in rhesus monkey or humans, despite plasma drug levels in these species that are equivalent to those found in mice. The oral LD_{50} values for ivermectin in dog, mouse, and rat vay from approximately 11.6 to 80.0 mg/kg, whereas in monkeys the minimum acute lethal dose is greater than 24 mg/kg. Plasma-level data show that the tolerance of these high doses by monkeys is not due to decreased absorption with increased doses. It appears that primates, in general, possess a relatively lower degree of sensitivity to the potential toxicity of ivermectin.

C. Subchronic Toxicity

The toxicity of ivermectin was assessed in 3-month studies in Crl:CD(BR) SD rats and beagle dogs and in a 2-week study in rhesus monkeys. In addition, a 2-week oral study in neonatal rhesus monkeys was conducted, since a previous study in neonatal rats (see Section II A above) suggested that neonates may be more sensitive to ivermectin toxicity. The results of these studies are summarized in Table 6.3.

A 3-month oral toxicity study in rats with in utero exposure at dosage levels of 0.4, 0.8, and 1.6 mg/kg/day was conducted in which offspring from dams treated with ivermectin for 2 weeks prior to mating and during pregnancy were selected at weaning for continuation on treatment. There were no abnormal physical signs or mortality attributable to treatment. Also, there were no ocular abnormalities and no changes in body weight gain, routine hematologic, or serum biochemical parameters which were related to treatment.

The spleens of 4 rats (3 at 1.6 mg/kg/day and 1 at 0.8 mg/kg/day) were enlarged. On microscopic examination there were varying degrees of congestion of the red pulp and varying amounts of extramedullary hematopoiesis. These rats also had iron-positive pigment in the renal tubular epithelium. These changes suggest a possible drug-related intravascular hemolysis, but the mechanism is unknown. There was reactive hyperplasia of the bone marrow in these rats, probably related to intravascular hemolysis. There were no other microscopic changes related to treatment at these dosage levels. A 0.4 mg/kg/day no-observed-

TABLE 6.3. Summary of results of subchronic oral toxicity studies with ivermectin.

Species	Duration	Dose levels (mg/kg/day)	Results
Rats	3 months	0.4, 0.8, and 1.6	Splenic enlargement and reactive hyperplasia suggestive of intravascular hemolysis at 0.8 mg/kg/day and above. NEL[a] = 0.4 mg/kg/day
Dogs	3 months	0.5, 1.0, and 2.0	Mydriasis at 1.0 mg/kg/day and above. Tremors, ataxia, and anorexia at 2.0 mg/kg/day. NEL = 0.5 mg/kg/day
Rhesus monkeys (*Macaca mulatta*)	2 weeks	0.3, 0.6, and 1.2	No treatment-related effects up to 1.2 mg/kg/day. NEL > 1.2 mg/kg/day
Neonatal rhesus monkeys (*Macaca mulatta*)	2 weeks	0.04 and 0.1	No treatment-related effects up to 0.1 mg/kg/day. NEL > 0.1 mg/kg/day

[a] NEL: No-effect level

effect level was established in this study. Similar changes were not seen in 3-month, 1-year, or 2-year studies with abamectin in rats at comparable and higher dose levels, nor in other species given ivermectin.

In a 3-month oral toxicity study in beagle dogs the compound was administered as a solution in sesame oil by gavage at doses of 0.5, 1.0, or 2.0 mg/kg/day. Mydriasis and slight weight loss were observed at doses of 1.0 and 2.0 mg/kg/day. Four of 8 dogs in the 2.0 mg/kg/day group developed tremors, ataxia, anorexia, and dehydration, and were sacrificed prior to the scheduled necropsy. No gross abnormalities were observed in these dogs. Mydriasis was observed in dogs receiving 1.0 or 2.0 mg/kg/day. No other treatment-related effects were found.

Postmortem studies conducted on all animals disclosed no treatment-related gross, microscopic, or organ weight changes. A no-effect level of 0.5 mg/kg/day was established for this study.

A 16-day oral toxicity study with ivermectin was conducted to determine its toxicity in immature domestic-bred rhesus monkeys (approximately 1 to 1.5 years old). Each of the 3 treatment groups were dosed daily via nasogastric intubation at dosage levels of 0.3, 0.6, and 1.2 mg/kg/day. These dosage levels were arbitrarily chosen to provide an approximate sixfold safety margin relative to the human clinical dose of ivermectin; based on the acute toxicity in rhesus monkeys, these doses would not be expected to produce clinical signs of toxicity. The control group received the vehicle, sesame oil, at the same 1.0 ml/kg dose volume as the treated groups.

No drug-related physical signs were noted in any of the treated animals. All animals survived the duration of the study with similar body weight gains for all treated groups as compared to the controls. No treatment-related ocular lesions or changes in hematology or serum biochemical parameters were found during the study. There were no organ weight, gross, or microscopic changes attributed to treatment. Therefore, treatment of immature monkeys with 1.2 mg/kg/day for 14 days failed to produce any treatment-related effects.

Because ivermectin is excreted in the milk of lactating animals, it was necessary to generate appropriate preclinical data on the safety of low-level exposure to nursing infants via maternal milk. Based on a clinical study in lactating women treated with ivermectin, a maximum milk level of the drug of 23 ng/ml was found on the day following treatment, with levels depleting to below the 0.1 ng/ml detection limit by approximately 1 week after treatment (M. Dobrinska, personal communication). This level of drug in human milk would result in an estimated maximum-acute dosage of about 3 to 4 ug/kg in a nursing infant.

To assess the potential significance of a low-level neonatal exposure to ivermectin, a study of neonatal rhesus monkeys was conducted. At initiation of the study all animals were 7 to 13 days old. The animals were divided into 2 treatment groups of 5 males and 3 females each; they received ivermectin dissolved in sesame oil via nasogastric intubation at dosage levels of either 40 or 100 μg/kg/day for 14 days.

Results of the physical examinations revealed no treatment-related physical signs. The results of the ophthalmic examinations and the daily check for mydriasis and pupillary light response indicated no treatment-related differences between the treated and control groups. Body weight changes were similar between control and treated animals, and the results of the hematologic and serum biochemical examinations indicated no treatment-related effects. Similarly, there were no treatment-related changes in organ weights and no gross postmortem or microscopic changes related to ivermectin administration at doses up to 100 μg/kg/day. Based on the results of this study, exposure of nursing infants to low levels of ivermectin is unlikely to produce toxicity.

D. Developmental and Reproductive Toxicity

The developmental toxicity of ivermectin was assessed by daily administration throughout the major period of organogenesis in mice, rats, and rabbits. The reproductive toxicity of the drug was determined by conducting a rat multigeneration study. The results of these studies are summarized in Table 6.4.

Table 6.4. Summary of results of developmental and reproductive toxicity studies with ivermectin.

Species	Dose (mg/kg)	Observations	NEL[a] (mg/kg)	
Mouse	0.1, 0.2, 0.4, 0.8	Mortality, tremors, convulsions, coma at 0.2, 0.4, and 0.8 mg/kg; cleft palate at 0.4 and 0.8 mg/kg	Maternotoxicity developmental toxicity	0.1 0.2
Rat	2.5, 5.0, 10.0	Sedation, cleft palate at 10 mg/kg	Maternotoxicity and developmental toxicity	5.0
Rabbit	1.5, 3.0, 6.0	Sedation and decreased body weight at 6 mg/kg; decreased fetal weights, increased number of fetal deaths, cleft palate, and clubbed forepaws at 3.0 and 6.0 mg/kg	Maternotoxicity developmental toxicity	3.0 1.5
Rat Multi-generation	0.05, 0.1, 0.2, 0.4	Neonatal mortality at 0.4 mg/kg/day	Neonatal and developmental toxicity	0.2

[a] NEL: No-effect level

To determine the potential for developmental toxicity in mice, ivermectin was administered orally in sesame oil to pregnant mice on days 6 through 15 of gestation. The dosage levels used were 0.1, 0.2, 0.4, and 0.8 mg/kg/day. There was treatment-related mortality in each of the 3 highest dosage levels, as shown in Figure 6.2. Deaths occurred after 1 to 8 doses. An increased incidence of cleft palate was found in fetuses from dams receiving either 0.4 or 0.8 mg/kg/day. There were no treatment-related abnormalities among fetuses at 0.1 or 0.2 mg/kg/day, despite the fact that doses of 0.2 mg/kg/day and above produced tremors, convulsions, coma, and death in some maternal animals.

The developmental toxicity of ivermectin in rats was determined by oral drug administration as a sesame oil solution to dams on days 6 through 17 of gestation. Dosage levels were 2.5, 5.0, and 10.0 mg/kg/day. Maternotoxicity, characterized by sedation, was observed in rats in the 10 mg/kg/day group and a low incidence of cleft palate was found in fetuses in the high dose group (Table 6.4). There were no other treatment-related malformations or evidence of maternotoxicity in this or any other treatment group.

In a developmental toxicity study pregnant rabbits were orally administered invermectin on days 6 through 18 of gestation at dose levels of 1.5, 3.0, and 6.0 mg/kg/day. Slight to marked sedation was present in the 6.0 mg/kg/day females 24 hours after the seventh dose, and slight

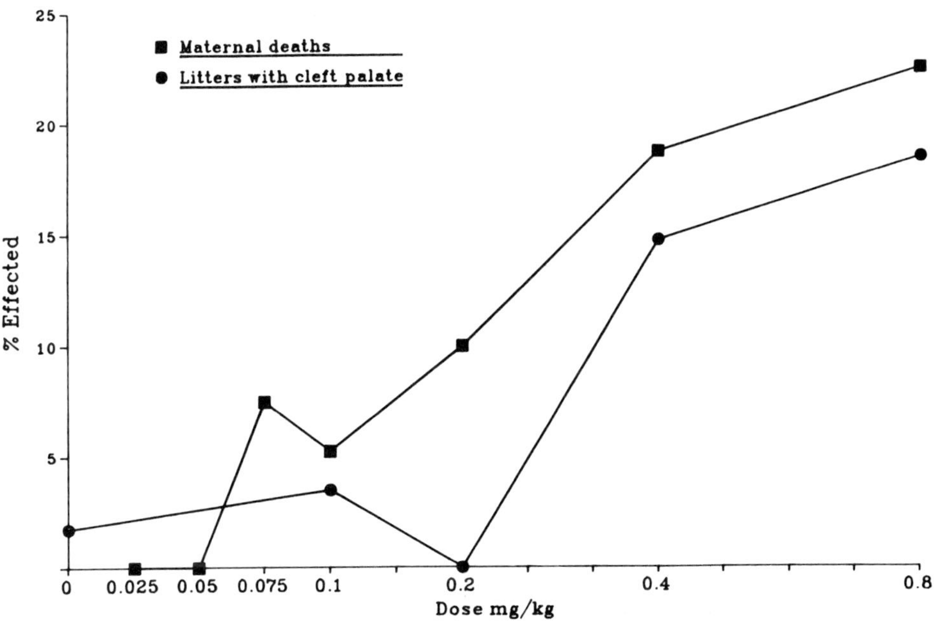

FIGURE 6.2. Ivermectin: comparison of maternal mortality and incidence of cleft palate in CF_1 mice.

sedation persisted in some females up to 8 days after cessation of dosing. No clinical signs of toxicity were present in females at 1.5 or 3.0 mg/kg/day. In the 6.0 mg/kg/day group, there was a significant ($P \leq 0.05$) decrease in mean maternal body weight during the period of drug administration; this was probably related to the sedation and likely lower food consumption in dams in this group. There were no treatment-related effects on mean maternal body weights in the 1.5 and 3.0 mg/kg/day groups.

There was a low but dose-related incidence of cleft palate and clubbed forepaws among fetuses in the 3.0 and 6.0 mg/kg/day dosage groups. At 3.0 mg/kg/day 1 fetus had cleft palate and 5 fetuses from 1 litter had clubbed forepaws. Eight fetuses from 3 litters at 6.0 mg/kg/day had cleft palate, and clubbed forepaw was observed in 6 fetuses from 3 litters. There were no malformations observed among fetuses at 1.5 mg/kg/day.

The results of the developmental toxicity studies with ivermectin demonstrate that a low incidence of abnormalities was produced only at dosage levels at or near those producing severe signs of maternotoxicity—including death—in some dams. Therefore, ivermectin is not considered to be selectively embryotoxic. Years of widespread clinical use of ivermectin in pregnant animals of a variety of species have failed to produce any evidence of developmental toxicity, further supporting the above conclusion.

Results of initial multigeneration studies of ivermectin in rats indicated increased pup mortality several days after parturition and decreased pup weights at maternal doses as low as 0.4 mg/kg/day. In an attempt to determine the threshold dose for neonatal toxicity, a multigeneration study was conducted in which ivermectin was administered to male and female rats once daily throughout the production of 2 litters in each of 3 successive generations at dose levels of 0.05, 0.1, 0.2, and 0.4 mg/kg/day.

There was no treatment-related mortality, nor were there physical signs of toxicity or effects on reproduction among parents or offspring in any dosage group throughout the production of 2 litters in each of the F0, F1b, and F2b generations. The body weights of offspring (F1a through F3b) during lactation (days 1 to 21 postpartum) were not adversely affected by drug administration. Treatment-related effects on body weight gain were limited to a slight but statistically significant ($P \leq 0.05$) decrease in mean body weight gain among F1b females in the 0.4 mg/kg/day group in the postweaning period. Comparable effects were noted among weanling male and female rats at the same dose level in a previous ivermectin multigeneration study. On the basis of this study, and other multigeneration studies in rats at higher dosage levels, 0.4 mg/kg/day appears to be near the threshold dose in dams for producing neonatal toxicity. Doses $\leq$ 0.2 mg/kg/day produced no neonatal toxicity or other reproductive effects.

The results of the multigeneration study and the acute toxicity study in infant rats (see Section II B above) indicated that noenatal rats were more sensitive to the drug than parental animals. To determine the reason for this difference in sensitivity, female rats were administered tritium-labeled ivermectin B1a at a dosage level of 2.5 mg/kg/day continuously for 61 days prior to mating and during mating, gestation, and lactation. Plasma and milk samples from dams and plasma samples from offspring were analyzed for total radioactivity on days 1, 4, and 6 postpartum. On day 10 postpartum all dams and offspring were sacrificed and total radioactivity determined in plasma and brain samples.

The total drug residues in plasma and milk of dams and plasma from their offspring are shown in Figure 6.3. The increase in maternal plasma radioactivity at parturition relative to days 4 to 10 postpartum is likely due to increased utilization of fat at parturition in the rat (Amano 1967; Scow *et al.* 1964), resulting in release of ivermectin from adipose tissue (Chiu *et al.* 1986). The concentrations of ivermectin in milk were consistently three- to fourfold higher than those obtained from maternal plasma samples on comparable days postpartum. Plasma drug levels in offspring were relatively low on day 1 postpartum but increased rapidly from days 6 to 10 such that they equaled or exceeded the values in the dams. It should be noted that the 0.8 ug/ml mean plasma concentration in offspring on day 10 postpartum is approximately 40 times the therapeutic plasma concentration in humans and other species. Of greater importance is the finding that the brain concentrations of ivermectin residues in offspring by day 6 postpartum were approximately tenfold the maternal brain concentrations (Figure 6.4).

The results of this study indicated that the high drug concentrations in milk from lactating dams chronically administered the drug were probably responsible for the toxicity observed among neonatal offspring in multigeneration studies. This conclusion is supported by the high drug levels found in the plasma and brain of offspring relative to adult rats. In particular there was a greater concentration of drug in the brain of neonatal rats during the early neonatal period of enhanced sensitivity, and this may explain the increased toxicity. This early neonatal period of increased sensitivity to ivermectin toxicity in rats correlates with the postnatal completion of the blood-brain barrier in this species (in humans it is formed prenatally; Betz and Goldstein 1981; Bohr and Mollgard 1974; Saunders 1977). Further support for the importance of postnatal exposure in the toxicity observed in neonatal rats is derived from a cross-fostering study, in which control pups cross-fostered to ivermectin-treated dams exhibited the same degree of neonatal mortality and toxicity as rats exposed in utero and fostered to drug-tested dams (R.T. Robertson, personal communication). Therefore, postnatal exposure via milk—not a combination of prenatal and postnatal exposure—explains the neonatal toxicity observed in multigeneration studies conducted with ivermectin.

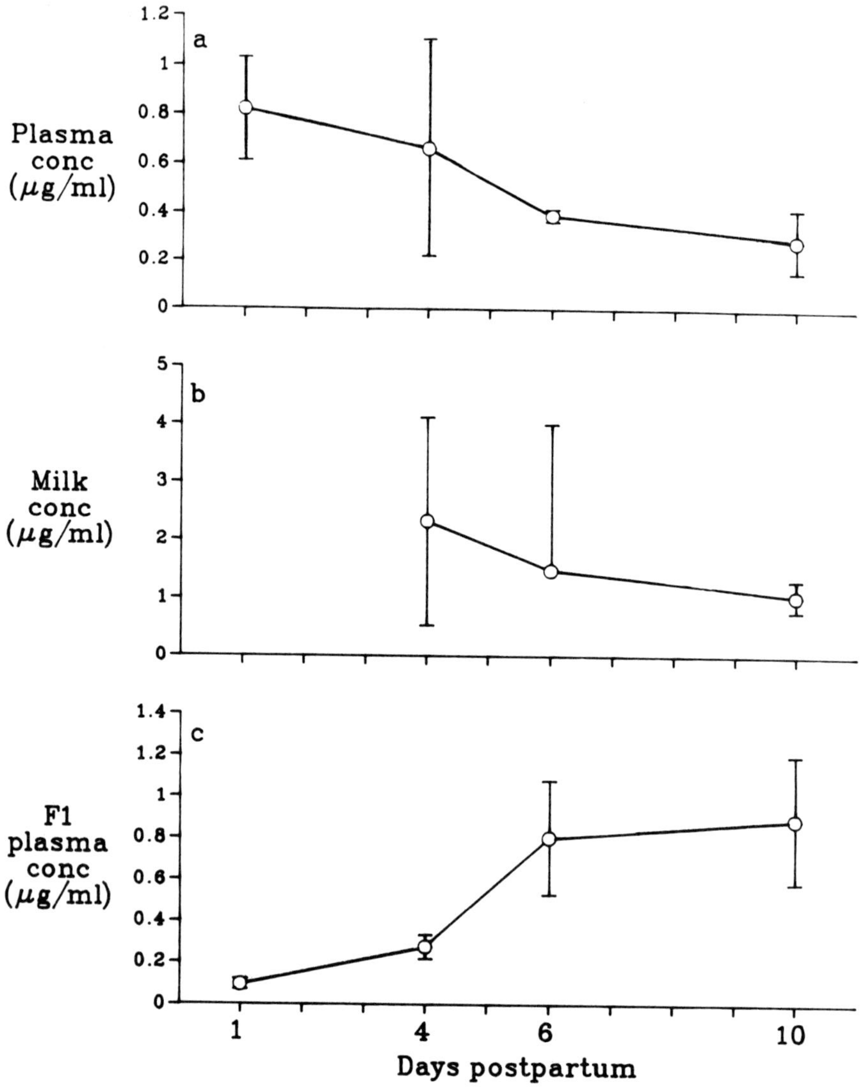

FIGURE 6.3. Mean concentrations of 3H-ivermectin in (a) plasma, (b) milk from lactating rats, and (c) plasma from offspring of treated dams. Error bars = ± standard deviation.

III. Toxicity Studies with Abamectin

Abamectin differs from ivermectin by a single double-bond at the C22-23 position. Abamectin is a pesticide with many different agricultural uses. It has been tested in acute, subacute, and genotoxicity assays similar to those for ivermectin with similar results, except that abamectin is slightly more toxic than ivermectin (Tables 6.5 and 6.6). Neither compound

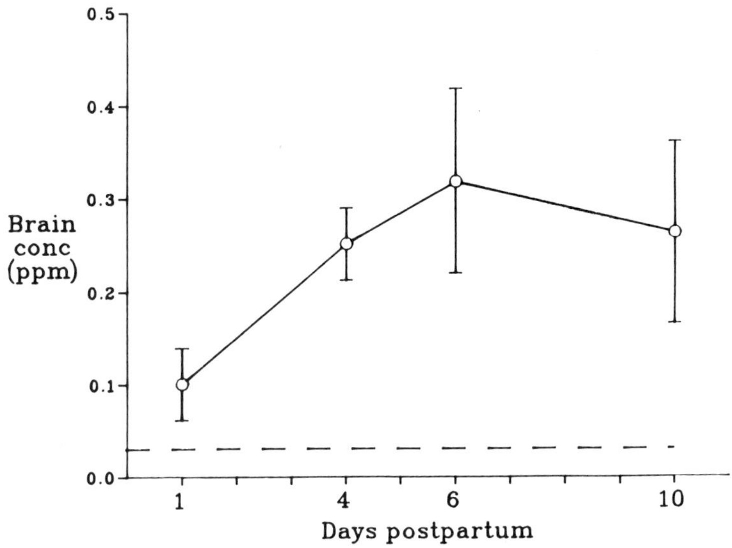

FIGURE 6.4. Mean 3H-ivermectin levels in brain from dams and offspring. Dashed line represents steady state brain concentration of dams measured on day 10 postpartum. Error bars = ± standard deviation.

is genotoxic. The oral LD_{50} in mice is 14–24 mg/kg for abamectin and 25–40 mg/kg for ivermectin; the minimal effect level for toxicity in dogs is 0.50 mg/kg/day for abamectin and 1.0 mg/kg/day for ivermectin. In developmental toxicology studies on abamectin, as for ivermectin, cleft palates were seen at or near maternotoxic doses. In multigeneration

TABLE 6.5. Comparative toxicity of abamectin and ivermectin in laboratory animals.

Type of Study	Species	Abamectin (mg/kg/day)	Ivermectin (mg/kg/day)
Oral LD50	CF1 mouse	13.6–23.8	24.6–40
Oral LD50	CRCD rat	10.6–11.3	42.8–52.8
Oral LD50	CRCD neonatal rat	1.52	2.3
Acute toxicity	Monkeys	MEL = 2 mg/kg	MEL = 2 mg/kg
		Minimum Effect Level (MEL) (mg/kg/day) Abamectin	Ivermectin
Suckling neonatal pup	CRCD rat	0.12	0.4
Subacute oral	Beagle dog	0.50	1.0
Chronic and subchronic	CRCD rat	2.0[a]	0.8

[a] 105-week study

TABLE 6.6. Results of teratology studies with abamectin and ivermectin in three species.

	Mouse		Rabbit		Rat	
	Abamectin	Ivermectin	Abamectin	Ivermectin	Abamectin	Ivermectin
Maternotoxicity						
NEL[a]	0.05	0.1	1.0	3.0	1.6	5.0
MEL[b]	0.075	0.2	2.0	6.0	2.0	10.0
Fetotoxicity						
NEL	0.2	0.8	1.0	1.5	1.6	10.0
MEL	0.4	[c]	2.0	3.0	[c]	[c]
Developmental toxicity						
NEL	0.2	0.2	1.0	1.5	1.6	5.0
MEL	0.4	0.4	2.0	3.0	[d]	10.0

[a] NEL = No effect level (mg/kg/day)
[b] MEL = Minimal effect level (mg/kg/day)
[c] No adverse effects
[d] No cleft palates seen at the maternotoxic dose of 2.0 mg/kg/day

studies pup toxicity was the most sensitive parameter, with minimum effect levels of 0.4 mg/kg/day for both compounds. Additional long-term studies of abamectin are discussed below (Table 6.7).

A. One-Year Oral Toxicity Study in Dogs

In a 1-year oral toxicity study in dogs there was no cumulative toxicity. Four groups of 6 male and 6 female 20 to 24-week-old beagle dogs were given abamectin in the feed at doses of 0, 0.25, 0.50, and 1.0 mg/kg/day.

One dog in the high-dose group died and 2 were killed in moribund condition. Clinical signs included mydriasis, weight loss, lethargy, tremors, and recumbency. All of these deaths were attributed to abamectin toxicity.

Mydriasis was seen in dogs in the middle (3% incidence) and high (15% incidence) dose groups. Mydriasis has been a consistent finding in other species—dogs, horses, monkeys—exposed to increased doses of ivermectin as well. No treatment-related changes in the structure of the eye were seen at the routine ophthalmologic examination nor by histopathology.

There were no gross or microscopic changes attributed to treatment even in the 3 high-dose dogs that died or were killed with treatment-related clinical signs. This has been true in other studies in dogs as well as in mice and rats. The no-effect level for abamectin given in the diet to dogs was 0.25 mg/kg/day.

B. Chronic Toxicity and Carcinogenicity Data in Rats and Mice

In a chronic toxicity and carcinogenicity study with a 1-year intermin necropsy, 5-week-old Crl:CD(SD) BR rats were assigned to 5 groups of 65

TABLE 6.7. Chronic studies with abamectin.

Species	Duration	Dose mg/kg/day	Findings
Rat	14 weeks	0.1, 0.2, and 0.4 (in sesame oil gavage)	No treatment-related signs of toxicity. NEL[a] = 0.4 mg/kg/day
Rat	8 weeks	1.4–5.8 mg/kg/day: (diet)	75% deaths at 60 ppm; 50% deaths at 40 ppm (about 5 mg/kg/day). No effect at 5 and 10 ppm (1.4 mg/kg/day). At 2.1 mg/kg, 2/20 had tremors; at 2.7 mg/kg, 8/20 had tremors. NEL = 1.4 mg/kg/day. MTDb estimated at 2.0 mg/kg/day
Rat	53 weeks	0.75, 1.5, and 2.0/2.5/2.0 (diet)	When high dose was increased to 2.5 mg/kg/day a few animals developed tremors so the dose was reduced to 2.0 mg/kg/day No treatment-related gross or microscopic changes. No oncogenic effect seen. NEL = 1.5 mg/kg/day
Mouse CD-1	up to 84 d	Initial study up to about 4 mg/kg/d caused no tox. Doses were increased in some groups and more dose groups were added to 12 mg/kg/d (diet)	Body weight decrease seen at 40 ppm (about 8 mg/kg/day) and 60 ppm (about 12 mg/kg/day) (−11% and −29% respectively). No tremors or convulsions. NEL = 4 mg/kg/day. MTD = 8 mg/kg/day
Mouse CD-1	94 weeks	2, 4, 8 mg/kg/d (diet)	Body weight gain depression at high dose (males 7%, females 21%) ($P < 0.05$). No treatment-related gross or microscopic changes. No oncogenic effect. NEL = 4 mg/kg/d
Dog	12 weeks	0.25, 0.5, 1.0, 2.0/4.0 (diet)	Extreme weight loss at 2.0 and 4.0—discontinued dosing. Mydriasis ≥ 1.0 mg/kg/day. NEL = 0.5 mg/kg/day
Dog	53 weeks	0.25, 0.5, 1.0 (diet)	Mydriasis seen at 1 mg/kg/day. Intermittent mydriasis at 0.5 mg/kg/day. No treatment-related gross or microscopic changes. NEL = 0.25 mg/kg/day

[a] NEL = No Effect Level
[b] MTD = Maximum tolerated dose

male and 65 female rats each: Control I, Control II, and abamectin given in the feed at 0.75, 1.50, and 2.0 mg/kg/day. The levels of abamectin in the feed were adjusted and mixed biweekly to attain the targeted dose levels.

Treatment-related increases in body weight gain were seen in both males and females in all dosage groups during the first year on study. At drug week 60, when the peak difference in body weight gain was apparent between treated and control rats, the treated females had 30%, 14%, and 13% increased body weight gain in the 0.75, 1.5, and 2.0 mg/kg/day groups, respectively, when compared with controls. By the end of the study (drug week 105) there were comparable mean body weight gain values for all groups of females when averaged over the entire study ($P > 0.05$); however, the increases in body weight gain over the combined controls among the treated males were still statistically significant ($P \leq 0.05$) (Robson 1959) at drug week 105 (21%, 9%, and 6% increases in the 0.75, 1.5, and 2.0 mg/kg/day groups, respectively).

Clinical signs of toxicity were limited to tremors seen in a few rats in the high-dose group and an occasional rat in the mid-dose group that consumed enough feed to exceed the 2.0 mg/kg/day dose of the high-dose group. Although some of the rats died with tremors, there were no gross or microscopic changes seen in the nervous or muscular systems to account for these tremors. This has been true for other species as well.

Abamectin was not carcinogenic in rats when given in the diet at doses of 0.75, 1.5, and 2.0 mg/kg/day for 105 weeks. There was no statistically significant ($P > 0.05$) increase in tumor incidence resulting from treatment with abamectin (Mantel 1963, 1980; Mantel *et al.* 1982; Peto 1974; Peto *et al.* 1980; Harter 1957; Cutler and Ederer 1958; Tukey, Ciminera, and Heyse 1985). There were also no treatment-related nonneoplastic histopathologic changes in this study. The no-effect level for toxicity was 1.5 mg/kg/day.

In a chronic toxicity and carcinogenicity study, Crl:CD-1 (ICR) BR mice, about 6 weeks old, were assigned to 5 groups: Control I, Control II, 2, 4, and 8 mg/kg/day of abamectin in the feed.

Treatment-related tremors were seen in drug weeks 89 and 91 in 2 female mice in the high-dose group.

Increased mortality was seen among the high-dose males ($P < 0.05$) but not the females (Mantel and Ciminera 1979). Dosing was stopped among the high-dose males in drug week 90 due to the low number of survivors (40%). All other mice were treated until sacrifice in drug week 94.

Treatment-related decreases in body weight gain ($P < 0.05$) were seen among both the high-dose males and females (7% and 21%, respectively) (Robson 1959). A dose-related trend toward increased food consumption (g/kg) was seen among the females but not the males, and the high-dose females had 20% decreased feed efficiency compared to controls (Tukey, Ciminera, and Heyse 1985).

There were no treatment-related ophthalmic changes. There were no effects of treatment on the hematologic or serum biochemical findings. There were no treatment-related organ weight changes or gross lesions.

Abamectin was not carcinogenic to mice when given in the diet for 94 weeks at doses of 2, 4, and 8 mg/kg/day. There was no statistically significant ($P > 0.05$) increase in tumor incidence resulting from abamectin treatment (Mantel 1963, 1980; Mantel *et al.* 1982; Peto 1974; Peto *et al.* 1980; Harter 1957; Cutler and Ederar 1958; Tukey, Ciminera, and Heyse 1985). The no-effect level for clinical evidence of toxicity is 4 mg/kg/day. These results demonstrate that abamectin, the close structural analog of ivermectin, is not carcinogenic in rodents when administered at maximum tolerated doses for 22 to 24 months.

C. Dermal Penetration Study in Monkeys

Because the main potential route of exposure to abamectin's pesticidal use on crops is dermal, a study was conducted to determine the amount of dermal absorption of abamectin. The forearms of monkeys were exposed to the concentrated emulsifiable concentrate (E.C.) of abamectin, the diluted E.C. of abamectin, and a suspension of abamectin in alcohol. Each of these 3 exposures represents a possible way humans working with the product could be exposed. The mixer/loader could be exposed to the concentrate, the applicator could be exposed to the dilute E.C., and the harvester could be exposed to the powder (suspension). The monkey was chosen as the most appropriate model to mimic skin absorption in humans (Wester and Maibach 1975, 1983).

Tritium-labeled abamectin was used to quantitate the excretion of the compound after i.v. and dermal administration. The tritium label is stable in this biological matrix in the 5 position and does not significantly exchange. By the i.v. route 95% of the 6-mg dose and 97% of the 300-mg dose were excreted in the urine and feces. Greater than 90% of the radioactivity was excreted in the feces within 7 days of the i.v. dosing. After dermal exposure > 99% of the radioactivity was recovered from the application site. Dermal penetration of abamectin was extremely low (0.17%–0.55% of applied dose) based on plasma levels and recovery from application site (see Table 6.8). Generally the dermal absorption of abamectin was < 1% of applied dose. Because abamectin does not readily penetrate the skin, perhaps because it is a high molecular-weight compound, the hazard to agricultural workers is significantly less than it would be otherwise. For the same reasons dermal penetration of ivermectin should also be very low.

IV. Summary and Conclusions

Acute oral toxicity studies with ivermectin in mice, rats, and monkeys have shown clear species differences in sensitivity, with rodents being uniquely sensitive to ivermectin's CNS toxicity. This conclusion is based upon the observation that doses of 0.2 mg/kg in mice, and slightly higher doses in rats, have produced clinical signs of drug effect (tremors and ataxia); this same dose has been shown to be without adverse effect in

TABLE 6.8. Percent dermal absorption of abamectin in rhesus monkeys.

Treatment	Average percent absorbed (excreta)[a]	Average percent absorbed (plasma)[b]
6 ug EC[d] 1 hr diluted	0.23	0.26
6 ug EC 10 hr diluted	0.55	0.19
300 ug 1 hr technical suspension[e]	0.17	1.22
300 ug 10 hr technical suspension	0.29	nd[c]
300 ug EC 1 hr	0.23	0.19
300 ug EC 10 hr	0.52	nd[c]

[a] % excreted (topical)
% excreted (i.v.)
[b] normalized AUC (topical)
normalized AUC (i.v.)
The amounts of radioactivity excreted or in the plasma were normalized to the treatment group since the amount of radioactivity dosed in each treatment was not identical. AUC = area under the curve
[c] The percent could not be determined because the level of radioactivity in the plasma samples was below the background level
[d] EC = emulsifiable concentrate of abamectin
[e] Technical suspension = abamectin powder in water

clinical studies in a variety of other species, including humans. In addition, an acute oral study in monkeys demonstrated that the minimum toxic dose in this species was 2.0 mg/kg or approximately tenfold the human clinical dose, which resulted in plasma drug levels 5.5 times greater than those in humans following treatment with 0.2 mg/kg of the drug. Doses up to 24.0 mg/kg in monkeys produced only slight increases in the observed toxic effects (emesis, mydriasis, and sedation), indicating a much flatter dose-response curve in this species compared to rodents. The finding that an acute overdose of ivermectin in a child exposed to approximately 8.0 mg/kg orally produced clinical signs similar to those produced in monkeys and that these effects rapidly reversed suggests that monkeys, and not mice, are the most appropriate model for predicting the acute toxic effects of ivermectin in humans.

Toxicity studies of 14 weeks duration in rats and dogs indicated no adverse effects at doses of 0.4 and 0.5 mg/kg/day, respectively. At doses of 0.8 mg/kg/day and above in rats a low incidence of splenic enlargement was found. In dogs 1.0 mg/kg/day and above produced mydriasis, but tremors, ataxia, and anorexia were produced only at the highest dose level of 2.0 mg/kg/day.

A 2-week oral toxicity study in immature rhesus monkeys (approximately 1 to 1.5 years old) at doses up to 1.2 mg/kg/day demonstrated no adverse effects, indicating no increase in sensitivity and little or no drug accumulation in immature monkeys in view of the 1.0 mg/kg no-effect level in the acute oral toxicity study in more mature monkeys.

A 2-week oral toxicity study in neonatal monkeys—with all animals less than 2 weeks old at initiation of the study—produced no evidence of toxicity with doses up to 100 ug/kg/day. Therefore, low-level human neonatal exposure to < 100 ug/kg of ivermectin is unlikely to produce toxicity.

In 3 laboratory species, developmental toxicity with ivermectin was found only at dosage levels at or near those which also produced signs of severe maternotoxicity. This indicates that ivermectin is not a selective developmental toxin (Khera 1984; Brent 1986). In the mouse, the most sensitive species tested, ivermectin was both maternotoxic and produced fetal cleft palate at dosage levels of 0.4 mg/kg/day and above. Maternotoxicity, characterized by tremors and death, without teratogenicity, was also observed at dosage levels as low as 0.2 mg/kg/day, the safe human therapeutic dose, clearly demonstrating that the mouse is an inappropriate model for predicting the toxicity of ivermectin. In the rat developmental toxicity study, dosages of 10 mg/kg/day, the highest dose tested, produced maternotoxicity characterized by sedation and an unthrifty appearance and cleft palates in affected offspring. At dosage levels of 5 mg/kg/day no maternotoxicity or fetal abnormalities were observed. In rabbits, maternotoxicity, including sedation and weight loss, resulted at a dosage level of 6.0 mg/kg/day. Cleft palate and clubbed forefeet were found at dosages of 3.0 mg/kg/day and above. No evidence of maternotoxicity or developmental toxicity was observed in rabbits receiving 1.5 mg/kg/day. The developmental toxicity data in laboratory animals with ivermectin suggest that the drug is not selectively toxic to the developing embryo and adverse effects are unlikely to occur at dose levels which are nonmaternotoxic. This conclusion is further supported by the widespread use of the drug in a variety of domestic animal species with no adverse effects on development reported, even when used at severalfold the 0.2 mg/kg therapeutic dose (Campbell and Benz 1984).

In an extensive series of multigeneration studies in rats no effects on mating, fertility, pregnancy, or gestation length were found at doses up to 3.6 mg/kg/day, the highest dose tested. At doses $\geq$ 1.2 mg/kg/day decreases in body weight gain were found in treated dams compared to controls. Postnatal toxicity characterized by decreased weight gain and pup mortality was found in F1 offspring at doses $\geq$ 0.4 mg/kg/day. These effects were found to be related not to in utero exposure but to postnatal exposure via maternal milk. The three- to fourfold higher levels of ivermectin in maternal milk compared to plasma resulted in significantly higher brain and plasma levels of the drug in nursing offspring. The period of enhanced neonatal sensitivity in rats (up to approximately day 10 postpartum) correlates with the completion of the blood-brain barrier in this species. No adverse reproductive or postnatal effects were found at doses $\leq$ 0.2 mg/kg/day.

Ivermectin has been used extensively in humans at an oral dose of

0.2 mg/kg for the treatment of onchocerciasis without any adverse drug-related effects (Greene *et al.* 1985). In addition, more limited clinical safety data are available in humans receiving 0.2 mg/kg/day on 2 consecutive days, demonstrating no adverse effects (K. Brown, personal communication). In contrast to humans, single doses of 0.2 mg/kg in mice have produced severe signs of toxicity and death in some animals. Therefore, the mouse is clearly inappropriate for human risk assessment of toxicity to ivermectin.

Comparative studies with abamectin and its semisynthetic analog, ivermectin, in primates and other species have shown that the 2 compounds produce virtually identical effects at the same or very similar dosage levels. Carcinogenicity studies with abamectin at maximum tolerated dosage levels for 22 and 24 months duration in mice and rats, respectively, have demonstrated the lack of carcinogenicity of this compound. The lack of genotoxic activity with ivermectin in a variety of bacterial and mammalian genetic toxicity assays, along with its close chemical structure and biological activity with abamectin, supports the conclusion that ivermectin should also be noncarcinogenic.

In using these data for the establishment of acceptable levels of human exposure to ivermectin in food residues, it must be remembered that there are clear species differences regarding ivermectin toxicity. Primates, including humans, are clearly less sensitive than rodents, particularly mice. Therefore, the use of the lowest no-effect level (NEL) in the most sensitive species (0.2 mg/kg in the mouse teratology study) provides an even greater safety margin when calculating the acceptable daily intake of ivermectin residues. Further safety margins are evident by recognizing that ivermectin levels in muscle are extremely low compared to liver, the target tissue used in establishing appropriate withdrawal periods in most animal species (see Chapter 10). The extremely low therapeutic dose level of 0.2 mg/kg in most species and limited number of treatments per year result in extremely low total drug residues. Therefore, the very low human exposure to ivermectin residues relative to the toxicity and safety data accumulated in a variety of animal species, including humans treated for onchocerciasis, supports the continued safe use of ivermectin in veterinary practice.

References

Amano Y (1967) Changes of the levels of blood glucose during pregnancy in the rat. *Jap. J. Pharmacol.* 17:105–114

Ames BN, McCann J, Yamasaki E (1975) Methods for detecting carcinogens and mutagens with the Salmonella/mammalian microsome mutagenicity test. *Mutat. Res.* 31:347–364

Betz L, Goldstein GN (1981) Developmental changes in metabolism and transport properties of capillaries isolated from rat brain. *J. Physiol.* 312:365–376

Bohr V, Mollgard K (1974) Tight junctions in human fetal choroid plexus visualized by freeze-etching. Brain Res. 81:314–318

Brent RL (1986) Definition of a teratogen and the relationship of teratogenicity to carcinogenicity. *Teratol.* 34:359–360

Campbell WC, Benz GW (1984) Ivermectin: a review of efficacy and safety. *J. Vet. Pharm. & Therap.* 7:1–16

Chiu SH, Sestokas E, Taub R, Buhs RP, Green M, Sestokas R, Vandenheuval WJ, Arison BH, Jacob TA (1986) Metabolic disposition of ivermectin in tissues of cattle, sheep, and rats. *Drug Metab. & Dispos.* 14:590–600

Clive D, Flamm W, Machesko M, Bernheim J (1972) A mutational assay system using the thymidine binase locus in mouse lymphoma cells. *Mutat. Res.* 16:77–87

Clive D, Spector JASF (1975) Laboratory procedure for assessing specific locus mutations at the TK locus in cultured L5178Y mouse lymphoma cells. *Mutat. Res.* 31:17–29

Cooper JR (1982) Amino acids. In Cooper JR, Bloom FR, Roth RH (eds), *The Biochemical Basis of Neuropharmacology,* 4th ed., Oxford University Press, p 250

Cutler SJ, Ederer F (1958) Maximum utilization of the life table method in analyzing survival. *J. Chron. Dis.* 8:699–712

Greene BM, Taylor HR, Cupp EW, Murphy RP, White AT, Aziz MA, Schulz-Key H, D'Anna SA, Newland HS, Goldschmidt LP, Auer C, Hanson AP, Freeman SV, Reber EW, Williams PN (1985) Comparison of ivermectin and diethylcarbamazine in the treatment of onchocerciasis. *New Eng. J. Med.* 313:133–138

Harter HL (1957) Error rates and sample sizes for range tests in multiple comparisons. *Biometrics* 13:511–36

Khera KS (1984) Maternal Toxicity—A possible factor in fetal malformation in mice. *Teratol.* 29:411–416

Mantel N (1963) Chi-square tests with one degree of freedom; extensions of the Mantel-Haenszel procedure. *J. Am. Stat. Assoc.* 58:690–700

Mantel N (1980) Assessing laboratory evidence for neoplastic activity. *Biometrics* 36:381–99

Mantel N, Ciminera J (1979) Use of log-rank scores in the analysis of litter-matched data on time to tumor appearance. *Canc. Res.* 39:4308–4315

Mantel N, Tukey JW, Ciminera JL, Heyse, JF (1982) Tumorigenicity assays, including use of the jackknife. *Biomet. J.* 24:579–596

Peto R (1974) Guidelines on the analysis of tumor rates and death rates in experimental animals. *Brit. J. Canc.* 29:101–105

Peto R, Pike MC, Day NE, Gray RC, Lee PN, Parish S, Peto J, Richards S, Wahrendorf J (1980) Guidelines for simple, sensitive significance tests for carcinogenic effects in long term animal experiments. In *International Association for Research on Cancer Monographs, Supplement 2,* Lyon, France, pp. 365–367

Robson DS (1959) A simplified method for constructing orthogonal polynomials when independent variable is unequally spaced. *Biometrics* 15:187–191

Saunders NR (1977) Ontogeny of the blood-brain barrier. *Exper. Eye Res.* (Suppl.), pp 523–550

Scow RO, Chernick SS, Brinley MS (1964) Hyperlipemia and ketosis in the pregnant rat. *Am. J. Physiol.* 206:796–804

Setlow RB, Carrier WL (1964) The disappearance of thymine dimers from DNA: An error correcting mechanism. *Proc. Natl. Acad. Sci. USA* 51:226–231

Tukey JW, Ciminera JL, Heyse JF (1985) Testing the statistical certainty of a response to increasing doses of a drug. *Biometrics* 41:295–301

Wester RC, Maibach HI (1975) Percutaneous absorption in the rhesus monkey compared to man. *Toxicol. & App. Pharm.* 32:394–398

Wester RC, Maibach HI (1983) Cutaneous pharmacokinetics. 10 steps to percutaneous absorption. *Drug Metab. Rev.* 14(2):169–205

Wilkins RJ, Hart RW (1973) Preferential DNA repair in human cells. *Nature* 247:35–36

Williams GM, Laspia MF, Dunkel, VC (1982) Reliability of the hepatocyte primary culture/DNA repair test in testing coded carcinogens and non-carcinogens. *Mutat. Res.* 97:359–370

CHAPTER 7

Pharmacokinetics of Ivermectin in Animals and Humans

David W. Fink and Arturo G. Porras

Introduction

The pharmacokinetic properties of ivermectin are a function of the species in which the compound is studied. Ivermectin is effective against parasites in a wide variety of hosts—including cattle, sheep, dogs, swine, and horses. A previous review of ivermectin has described the effects of formulation and route of administration on its pharmacokinetic properties in animals (Lo *et al.* 1985). That publication included examples of formulation modifications directed toward the development of oral and parenteral dosage forms; it also illustrated the use of drug plasma concentrations for characterizing the drug and for modifying formulations for specific efficacy. The following summary presents the results of representative pharmacokinetic and bioavailability studies of this drug in different animal species and in humans. It includes descriptions of the experimental procedures as well as the various measurement techniques used in these studies to describe the pharmacokinetic properties of ivermectin.

Cattle

Commercially, ivermectin is most widely used for treating cattle. Bioavailability studies have been run in this species using intravenous and subcutaneous injectable formulations. To measure the intrinsic pharmacokinetic properties of ivermectin in cattle, the tritium-labeled compound was formulated in a solution of 0.07 mCi/mg specific activity at a concentration of 10.0 mg/ml; the solvent consisted of 60% (v/v) propylene glycol and 40% (v/v) glycerol formal (Hibbert and Carter 1928) containing 5% polyvinylpyrrolidone. This solution was administered to cattle in a single intravenous bolus at a dose of 300 μg/kg body weight.

The pharmacokinetic results are shown in Figure 7.1. The data exhibit a typical biexponential decay based upon the usual 2-compartment open model.Figure 7.1 is a plot of the total concentration in plasma over time following IV administration as determined by HPLC and radiochemical analyses. The close agreement between the radioactivity data and the HPLC data (the average relative difference is 5%) confirms that there are no metabolites of ivermectin in the plasma over this time interval. This is important in bioavailability studies, because the intact drug must be discriminated in the plasma from possible degradates and metabolites of similar structures. This selectivity is especially important for ivermectin, because the structure is so complex that there are many structural changes and degradation processes that can occur. For example, one metabolic transformation of ivermectin (resulting from incubation at 37°C with rat or steer liver microsomes) is the formation of the C(24)-hydroxymethyl compounds and their respective monosaccharides (Miwa *et al.* 1982).

The bioavailability analyses in this study used a sensitive high-pressure liquid chromatographic (HPLC) analytical method. This method uses fluorescence detection after preliminary sample preparation by liquid-liquid partitioning and conventional gravity-fed column chromatography (Tolan *et al.* 1980; Fink 1982). The potency of ivermectin requires the use of extremely sensitive analytical procedures. This derivatization technique was developed to increase sensitivity for detection by forming an intensely fluorescent compound based upon an analytical aromatization reaction.

The results of the experiment depicted in Figure 7.1, in addition to the biexponential decay, reveal a very short distributive phase in cattle, k = 6 day^{-1}, a biological half-life $t_{1/2}$ of 2.8 days, a very large volume of distribution, 1.9 l/kg (consistent with the lipophilicity of this compound), and an area under the curve (AUC) of about 700 day-ng/ml. In an independent study, application of a 3-compartment model to the data obtained from 6 cattle also yielded an equal biological half-life $t_{1/2}$ = 2.7 days. In this study, the 3-compartment (triexponential) model provided a statistically significantly closer fit to the data than the 2-compartment

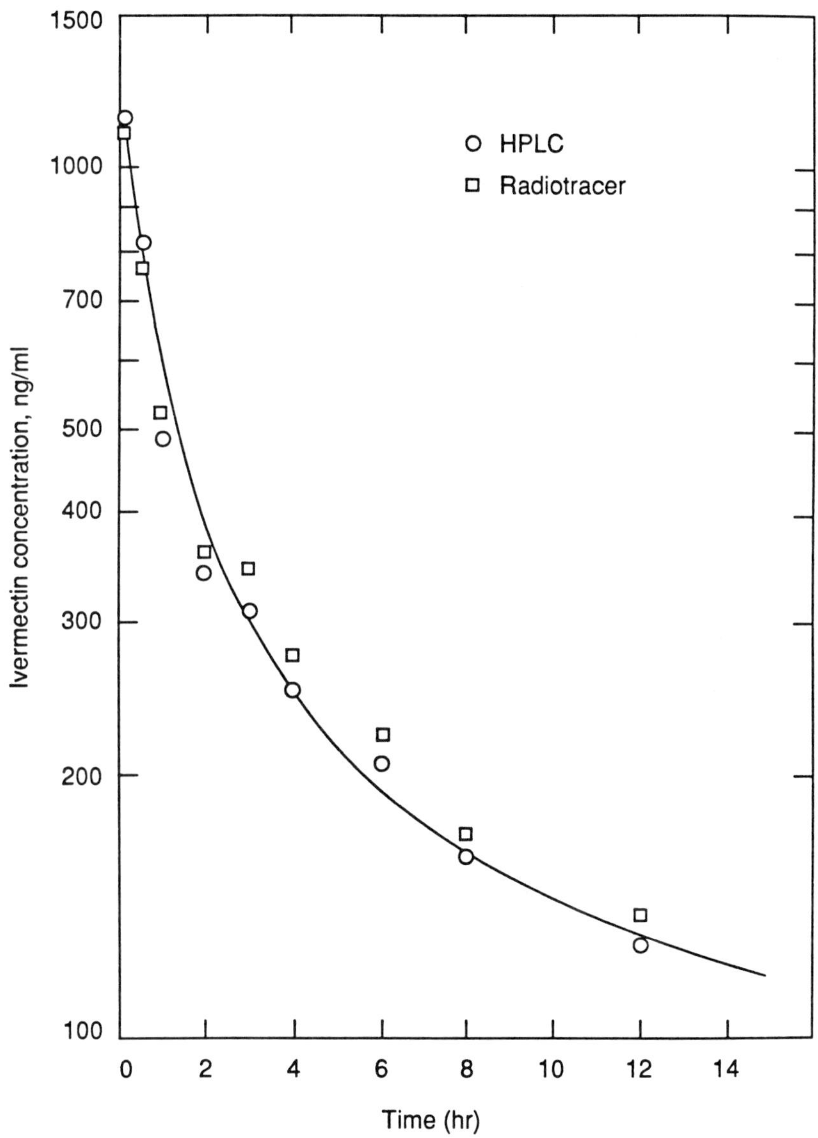

FIGURE 7.1. Comparison of bioavailability analyses and radiotracer counts in cattle plasma following intravenous dose. Data for 0.5 day following injection. Dose rate: 300 μg/kg body weight. Specific Activity: 0.07 mCi/mg.

(biexponential) model in 3 of the 6 animals (Wilkinson, Pope, and Baylis 1985). Schnitzerling and Nolan (1985) also found that the biological half-life of ivermectin is 3 days in cattle, using a normal-phase chromatographic system that does not resolve the 2 components of ivermectin. These workers studied the binding of ivermectin to plasma protein: they demonstrated that the drug is carried mainly in the plasma (80%), and that this distribution equilibrium between plasma and red blood cells remains relatively constant with time.

Figure 7.2 depicts the results of a replicate study in 2 cattle measured by chemical analysis and extending out to 4 weeks following the intravenous dose. The plasma samples again were collected at specific time intervals and analyzed as described previously (Tolan *et al.* 1980). The insert in this figure shows the rapid distribution phase in cattle: the biexponential decay mode is more clearly evident in this expanded scale.

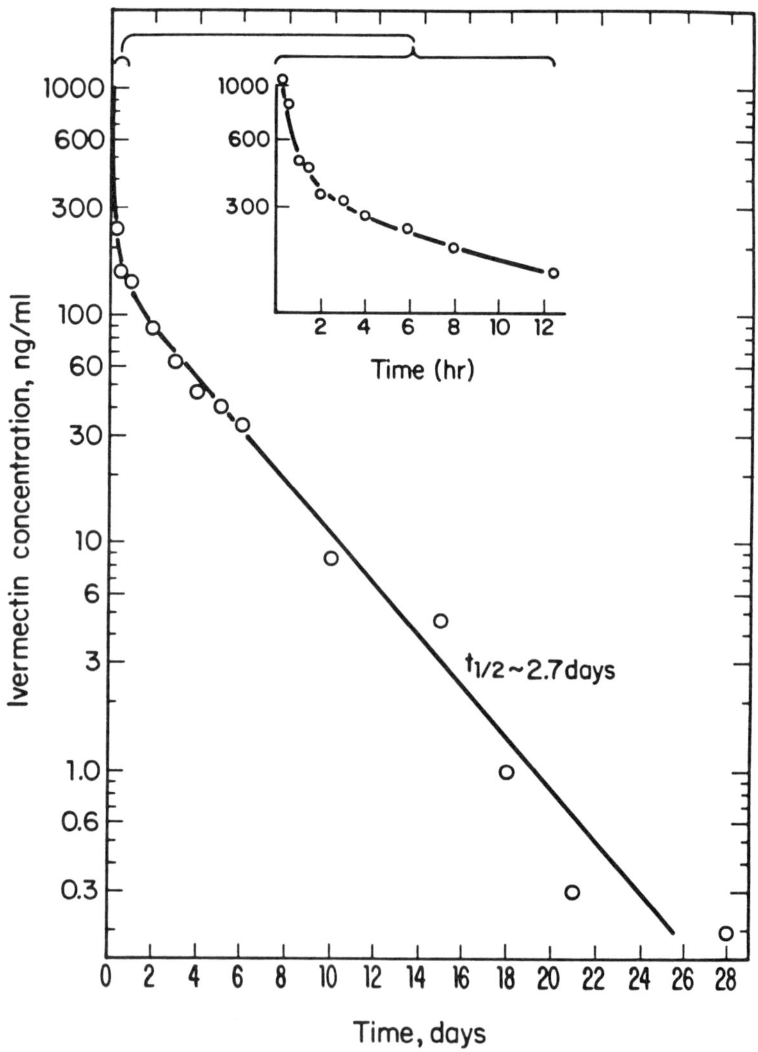

FIGURE 7.2. Plasma concentration of ivermectin in cattle for 1 month following intravenous administration. Mean of 2 cattle.

The plasma profile of the commercially available ivermectin cattle injectable formulation (IVOMEC) is shown in Figure 7.3. The dosage form is a 1% (w/v) solution of the drug in a mixed solvent vehicle of 60% (v/v) propylene glycol and 40% (v/v) glycerol formal. As shown in Figure 7.3, a subcutaneous injection, administered at a dose of 200 μg/kg body weight, attains a peak plasma concentration, C_p, of 44 ng/ml ivermectin within a time t_p of 1 day. It is striking that the biological half-life afforded by this injectable formulation, 8.3 days, is significantly longer than the intrinsic half-life of the drug, 2.8 days. This effect has been attributed to a slow absorption (k_a) process that dominates the pharmacokinetics of the nonaqueous injectable product (Lo *et al.* 1985). The clinical significance was noted by Campbell and Benz (1984) in a review of the efficacy and safety of ivermectin: these workers reported that the anthelmintic efficacy of this product persisted for 2 weeks after the treatment of cattle, and that this prolonged effect was consistent with these plasma levels of the drug (Figure 7.3).

Formulation modifications, based on the solubility properties of the drug, can have a significant effect on the bioavailability of ivermectin in cattle following subcutaneous administration. For example, changes in

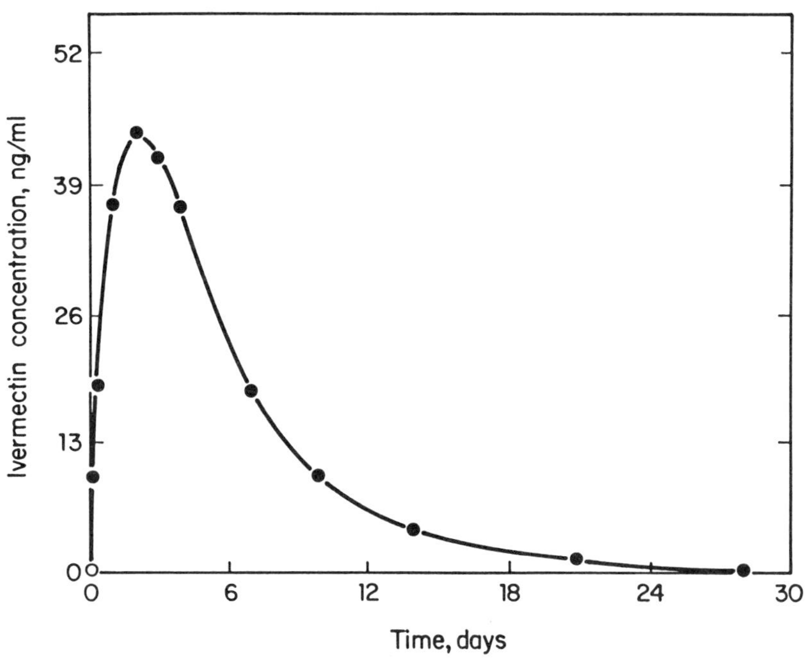

FIGURE 7.3. Bioavailability of ivermectin in cattle dosed subcutaneously with IVOMEC propylene glycol-glycerol formal [60 : 40 (v/v)] vehicle at 200 μg/kg body weight. Formulation concentration: 10 mg/ml ivermectin. Each point is the average plasma concentration obtained from 10 cattle.

solvent composition can be used to achieve prolonged blood levels. As illustrated in Figure 7.4, the bioavailability method was used to compare two experimental formulations, labeled 4-1 and 4-2. Formulation 4-1 is an aqueous micellar solution of ivermectin formulated to overcome its solubility limitations in water (Lo and Williams 1983). A micelle is formed with a surface-active agent, such as polyoxyethylene sorbitan monooleate (polysorbate 80, Tween 80), and a cosolvent such as glycerol formal in the presence of other substrates, such as benzyl alcohol. Formulation 4-2 is modified from 4-1 by mixing it with glycerol formal solvent; Formulation 4-2 is designed for prolonged absorption following subcutaneous dosing. The plasma concentrations achieved (Figure 7.4) with the aqueous product (4-1) are significantly higher than with the modified formulation (4-2); the former vehicle affords a much greater bioavailability (AUC) than the latter. The aqueous formulation (4-1) is more rapidly and

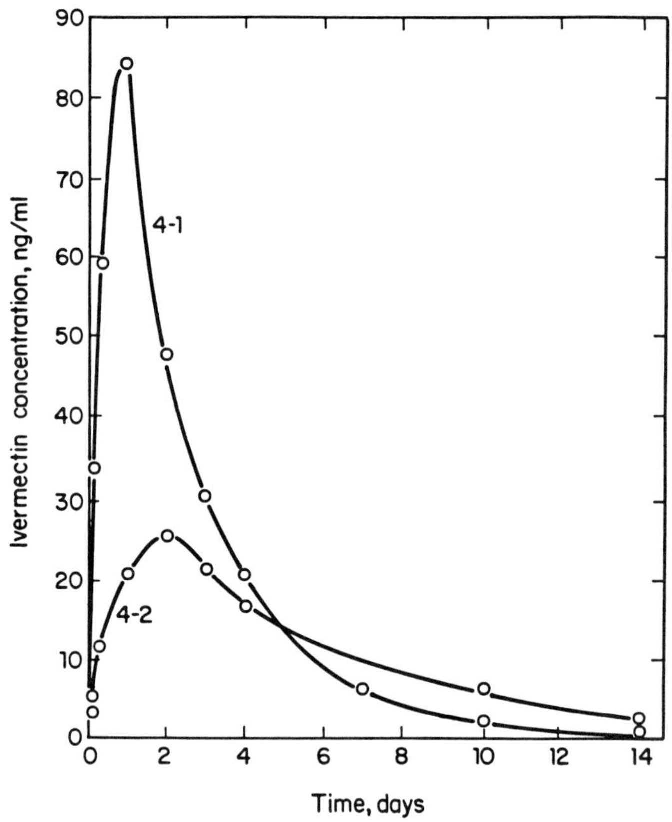

FIGURE 7.4. Effect of aqueous/nonaqueous solvent ratio on bioavailability of ivermectin following subcutaneous administration to cattle at 200 μg/kg body weight. Formulation 4-1 is an aqueous (micelle) solution; 4-2 is an aqueous-glycerol formal 50 : 50 (v/v) mixed solvent vehicle. (Modified from Lo *et al.* 1985.)

TABLE 7.1. Effect of injection vehicle on the bioavailability of ivermectin in cattle dosed subcutaneously at 200 μg/kg body weight. (Adapted from Lo *et al.* 1985.)

Parameter	Formulation[a] 4–1	4–2
Mean plasma peak time (days)	1	2
Peak plasma concentration (ng/ml)	84 ± 7	25 ± 14
Biological half-life (days)	2.0 ± 0.3	3.7 ± 0.7
AUC (day-ng/ml)	246 ± 46	186 ± 81
Fraction of drug absorbed (%)	55	41

[a] 4–1: aqueous (micelle): 4–2: Mixed aqueous (micelle)-glycerol formal 50% (v/v)

extensively absorbed and, in the traditional sense, is actually the more efficient delivery system of the two.

Table 7.1 is a summary of the pharmacokinetic data of Figure 7.4. A significant difference in peak plasma concentration between the two formulations is evident. The biological half-lives are also significantly different, resulting from the slow absorption process that dominates the pharmacokinetics in nonaqueous injectable products. The biological half-life of the aqueous micellar product, 2.0 ± 0.3 days, is in the range of the half-life calculated from the intravenous data (Figure 7.2), and results from the rapid k_a offered by this injection. Finally, it is seen that the area under the curve (AUC) from the micellar solution is 246 day-ng/ml, which is at least 25% greater than that obtained from the modified formulation. It is apparent that the modified micellar solution (4-2)—with its intermediate mixed-solvent system—exhibits pharmacokinetic properties that are intermediate between those of the aqueous micellar product (4-1) and the commercial nonaqueous solution (Figure 7.3).

Sheep

For administration to sheep, ivermectin was dissolved in a mixed solvent of 60% (v/v) propylene glycol–40% (v/v) glycerol formal containing 5% polyvinylpyrrolidone; it was given as a single intravenous bolus. The concentration of the solution for this species was 2 mg/ml ivermectin and the dose rate was 300 μg/kg body weight. Plasma samples were collected at specific time intervals and analyzed for ivermectin.

The points shown in Figure 7.5 are the averages over 4 animals. At each sampling point the range of results was ±15% or less. The results in sheep were analogous to those for cattle. Plasma concentration as a function of time clearly exhibited a biexponential decay for sheep. The biological half-life was again 2.7 days, very similar to that obtained in cattle. However, there is a significant difference in the volume of distribution of ivermectin between the 2 species. Volume of distribution, V_d, was

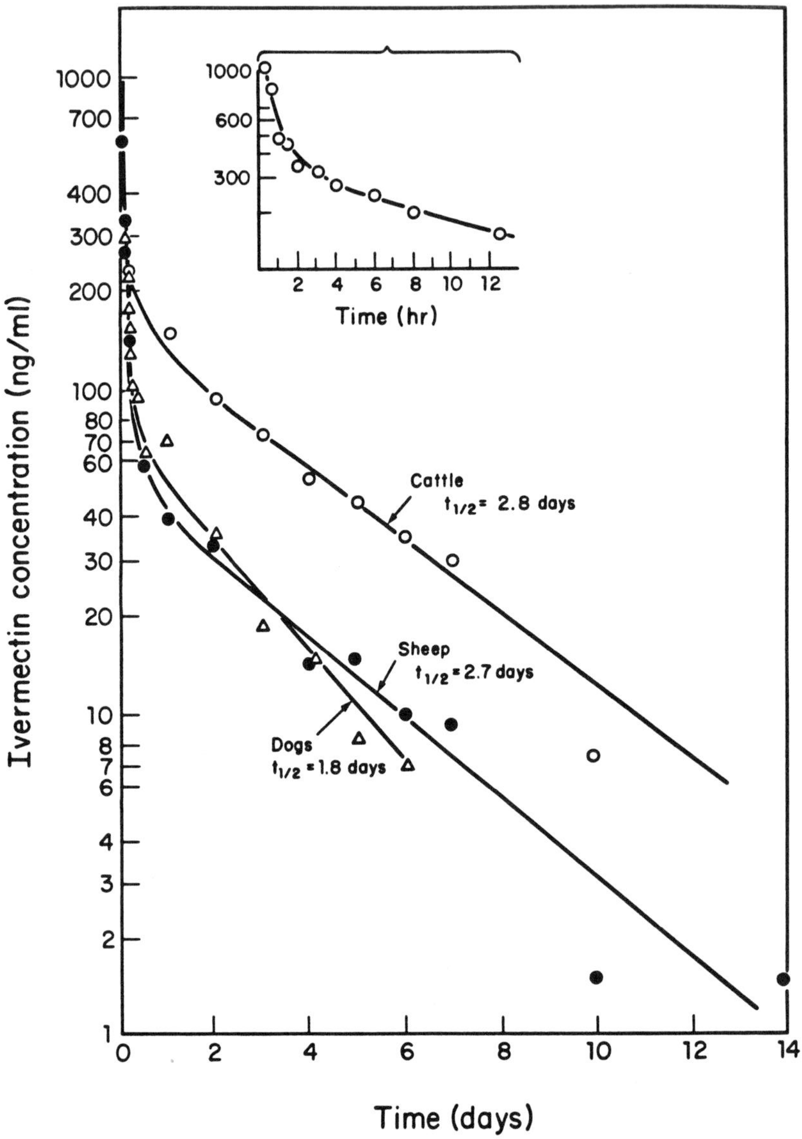

FIGURE 7.5. Biexponential decay of ivermectin concentration in plasma following intravenous administration to cattle (○), sheep (●), and dogs (△). Dose rates: 300 μg/kg body weight for cattle and sheep; 200 μg/kg for dogs. Insert depicts the rapid distribution phase in cattle. (Points are average from: 2 cattle, 4 sheep, and 5 dogs, respectively.) (Reproduced, with permission, from Lo *et al.* 1985.)

calculated by dividing the total dose by the plasma concentration at injection, which is obtained by extrapolation of the lines of Figure 7.5 to time t = 0. In sheep, the volume of distribution, V_d = 4.6 l/kg, is greater than that in cattle. And, as in cattle, the distributive phase is very rapid, k_d = 10 day^{-1}.

The bioavailability analyses in this species were obtained using the fluorescence-derivatization technique described for cattle. (Tolan *et al.* 1980). The responses of the known acid- and base-catalyzed hydrolysis products of ivermectin (Fink, in press) were recorded to demonstrate that the fluorescence-derivatization reaction furnishes efficient resolution of ivermectin in plasma from its possible hydrolysis products.

Other workers have also evaluated the pharmacokinetics of ivermectin in sheep. In contrast to the data described previously,Prichard and colleagues (1985) reported a longer ivermectin biological half-life in sheep, of 7.42 days. For plasma analyses, these workers used a diacetylated derivative of ivermectin as an internal standard in a method based upon direct ultraviolet absorption detection in lieu of fluorogenic derivatization. In another study, Marriner, McKinnon, and Bogan (1987) reported that the biological half-life in sheep was 61 hours, which is in close agreement with the measurement of 65 hours shown in Figure 7.5. These authors also attribute the low plasma concentrations found in sheep to the large volume of distribution in this species.

Further confirmation of the intrinsic pharmacokinetic properties of ivermectin in sheep can be found following drug administration by other routes of administration. Two groups of 5 sheep were each treated with an oral formulation of ivermectin at a dose of 200 μg/kg body weight using a dosing syringe. One of the groups received a solution containing 0.8 mg/ml ivermectin in propylene glycol, and the other group was given an aqueous micelle product (Lo and Williams 1983) containing the same concentration of the anthelmintic. As usual, plasma samples were collected from the sheep at appropriate time intervals for chemical analysis. The results showed that when ivermectin was administered orally to sheep (in either formulation), the biological half-life obtained from the terminal portion of the bioavailability curve ranged from 3 to 5 days. These data are in good agreement with the intravenous data mentioned previously and the results of Marriner and colleagues (1987).

A replicate study by oral dosing in sheep has also demonstrated that the aqueous micelle solution of ivermectin is bioequivalent to the propylene glycol solution. Both formulations exhibited a peak plasma concentration within 1 day and exhibited a terminal portion with a $t_{1/2}$ in the range of 3 to 5 days. Compared to the subcutaneous injectable route, this $t_{1/2}$ of the nonaqueous oral solution reflects the elimination of injection-site absorption processes attendant with nonaqueous vehicles as previously described (Lo *et al.* 1985). The fraction of the dose absorbed from each of these formulations was 50%.

Dogs

The dosing solution for intravenous administration to dogs was a 4-mg/ml solution of ivermectin in the aqueous micellar formulation, which uses a surface active agent to dissolve the drug (Lo and Williams 1983). This solution contained 8% (w/v) polyoxyethylene sorbitan monooleate surfactant, 20% (w/v) glycerol formal cosolvent, and 1% benzyl alcohol; pH was regulated to 6.2 with 1*N* HC1. The injection was given to 5 dogs, each at a dose of 200 μg/kg body weight.

The procedure used for these bioavailability studies in dogs was a direct method, based upon ultraviolet photometric detection of the drug using a chemical derivative (the Δ^2 isomer) of ivermectin as an internal standard (Pivnichny, Shim, and Zimmerman 1983). This procedure was adapted to a laboratory robotic system to increase the number of data points available in these pharmacokinetic studies (Pivnichny, Lawrence, and Stong 1987).

The curve obtained for the plasma concentration in dogs over time (Figure 7.5) shows a greater slope than that obtained from the ruminants. The results in dogs reveal a significant species difference in that ivermectin is eliminated (biotransformation, distribution, and excretion) more rapidly ($t_{1/2}$ = 1.8 days) than in either cattle or sheep. This measurement of the terminal half-life in dogs is in accord with results recently reported by Dainippon in Japan, which yielded a $t_{1/2}$ = 1.6 days in dogs (Kojima, Yamamoto, and Nakanishi 1987). The pharmacokinetic properties between species are summarized for comparison in Table 7.2.

The widespread use of ivermectin in a tablet formulation (HEARTGARD-30) to prevent heartworm disease in dogs in a monthly dosage regimen of only 6 μg/kg is a dramatic illustration of the potency of this drug. Bioavailability studies of these tablets document the rapid oral absorption achieved by this dosage form. The results, shown in Figure 7.6, demonstrate that the plasma level obtained from the tablets peaks within 2 to 4 hours and decays exponentially beyond the peak. The dose used for this study was 100 μg/kg, to provide sufficient precision of the replicates relative to the sensitivity of the measurement process.

TABLE 7.2. Intrinsic pharmacokinetic properties of ivermectin in three animal species. (Reproduced, with permission, from Lo *et al.* 1985.)

	Pharmacokinetic property		
Species	K_d(day^{-1})	$t_{1/2}$(day)	V_d(l/kg)
Cattle	6	2.8	1.9
Sheep	10	2.7	4.6
Dog	8.1	1.8	2.4

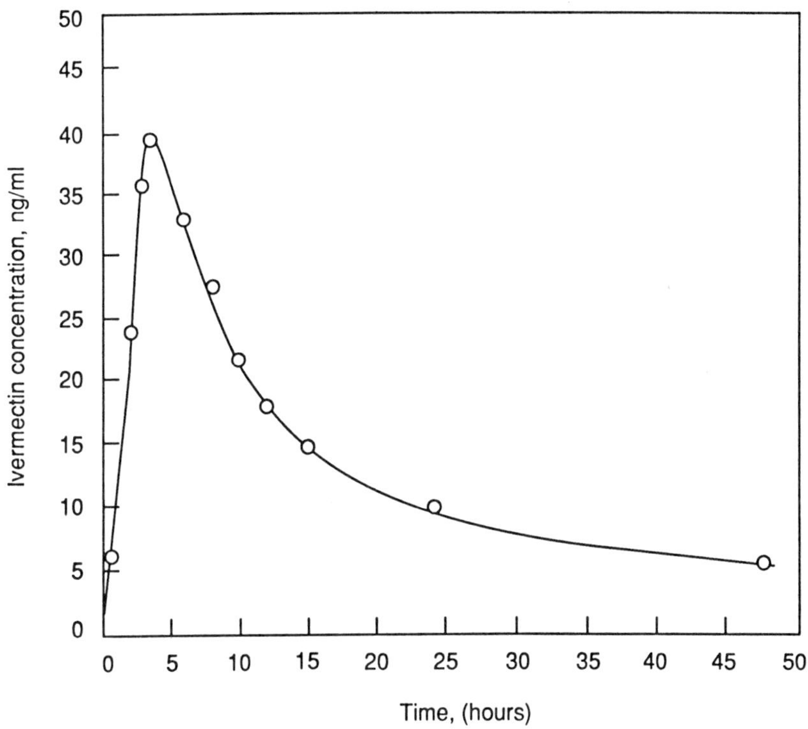

FIGURE 7.6. Bioavailability of ivermectin in dogs dosed with HEARTGARD tablet formulation at 100 μg/kg body weight. Each point is the average of 8 dogs.

The oral bioavailability achieved by this tablet formulation in dogs has been measured over a range of 3 dose rates using 3 different measurement techniques, as shown in Table 7.3. The concentration at the peak (C_p) increases directly with the dose, suggesting a linear relationship between the amount of drug absorbed and the dose administered. Further, the rate of absorption was equal in the 3 studies, as evidenced by the t_p observed

TABLE 7.3. Bioavailability in dogs of ivermectin from tablet formulation at three dose levels.

Dose administered	Measurement technique	Peak plasma concentration
6 μg/kg	Radiotracer counting	3.3 ng/ml
27 μg/kg	Fluorogenic derivatization[a]	19.1 ng/ml
100 μg/kg	Direct photometric[b]	40 ng/ml

[a] From Kojima Yamamoto, and Nakanishi 1987.
[b] From Pivnichny Shim, and Zimmerman 1983.

at 3 to 4 hours; this is additional evidence of the dose-independent pharmacokinetics obtained from this tablet formulation for dogs. A recent study has also demonstrated the bioequivalence of ivermectin when the total dose is administered to dogs either (a) in tablets, each containing 46 micrograms of the drug, or (b) in twice as many tablets, each of which is formulated to contain 23 micrograms of ivermectin (Kojima *et al.* 1987).

Swine

One marked example of the effect of route of administration on bioavailability can be found in a bioequivalence study in swine treated with ivermectin by subcutaneous injection and by oral administration. Two groups of 4 pigs were each given ivermectin at a dose of 200 μg/kg parenterally in a propylene glycol-glycerol formal (60 : 40 v/v) vehicle or orally in propylene glycol solution. The drug concentration in these dosing solutions was 10 mg/ml ivermectin. Plasma samples were collected at appropriate time intervals and analyzed using the fluorogenic-derivatization technique described previously (Tolan *et al.* 1980). The results are shown in Figure 7.7.

After either subcutaneous or oral administration of ivermectin to swine, the plasma concentration of the drug reached a peak and then declined exponentially with time. It is significant that the terminal portions resulting from these 2 dosing regimens are nearly parallel, suggesting that ivermectin is eliminated rapidly in swine following either route of absorption. The concentration of ivermectin in the plasma, however, attains its peak, t_p, faster following the oral dose than the parenteral: that these peaks appeared at 0.5 days and 2 days, respectively, demonstrates a higher absorption rate via oral administration than subcutaneous. These results in swine are in accord with the bioavailability obtained with subcutaneous injections in cattle and sheep. The slower absorption associated with the parenteral route has been attributed to precipitation of the drug at the injection site (Lo *et al.* 1985). The area under the plasma concentration-vs.-time curve (AUC) was larger after subcutaneous administration, indicating that a greater fraction of the dose is absorbed than after oral dosing. The bioavailability of ivermectin after oral administration, relative to that after subcutaneous administration, was estimated to be 41%.

The feed route offers another opportunity to study the bioavailability of ivermectin in swine following oral administration. Two groups of 6 Yorkshire barrows were each given a single oral dose of 400 μg/kg body weight ivermectin in premix formulations prepared for homogeneous distribution in the swine feed. One premix formulation was composed of 0.22% ivermectin adsorbed on ground corn cobs. The second premix was prepared to contain 0.6% ivermectin adsorbed on the same ground corn cob substrate. Plasma samples were collected from the pigs during 14

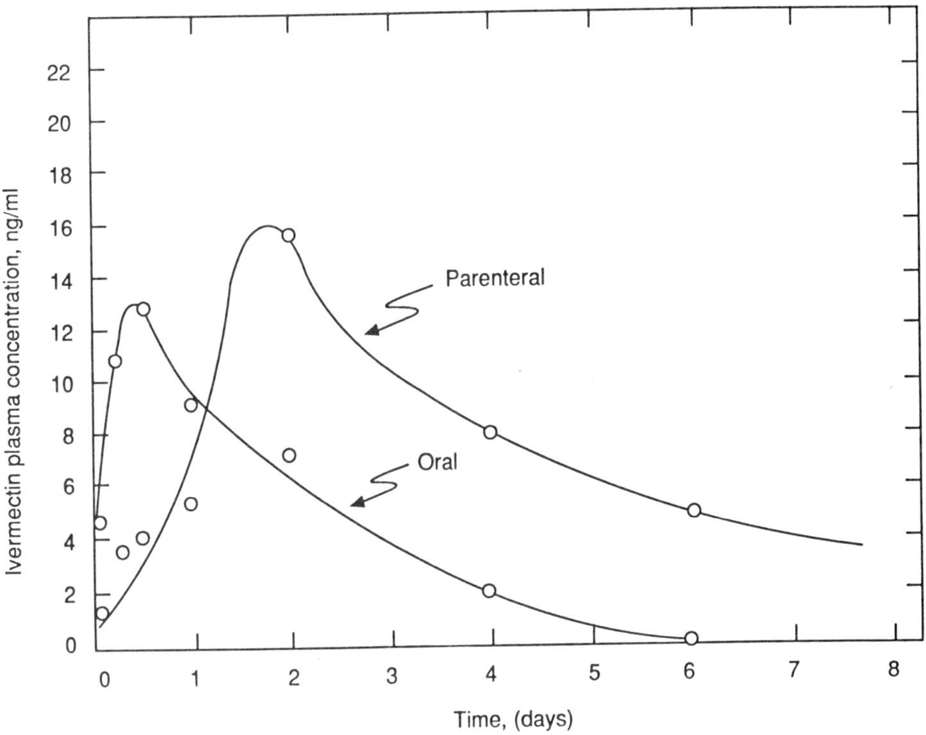

FIGURE 7.7. Bioavailability of ivermectin in swine administered orally and parenterally. Dose: 200 μg/kg. Vehicles: Oral: propylene glycol; parenteral: propylene glycol-glycerol formal mixed solvent (60:40 (v/v). Each point is the average of 4 animals.

days following the dosing, and these samples were analyzed for ivermectin. These bioavailability studies were also used to evaluate the efficacy of ivermectin in feed formulations. Two studies were run, with swine dosed at 400 μg/kg body weight in all the feed consumed: in both studies, the drug reached its peak concentration in the plasma within 4 to 8 hours, in agreement with the results of oral administration shown in Figure 7.7. These results are shown in Figure 7.8. Note that the drug is rapidly adsorbed by the oral route, that it is eliminated rapidly from swine ($t_{1/2} \sim 0.5$ day), and that good experimental agreement in the bioavailability results was found between these 2 independent swine oral studies.

Horses

One additional clear example of the significant effect of formulation and route of administration on the bioavailability of ivermectin has recently been reported in a study in pregnant mares. A paste formulation and an aqueous micellar formulation of this drug were administered (Asquith *et*

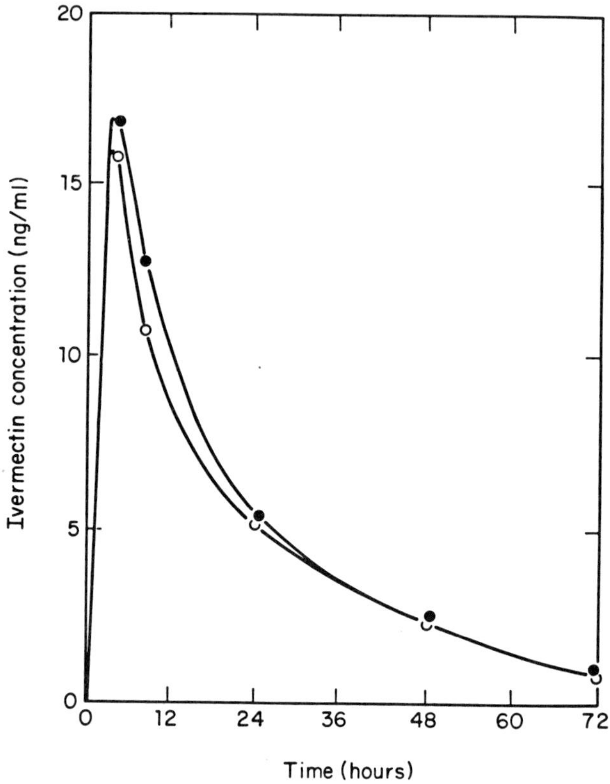

FIGURE 7.8. Bioavailability of ivermectin in swine following single oral administration of adsorbate feed premixes. Drug (0.6% or 0.22%) adsorbed on ground corn cobs. Dose: 400 μg/kg body weight. Closed and open circles designate two independent replicate bioavailability studies. The range of standard deviations from these 10 data points was 0.4 ng/ml to 5.9 ng/ml ivermectin. (Reproduced, with permission, from Lo *et al.* 1985.)

al. 1987). The dose for both treatments was 200 μg/kg, and the liquid micellar solution (1%) was administered by nasogastric intubation. A striking difference in bioavailability was found; the solution is absorbed much more rapidly than the paste product. Although the liquid formulation attained its peak concentration within 4 to 5 hours, the paste product took 15 hours to reach its maximum plasma concentration. Accordingly, the peak plasma concentration obtained from the solution was higher than that offered by the paste, and the bioavailability (AUC) was 20% higher following the nasogastric oral liquid dose.

Humans

Disposition of ivermectin in humans was studied in 4 healthy volunteers after an oral dose (no i.v. formulation exists) of ^{3}H-ivermectin labeled in the C(22) and C(23) positions. Concentrations of ivermectin in blood peaked at around 4 hours postdose and slowly decreased afterward (see Figure 7.9). Peak plasma concentrations of radioactive metabolites were about twice those of parent drug and occurred somewhat later (*ca.* 7h). The elimination phase of ivermectin does not consist of a simple exponential, and examination of individual plasma-concentration profiles reveals secondary peaks suggestive of enterohepatic recycling. The half-life was estimated at about 12 hours. Ivermectin and its metabolites seem to be excreted in bile with minimal ($\leq$ 1.0% of administered dose) urinary excretion. Secretion of ivermectin in human milk has been observed to a minor extent.

Urine, feces, and plasma of subjects given radioactive ivermectin were analyzed to establish the chemical identities of metabolites. Positive identification has been obtained for the presence of 3″-0-desmethyl-22,23-dihydroavermectin B_{1a}, and 22,23-dihydroavermectin B_{1a} monosaccharide in urine and feces, respectively. Plasma metabolites that are less polar than the parent drug have been tentatively characterized as fatty acid ester conjugates of the monosaccharides or aglycone of the drug (S.-H.L. Chiu, personal communication).

Some of the metabolites are, systemically, longer lived than the parent drug (see Figure 7.9). Monitoring the appearance and disappearance of radioactively labeled metabolites in plasma gives an apparent half-life of about 3 days.

The absolute bioavailability of ivermectin in humans is unknown. Twelve healthy volunteers were given single doses of the commercially available tablet, unformulated ivermectin in a capsule or a solution of

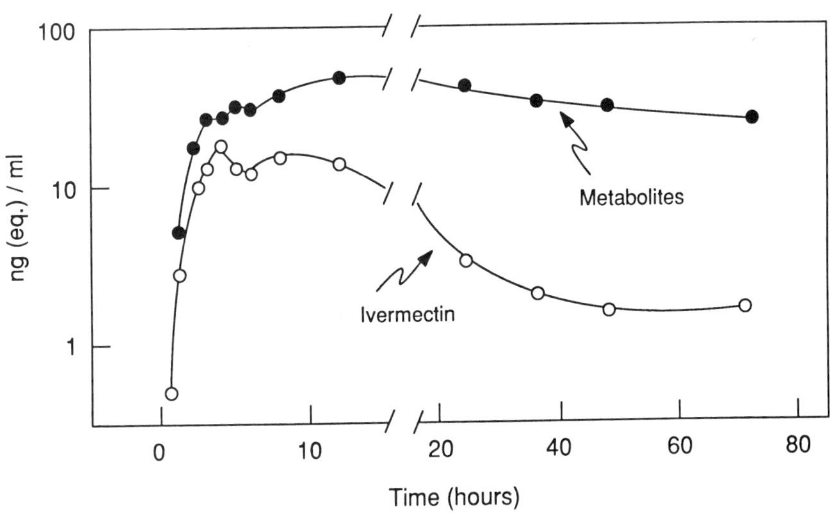

FIGURE 7.9. Mean concentrations of ivermectin and metabolites in human plasma after administration of a 14-mg dose of ^{3}H-labeled drug (average from 4 subjects).

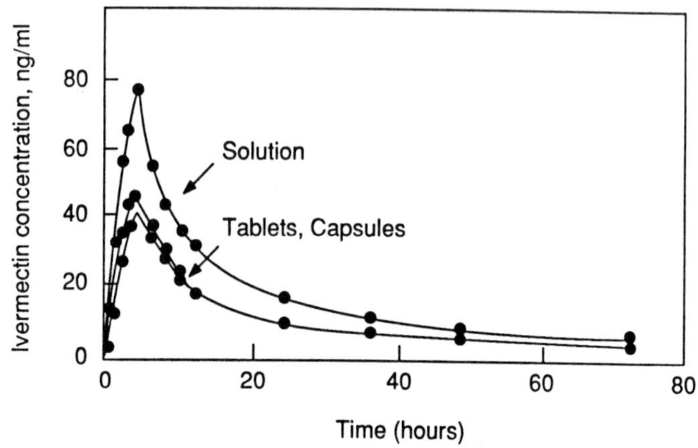

FIGURE 7.10. Mean plasma concentrations of ivermectin in humans after administration of 12-mg single doses to 12 healthy volunteers as either capsules, tablets, or a hydroalcoholic solution.

ivermectin (0.6 mg/ml) in 40% aqueous ethanol. Mean plasma concentration-vs-time curves are shown in Figure 7.10. The bioavailabilities of the two solid formulations were similar, while the alcoholic solution was substantially more bioavailable (mean AUC ratios of 1.73 and 1.96 relative to capsules and tablets, respectively). Formulation seems to have no effect on the time at which maximum concentrations in plasma are observed (*ca.* 4h). Such behavior is consistent with absorption of

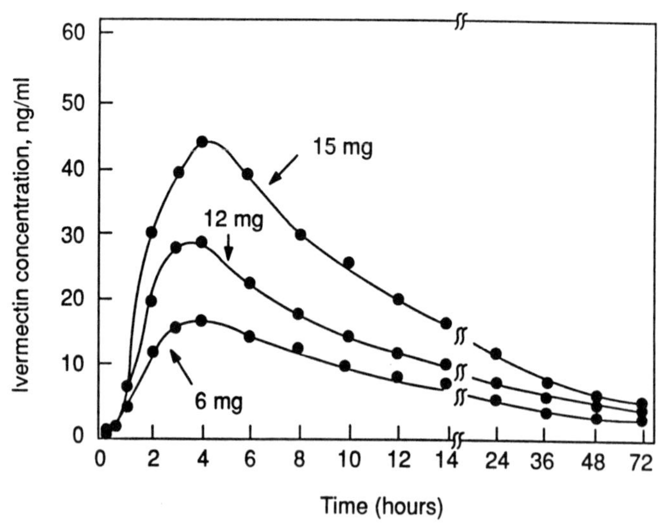

FIGURE 7.11. Mean concentrations of ivermectin in human plasma after administration of single doses of 6, 12, and 15 mg to 12 healthy volunteers.

ivermectin being limited by dissolution rate. These results put an upper limit of some 50% to 60% on the bioavailability of ivermectin from capsules and tablets (data from University of Liverpool and Merck and Co., Inc.).

Investigation of the effect of dose on observed plasma concentrations in 12 healthy volunteers (see Figure 7.11) indicated that, in the therapeutic range, the pharmacokinetics of the drug are concentration-independent (Porras *et al.* 1987). Observed AUC and C_{max} values increased significantly when the dose was increased from 6 to 12 to 15 mg (single doses). Ratios of dose-adjusted AUC estimates for the 12 versus 6 mg doses, the 15 versus 6 mg doses, and the 15 versus 12 mg doses were 0.81, 0.86, and 1.07, respectively. The corresponding C_{max} ratios were 0.88, 0.92, and 1.05. In all cases the 95% confidence interval included unity. There was no detectable effect of dose on the time taken to reach maximum plasma concentration. These results are strongly supportive of dose proportionality.

References

Asquith RL, Lane TJ, Plue RE, Seward RL, Kivipelto J (1987) The bioavailability of ivermectin in horses when administered in a liquid formulation by nasogastric intubation versus in an oral paste. *Equ. Vet. Sci.* 7:28–30

Campbell WC, Benz GW (1984) Ivermectin: a review of efficacy and safety. *J. Vet. Pharm. & Therap.* 7:1–16

Fink DW (1982) Some specific fluorogenic reactions in pharmaceutical and environmental applications. *Trends in Anal. Chem.* 1:254–258

Fink DW (in press) Ivermectin: analytical profile. In Florey K (ed) *Analytical Profiles of Drug Substances,* Academic Press, New York

Hibbert H, Carter NM (1928) Studies on the reactions relating to carbohydrates and polysaccharides. XVII. Structure of the isomeric methylidene glycerols. *J. Am. Chem. Soc.* 50:3120–3127

Kojima K, Yamamoto K, Nakanishi Y (1987) Determination of 22,23-dihydroavermectin B_{1a} in dog plasma using solid-phase extraction and high-performance liquid chromatography. *J. Chromatogr.* 413:326–331

Kojima K, Yamamoto K, Katae H, Nakanishi Y (1987) Bioavailability of oral ivermectin in dog [sic]. *Nippon Juigaku Zasshi* 49:899–900

Lo P-KA, Fink DW, Williams JB, Blodinger J (1985) Pharmacokinetic studies of ivermectin: effects of formulation. *Vet. Res. Commun.* 9:251–268

Lo P-KA, Williams JB (1983) Solubilization of ivermectin in water. U.S. Patent 4,389,397

Marriner SE, McKinnon I, Bogan JA (1987) The pharmacokinetics of ivermectin after oral and subcutaneous administration to sheep and horses. *J. Vet. Pharm. Therap.* 10:175–179

Miwa GT, Walsh JS, VandenHeuvel WJA, Arison B, Sestokas E, Buhs R, Rosegay A, Lu AYH, Walsh MAR, Walker RW, Taub R, Jacob TA (1982) The metabolism of avermectins B_{1a}, H_2B_{1a}, and H_2B_{1b} by liver microsomes. *Drug Metab. Dispos.* 10:268–274

Pivnichny JV, Lawrence AA, Stong JD (1987) A robotic sample preparation scheme for the high performance liquid chromatographic determination of ivermectin in animal plasma. *J. Chromatogr. Sci.* 25:181–186

Pivnichny JV, Shim J-SK, Zimmerman LA (1983) Direct determination of avermectins in plasma at nanogram levels by high-performance liquid chromatography. *J. Pharm. Sci.* 72:1447–1450

Porras AG, Chiou R, Kukovetz W, Hall-Gregg M, Stubbs RJ, Mesinger M, Beubler N, Jaeger A (1987) Dose proportionality of the anthelmintic ivermectin in man. Abstract presented at the 2nd National Meeting of the AAPS, June 5–12, 1987, Boston, Mass.

Prichard RK, Steel JW, Lacey E, Hennessy, DR (1985) Pharmacokinetics of ivermectin in sheep following intravenous, intra-abomasal or intraruminal administration. *J. Vet. Pharm. & Therap.* 8:88–94

Schnitzerling HJ, Nolan J (1985) Normal phase chromatographic determination of nanogram quantities of ivermectin in cattle blood or plasma. *J. Assoc. Offic. Anal. Chem.* 68:36–40

Tolan JW, Eskola P, Fink DW, Mrozik H, Zimmerman LA (1980) Determination of avermectins in plasma at nanogram levels using high-performance liquid chromatography with fluorescence detection. *J. Chromatogr.* 190:367–376

Wilkinson PK, Pope DG, Baylis FP (1985) Pharmacokinetics of ivermectin administered intravenously to cattle. *J. Pharm. Sci.* 74:1105–1107

CHAPTER 8

Metabolism and Tissue Residues

Shuet-Hing Lee Chiu and Anthony Y.H. Lu

I. Introduction

Ivermectin is used widely as an antiparasitic agent in food-producing animals. As in the case of any such drug, the residual tissue concentration of the therapeutic agent, or tissue residue, is a safety concern to the meat-consuming public. To evaluate the toxic potential of the residual tissue concentration of ivermectin and its metabolites, metabolism studies have been carried out in target species (cattle, sheep, swine) using the radiolabeled drug. Comparative metabolic studies were done in a laboratory animal, the rat, and in liver microsomes from various species.

Radiolabeled ivermectin was synthesized either by incorporating tritium atoms in the C5 position by oxidation of the C5-alcohol to ketone with manganese dioxide followed by reduction back to the alcohol with sodium borotritide, or in the C22-23 positions by catalytic tritiation of avermectin. In these synthetic reactions, the 2 components of ivermectin, dihydro-B_{1a} (H_2B_{1a}) and dihydro-B_{1b} (H_2B_{1b}) are synthesized and purified separately and then mixed in a ratio of 80 : 20 with respect to H_2B_{1a} to H_2B_{1b} for dose preparation. Most of the studies were carried out with C22-23–labeled drug (22,23-[^{3}H]ivermectin). The tritium label has been shown to be stable by volatility studies (Jacob *et al.* 1983).

This chapter addresses only those studies on ivermectin tissue residue and metabolism that employed the radiolabeled drug. For a review of those studies that used unlabeled ivermectin, the reader is referred to Chapter 9.

II. Tissue Residues in Cattle, Sheep, and Swine

Tissue residues are often assayed as total radioactivity in the tissue or body fluids after an animal is dosed with a radioactive drug. The total tissue residues include the free drug, its metabolites, and any tissue-bound residues as they are generally classified (Weber 1980; Dorough 1980). The "free" and "bound" residues are differentiated by their extractability by methods such as exhaustive extraction, denaturation, or solubilization (Weber 1980). While toxicological evaluation of the free drug residue is possible when the levels and structures of these residues are known, evaluating the bound residue is extremely difficult (Lu *et al.* 1987).

Ivermectin residues in animal tissues are essentially free residues; the total radioactivity in "edible" tissues (liver, kidney, muscle, and fat) of cattle, sheep, swine, and rats is nearly quantitatively extractable with organic solvents (Chiu *et al.* 1986, 1987). Thus, the bound residue is not a concern with ivermectin.

Tissue-residue studies were carried out on animals dosed once at 0.3 or 0.4 mg/kg body weight either subcutaneously (cattle, swine), intraruminally (cattle, sheep), or orally (rats). Animals were slaughtered over a period of 1 to 28 days after dosing (Campbell *et al.* 1983; Jacob *et al.* 1983). About 25 tissues and body fluids were collected from the target species and assayed to examine the distribution of the radioactive residue. Urine and feces were usually collected over the whole period of the study and assayed for the recovery of the radioactive dose. Radioactivity in tissues and feces was assayed by combustion of the aqueous homogenates followed by scintillation counting. Radioactivity in plasma and other fluids was analyzed directly by scintillation counting. Table 8.1 shows the tissue residue levels from 4 steers slaughtered 7, 14, 21, and 28 days after receiving a single subcutaneous dose of 22,23-[^{3}H]ivermectin at 0.3 mg/kg body weight. Among the 25 tissues and fluids analyzed, brain tissue showed the lowest residue levels (4 ppb 7 days after dosing). Of the edible tissues, liver and fat tissue levels were the highest, with depletion half-lives of 4.8 and 7.6 days, respectively. Similar tissue-residue distribution patterns exist in the sheep, swine, and rats, although the residue-depletion half-lives are much shorter in sheep and rats (1–2 days), reflecting more rapid metabolism in these animals (Table 8.2). The half-lives of the parent drug and total tissue residue are in close agreement in liver tissue in all species (except swine), suggesting equally efficient depletion of the parent drug and its metabolites. The parent drug depletes relatively faster in fat tissue than the total residue (about twofold) in cattle

TABLE 8.1. Total radioactive residue levels (ppb) in tissues and fluids from cattle dosed subcutaneously with 22,23-[^{3}H]ivermectin at 0.3 mg/kg body weight.[a]

Days post dose	7	14	21	28
Abomasum	44	17	10	1
Adrenals	29	6	7	2
Bile	273	54	22	1
Bone marrow	92	21	23	9
Brain	4	1	0	0
Cecum	33	9	3	0
Colon	44	11	9	0
Fat	270	83	69	29
Heart	41	8	3	0
Intestine (small)	22	5	6	1
Kidney	68	6	7	2
Liver	782	55	68	11
Lung	66	12	4	1
Lymph gland	41	13	20	6
Muscle	23	2	4	0
Pancreas	83	16	9	1
Plasma	45	11	6	3
Rumen	34	10	10	2
Rumen fluid	7	1	0	0
Spleen	38	8	5	3
Thymus	64	21	9	1
Thyroid	58	16	8	6
Tongue	27	4	4	0
Injection site	70	28	33	39

[a] Tissues and fluids were collected from 1 steer per time point. Radiolabeled ivermectin was at a specific activity of 0.1 mCi/mg. All samples except plasma were assayed by combustion of the tissue homogenate in water.

TABLE 8.2. Depletion half-lives of 22,23-[^{3}H]ivermectin total residue and unchanged drug in liver and fat tissues of cattle, sheep, swine, and rat.[a]

	$t_{1/2}$ (day)					
	Liver			Fat		
Species	Total residue	H_2B_{1a}	H_2B_{1b}	Total residue	H_2B_{1a}	H_2B_{1b}
Cattle	4.8	4.7	4.0	7.6	4.3	3.2
Sheep	1.2	1.2	1.0	1.8	1.1	0.9
Swine	5.2	3.8	3.2	5.1	3.8	4.0
Rat	0.95	0.90	—[b]	1.3	—[b]	—[b]

[a] Results are from studies in which all species except swine were dosed at 0.3 mg/kg body weight, subcutaneously (steers), intraruminally (sheep), or orally (male rat). Swine were dosed SC at 0.4 mg/kg body weight. Unchanged drug H_2B_{1a} and H_2B_{1b} were analyzed by RIDA.

[b] Not calculated due to insufficient data.

and sheep, probably because the fat tissues of these species eliminate nonpolar metabolite conjugates less efficiently. This phenomenon will be discussed at more length in the section on *In Vivo* Fat Metabolism of Ivermectin. There is no difference between liver and fat residue depletion in swine.

The distribution pattern of tissue residue remains unchanged when the drug is dosed via different routes. Of the 3 routes—subcutaneous, intraruminal, and percutaneous—in steers, the intraruminal dosing gives the lowest residue levels in liver and fat. The depletion half-lives, however, vary with the dosing method. Residue levels in the brain remain the lowest by all dosing routes (S.H.L. Chiu, M. Green, F.P. Baylis, D. Eline, and T.A. Jacob, unpublished results).

Radiolabeled ivermectin is excreted mainly in feces in all 4 species studied. Regardless of whether the drug was administered intraruminally or subcutaneously to cattle, only 0.5% to 2.0% of the dose was eliminated in urine; the remainder appeared in feces (Jacob *et al.* 1983). Recovery of the radioactive dose 7 days after dosing varies between 62% to 83% in cattle, sheep, and rats.

III. Absorption, Distribution, and Excretion of Ivermectin in Rats

To establish the relevance of rodent toxicology studies to human safety issues, comparative metabolism studies of ivermectin were also carried out in the rat. Total radioactivity in rat plasma was compared following 5 dosing routes: gavage, subcutaneous, intramuscular, intraperitoneal, or intravenous (Jacob *et al.* 1983). Orbital blood samples taken during the first 24 hours showed that by 4 hours after dose, total radioactivity in blood from all dosing routes converged to about 0.03 ppm. Furthermore, depletion rates of blood radioactivity during the subsequent 8 to 24-hour period were quite similar. Radioactive residue levels in "edible" tissues increased proportionately with the dose, ranging from 0.06 mg/kg to 7.5 mg/kg (125-fold dose increase). At the dose used in food-producing animals (0.3 mg/kg), the tissue-to-blood ratio is generally greater than 1. At 1 day post dose, the ratio is highest in testicular fat (24 : 1), followed by kidney (18 : 1), liver (11 : 1), and muscle (3 : 1). By oral dosing, plasma levels peaked between 4 to 8 hours post dose and depleted at a half-life of about 1 day in both plasma and liver at all dosage levels. Intravenous dosing resulted in a rapid distribution of radioactivity to lung, heart, liver, and kidney within 2 hours (Figure 8.1). During the first 24 hours after dosing, residues in these tissues deplete at half-lives of approximately 12 hours. Residue in the fat tissue, on the other hand, does not peak until 12 hours and depletes relatively slower, remaining as the highest residue concentration among tissues.

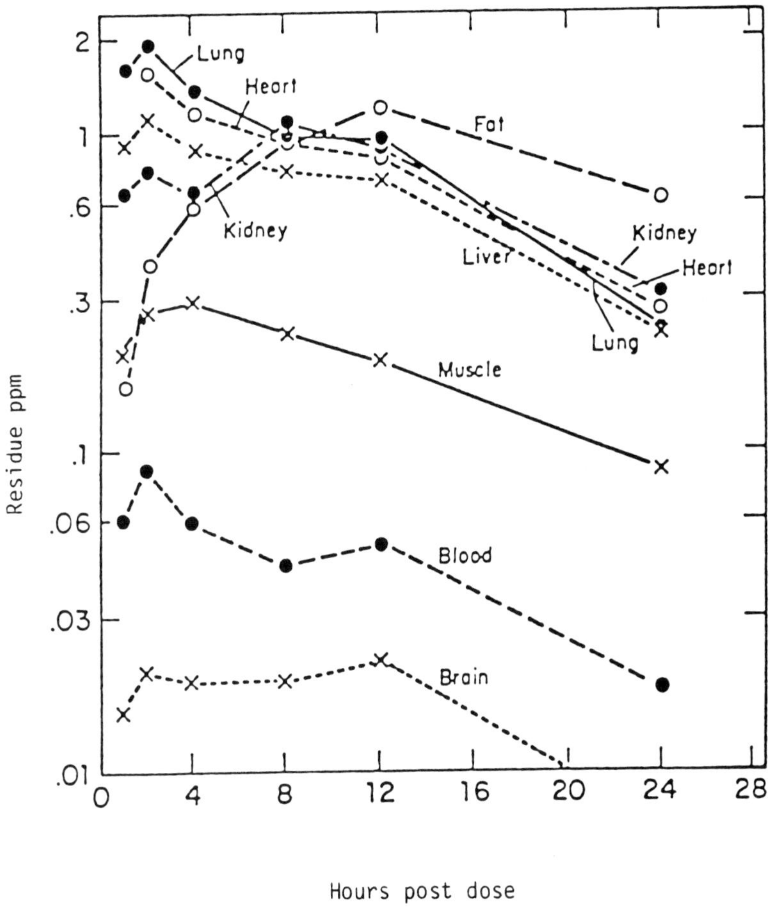

FIGURE 8.1. Depletion of total radioactive residues in tissues and blood of rats dosed intravenously at 0.3 mg/kg[a].

[a] Ivermectin was dissolved in 0.5 ml rat plasma for i.v. dosing.

Absorption and distribution of the 2 components of ivermectin are similar in rats. For all rat tissues analyzed, depletion of the major component H_2B_{1a} showed half-lives of 1 to 1.5 days. The minor component H_2B_{1b}, however, appears to deplete slightly faster, with half-lives of 0.4 to 0.8 day (Table 8.3). This phenomenon is also observed in cattle but not particularly noticeable in sheep and swine.

IV. *In Vitro* Liver Metabolism of Ivermectin

The toxicological evaluation of free drug or metabolite residue in animal tissues requires the elucidation of metabolites, structures, as well as quantification of the parent drug and its metabolites. Because of the low

TABLE 8.3. Total radioactive residues in blood and tissues of male Sprague Dawley rats dosed subcutaneously at 0.3 mg/kg with 22,23-[^{3}H]H_2B_{1a} or 22,23-[^{3}H]H_2B_{1b}.[a]

	Tissue residues (ppm)						Depletion $t_{1/2}$	
Post-dose	1 day		2 days		4 days		(day)	
Tissues	H_2B_{1a}	H_2B_{1b}	H_2B_{1a}	H_2B_{1b}	H_2B_{1a}	H_2B_{1b}	H_2B_{1a}	H_2B_{1b}
Liver	0.320	0.229	0.130	0.082	0.043	0.010	1.06	0.66
Kidney	0.220	0.185	0.118	0.068	0.041	0.009	1.25	0.69
Fat pad	0.493	0.497	0.274	0.168	0.110	0.027	1.40	0.72
Muscle	0.109	0.067	0.044	0.023	0.017	0.004	1.16	0.75
Lung	0.166	0.108	0.064	0.041	0.027	0.004	1.19	0.63
Heart	0.126	0.105	0.073	0.044	0.027	0.005	1.36	0.68
Blood	0.019	0.013	0.009	0.004	0.003	0.000	1.14	0.42
Plasma	0.023	0.017	0.012	0.005	0.004	0.001	1.20	0.75

[a] Three rats (200 g each) were dosed at each time point with radiolabeled drug at specific activity of 0.1 mCi/mg. Blood was collected by heart puncture. Fat pad was removed from the testicular areas of the animals.

tissue-residue levels in animals treated with ivermectin at normal slaughter time (14–28 days after dosing), it is extremely difficult to isolate directly from tissue sufficient amounts of pure metabolites for structural identification. In this regard, *in vitro* metabolism systems such as liver homogenates or liver microsomes are superior because conditions can be manipulated to maximize the formation of metabolites. The relatively "clean" system (compared to the *in vivo* tissue matrix) also facilitates the isolation and purification of metabolites (Lu *et al.* 1987). The *in vitro* metabolism of ivermectin was studied with 22,23-[^{3}H]H_2B_{1a} and 22,23-[^{3}H]H_2B_{1b} by incubation with liver microsomes from rat, steer, and swine in the presence of an NADPH-regenerating system (Miwa *et al.* 1982; Chiu *et al.* 1984). Using these systems, rat and cattle liver microsomes form 24-hydroxymethyl-H_2B_{1a} (V, Figure 8.2) and 24-hydroxymethyl-H_2B_{1b} (VI) as major metabolites,[1] while swine microsomes give rise to 3″-0-desmethyl-H_2B_{1a} (IX) and 3″-0-desmethyl-H_2B_{1b} (*X*) as major metabolites. Minor metabolites from cattle and rat in vitro systems include monosaccharides of the major metabolites (24-OH-H_2B_{1a}-MS, VII; 24-OH-H_2B_{1b}-MS, VIII). These compounds are used as references to characterize *in vivo* metabolites from tissues.

[1] Nomenclatures 24-hydroxymethyl-H_2B_{1a} and 24-hydroxymethyl-H_2B_{1b} were used for metabolites V and VI in all previous publications and abbreviated as 24-OH-H_2B_{1a} and 24-OH-H_2B_{1b}, respectively. These abbreviated nomenclatures are also used in this review. The correct nomenclatures are either 24a-hydroxy-H_2B_{1a} and -H_2B_{1b}; or 24-desmethyl-24-hydroxymethyl-H_2B_{1a} and -H_2B_{1b}.

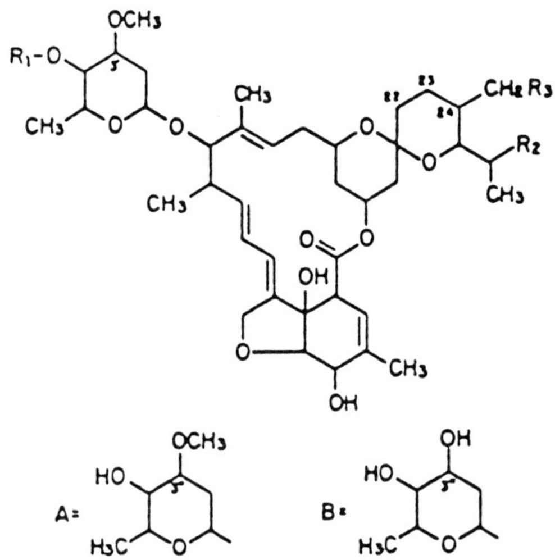

		R_1	R_2	R_3
I	H_2B_{1a}	A	CH_2CH_3	H
II	H_2B_{1b}	A	CH_3	H
III	H_2B_{1a}-Monosaccharide	H	CH_2CH_3	H
IV	H_2B_{1b}-Monosaccharide	H	CH_3	H
V	24-OH-H_2B_{1a}	A	CH_2CH_3	OH
VI	24-OH-H_2B_{1b}	A	CH_3	OH
VII	24-OH-H_2B_{1a}-Monosaccharide	H	CH_2CH_3	OH
VIII	24-OH-H_2B_{1b}-Monosaccharide	H	CH_3	OH
IX	3"-O-Desmethyl-H_2B_{1a}	B	CH_2CH_3	H
X	3"-O-Desmethyl-H_2B_{1b}	B	CH_3	H

FIGURE 8.2. Structures of ivermectin and derivatives.

V. *In Vivo* Liver Metabolism of Ivermectin

Despite the low concentration of ivermectin residues in tissues, they can be extracted by organic solvents nearly quantitatively, purified, and assayed chromatographically. Several methods have been reported for quantifying the parent drug at low levels in biological samples. These are analytical methods based on high-performance liquid chromatography either by direct UV detection (Pivnichny, Shim, and Zimmerman 1983) or by fluorescence detection of ivermectin derivatives (Tolan *et al.* 1980; Tway, Wood, and Downing 1981; Stong 1987). For assay of the radioactive parent compound in tissues, a microgram-scale reverse isotope dilution assay (RIDA) method is especially valuable (Chiu *et al.* 1985).

This method compares the specific activity of parent-drug residue in tissue before and after dilution of radioactivity with a known amount of unlabeled ivermectin during isolation. Thus, the assay provides an absolute amount of the parent drug in the tissue sample assayed, independent of losses during extraction and purification. Results of the analyses of unchanged parent drug in radioactive liver residue from cattle, sheep, swine, and rat are shown in Table 8.4 (Chiu *et al.* 1987). The unaltered drug (H_2B_{1a} and H_2B_{1b}) accounts for at least 50% of the total radioactive residue in tissues of cattle up to 14 days after dosing, in sheep 5 days after dosing, and in swine and rats, 7 and 3 days after dosing, respectively. The rest of the residue consisted of more polar metabolites.

The *in vivo* liver metabolism of ivermectin by cattle, sheep, swine, and rats correlates with that obtained by *in vitro* liver microsomes from the same species. Three polar metabolites—24-OH-H_2B_{1a}, 24-OH-H_2B_{1a}-MS, and 24-OH-H_2B_{1b}—account for 50%, 28%, and 39% of the total metabolites in liver tissue of cattle, rat, and sheep, respectively. The rest of the metabolites are complex mixtures of minor metabolites that are present in much lower concentrations. Similarly, 3″-0-desmethyl-H_2B_{1a} and -H_2B_{1b}, the major *in vitro* metabolites of swine liver microsomes,

TABLE 8.4. Total radioactive residue and unaltered 22,23-^{3}H-ivermectin in liver tissue of steers, sheep, swine, and rats.[a]

Species	Days	Total residue (ppb)	% of total residue	
			H_2B_{1a}	H_2B_{1b}
Steer	7	622 ± 223	56	7.7
	14	104 ± 43	49	3.4
	21	48 ± 17	36	3.9
	28	31 ± 18	37	2.5
Sheep	1	212 ± 69	54	21
	3	105 ± 44	51	27
	5	23 ± 9.9	56	12
	7	44 ± 31	ND	ND
Swine	1	194 ± 110	37	17
	7	110 ± 32	31	20
	14	22 ± 13	20	6.5
	28	2.7 ± 0.6	ND	ND
Rat	1	152	66	5.8
	3	47	56	9.0

[a] All animals except swine were dosed at 0.3 mg/kg body weight, subcutaneously (steer), intraruminally (sheep), or by gavage (rat). Swine were dosed subcutaneously at 0.4 mg/kg body weight. Three animals were dosed at each point and tissues collected separately for steer, sheep, and swine.Percentages of parent drug represent averages from RIDA of at least 2 animals at each point.Twenty-four rats were dosed and tissues composited for each time point. N.D., not determined.

account for 69% of total metabolites (or 45% of total residue) in composite liver-tissue samples from 7 and 14 days post dose animals. Confirmation of *in vivo* metabolite structures has been achieved by chromatographic comparison with *in vitro* metabolites either directly (in at least 2 modes of HPLC separation), or after chemical derivatization (such as acid hydrolysis or fluorescence derivatization) (Chiu *et al.* 1987). These rigorous comparative tests are carried out for the identification of all major metabolites and some of the minor metabolites from cattle, sheep, rat, and swine.

VI. *In Vivo* Fat Metabolism of Ivermectin

The radioactive residue levels of ivermectin in fat tissues are either higher than (rat, sheep, swine) or comparable to (cattle) those in the liver. Similar to what one obtains in liver tissue, the parent drug constitutes at least 50% of the total tissue residue during the early withdrawal periods, i.e., 14 days post dose in steers, 3 days post dose in sheep, 7 days post dose in swine, and 3 days post dose in rats. The percentage of parent drug, however, decreases rapidly at later time points (Table 8.5). With the

TABLE 8.5. Total radioactive residue and unaltered 22,23-^{3}H-ivermectin in fat tissue of steers, sheep, swine, and rats.[a]

			% of total residue	
Species	Days	Total residue (ppb)	H_2B_{1a}	H_2B_{1b}
Steer	7	220 ± 58	61	5.9
	14	88 ± 6	50	2.3
	21	45 ± 21	18	0.9
	28	33 ± 9	18	1.1
Sheep	1	245 ± 112	71	24
	3	153 ± 62	51	9.3
	5	63 ± 25	28	5.5
	7	73 ± 35	19	3
Swine	1	384 ± 234	43	16
	7	152 ± 43	50	13
	14	28 ± 15	25	10
	28	6.3 ± 3	ND	ND
Rat	1	232	50	13
	3	137	66	12

[a] All animals except swine were dosed at 0.3 mg/kg body weight, subcutaneously (steer), intraruminally (sheep), or by gavage (rat). Swine were dosed subcutaneously at 0.4 mg/kg body weight. Three animals were dosed at each point and tissues collected separately for steer, sheep, and swine. Percentages of parent drug represent averages from RIDA of at least 2 animals at each point. Twenty-four rats were dosed and tissues composited for each time point. ND, not determined.

exception of swine, a group of metabolites less polar than the parent drug is present in the fat tissue of these animals; they are particularly notable in tissues of sheep and cattle, accounting for 60% to 70% of total residue in the fat when these animals were withdrawn from dosing for a period of 5 or 28 days, respectively. Upon saponification or esterase treatment, these nonpolar metabolites regenerate polar products that resemble chromatographically the polar liver metabolites of ivermectin (e.g., 24-OH-H_2B_{1a}). Furthermore, the nonpolar metabolites give rise to products identical to monosaccharide and aglycone of 24-OH-H_2B_{1a} when subjected to p-toluenesulfonic acid–catalyzed methanolysis conditions (Figure 8.3). These results lead to the hypothesis that the polar ivermectin metabolites produced in the liver are esterified as fatty acid esters and stored in fat tissue as nonpolar entities. These nonpolar compounds can be converted back to the polar metabolites chemically or enzymatically, as shown in Figure 8.4 (Chiu *et al.*, 1988). Two approaches were taken to substantiate this hypothesis. First, the regeneration of polar metabolites from the nonpolar metabolites was studied with cholesterol esterase, and the structures of the hydrolysis products were confirmed as identical to known liver metabolites (24-OH-H_2B_{1a}, -H_2B_{1b}, -H_2B_{1a}-MS). Secondly, samples of fatty acid (oleic acid) esters of 24-OH-H_2B_{1a} and -H_2B_{1b} were synthesized and directly compared with the nonpolar metabolites isolated from a 2-kg fat sample from steers. These studies have established the general structural class of the ivermectin nonpolar metabolites as being the fatty acid conjugates of 24-hydroxymethyl derivatives of ivermectin.

The ivermectin metabolism pathway in fat tissue presents a rather uncommon, but not unique, phenomenon in xenobiotic metabolism. Although formation of less polar metabolites deviates from the most common metabolic pathway—in which more polar metabolites are formed for readiness of eliminations—several precedents have been reported in recent years (Caldwell and Marsh 1983). Formation of fatty acid esters of xenobiotics containing an alcoholic hydroxyl group, in particular, have been reported for tetrahydrocannabinol (Leighty, Fentiman, and Foltz 1976), pyridopyrimidine (Schmid *et al.* 1980), and etofenamate (Dell *et al.* 1982). The metabolic pathway of ivermectin is an interesting addition to these examples.

In contrast to cattle, sheep, and rat, swine do not follow the fat metabolism pattern observed in the other three species. The fat metabolite profile of swine resembles that of the liver tissue, i.e., 2 major metabolites slightly more polar than the parent drug are present. These are confirmed to be the 3″-0-desmethyl derivatives of H_2B_{1a} and H_2B_{1b} by chromatographic comparison with authentic samples generated by swine liver microsomes. The absence of ester conjugation of swine liver metabolites in fat tissue can probably be attributed to the fact that there is no primary hydroxyl functional group in these metabolite structures. As a result, these molecules are less favorable substrates for esterification compared to 24-hydroxymethyl- H_2B_{1a} and -H_2B_{1b} produced in the livers

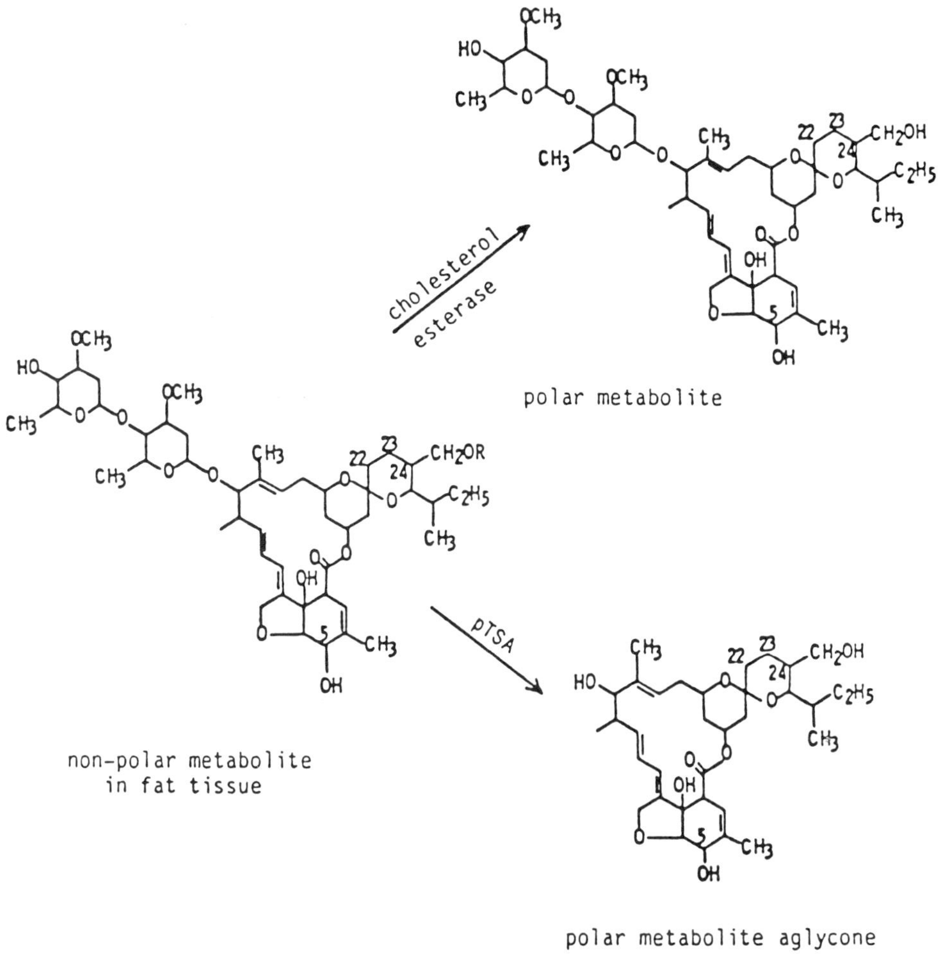

pTSA = p-toluenesulfonic acid
R = fatty acid acyl

FIGURE 8.3. Scheme of hydrolysis reactions of dihydroavermectin-B1a non-polar metabolites in fat tissue with p-toluenesulfonic acid (pTSA) or cholestrol esterase.

of the other 3 species. The similarity of liver and fat metabolite profiles in swine explains the close resemblance of the residue depletion half-lives in the two tissues of swine (Table 8.2).

VII. Conclusion

The absorption, excretion, distribution, and metabolism of tritium-labeled ivermectin have been studied in target food-producing species (cattle, sheep, swine) and a laboratory species (rat). The drug is absorbed rapidly via subcutaneous, intraruminal, or oral dosing routes. Fecal excretion is

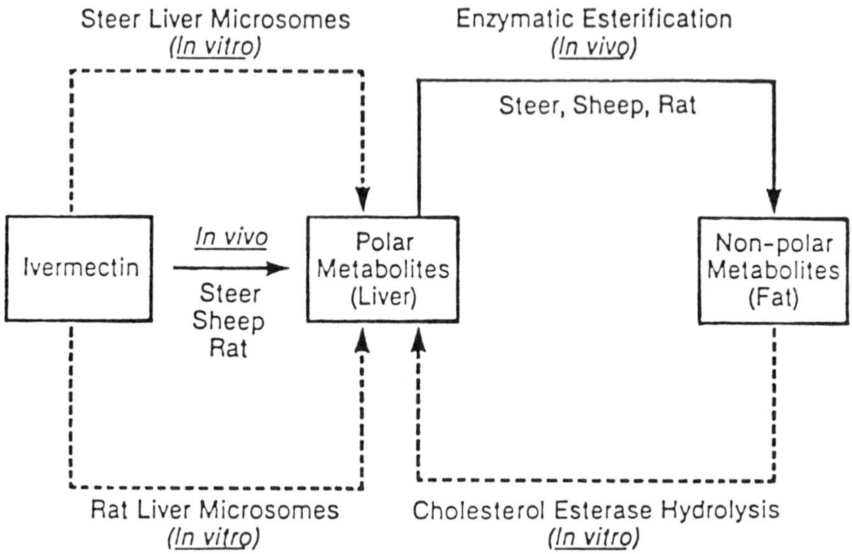

FIGURE 8.4. Relationship of ivermectin metabolites in the liver and fat tissues of sheep, rat, and steer with *in vitro* metabolites by steer and rat liver microsomes.

the major pathway of drug elimination in all species studied. Only about 2% of dose is excreted via urine. Highest residual tissue concentrations of radioactivity are present in the liver and fat tissues, while lowest levels are observed in the brain. Metabolism of radiolabeled ivermectin in liver and fat of cattle, sheep, and rat is similar. Some differences are noted in swine. The parent drug is the major liver residue in all four species in the early withdrawal time period. The major liver metabolite in cattle, sheep, and rat is 24-hydroxymethyl-H_2B_{1a}, which is further conjugated to fatty acids as esters and deposited in the fat tissue. The major liver metabolites in swine are 3″-0-desmethyl-H_2B_{1a} and 3″-0-desmethyl-H_2B_{1b}. These drug-like compounds are also present in fat tissue as major metabolites. *In vivo* metabolism of ivermectin has been found to correlate closely with that by *in vitro* liver microsomes of the same species.

REFERENCES

Caldwell J, Marsh MV (1983) Interrelationships between xenobiotic metabolism and lipid biosynthesis. *Biochem. Pharm.* 32:1667–1672

Campbell WC, Fisher MH, Stapley EO, Albers-Schonber G, Jacob TA (1983) Ivermectin: A potent new antiparasitic agent. Science 221:923–928

Chiu SHL, Buhs RP, Sestokas E, Taub R, Jacob TA (1985) Determination of ivermectin residue in animal tissues by high performance liquid chromatography-reverse isotope dilution assay. *J. Agric. Food Chem.* 33:99–102

Chiu SHL, Carlin JR, Taub R, Sestokas E, Zweig J, VandenHeuval WJA, Jacob

TA (1988) Comparative metabolic disposition of ivermectin in fat tissues of cattle, sheep, and rats. *Drug Metab. & Dispos.* 16:728–736

Chiu SHL, Sestokas E, Taub R, Buhs RP, Green M, Sestokas R, VandenHeuvel WJA, Arison BH, Jacob TA (1986) Metabolic disposition of ivermectin in tissues of steers, sheep, and rats. *Drug Metab. & Dispos.* 14:590–600

Chiu SHL, Sestokas E, Taub R, Smith JL, Arison B, Lu AYH (1984) The metabolism of avermectin-H_2B_{1a} and -H_2B_{1b} by pig liver microsomes. *Drug Metab. & Dispos.* 12:464–469

Chiu SHL, Taub R, Sestokas E, Lu AYH, Jacob TA (1987) Comparative in vivo and in vitro metabolism of ivermectin in steers, sheep, swine, and rat. *Drug Metab. Rev.* 18:289–302

Dell HD, Fiedler J, Kamp R, Gaug W, Kurz J, Weber B, Wuensche C (1982) Etofenamate fatty acid esters, an example of a new route of drug metabolism. *Drug Metab. & Dispos.* 10:55–60

Dorough HW (1980) Classification of radioactive pesticide residues in food-producing animals. *J. Environ. Path. Toxicol.* 3:11–19

Jacob TA, Buhs RP, Carlin JR, Chiu SHL, Miwa GT, Rosegay A (1983) The metabolism and tissue residue profiles of ivermectin. In *Proceedings of the MSD AGVET Symposium on Recent Developments in the Control of Animal Parasites,* XXII World Veterinary Congress, Perth, Australia

Leighty EG, Fentiman Jr AF, Foltz RL (1976) Long-chain metabolites of Δ^9- and Δ^8-tetrahydrocannabinols identified as novel fatty acid conjugates. *Res. Comm. Chem. Pathol. Pharm.* 14:13–28

Lu AYH, Wislocki PG, Chiu SHL, Miwa GT (1987) Tissue drug residues and their toxicological significance. *Drug Metab. Reviews* 18:363–378

Miwa GT, Walsh JS, VandenHeuvel WJA, Arison B, Sestokas E, Buhs R, Rosegay A, Avermitilis S, Lu AYH, Walsh MAR, Walker RW, Taub R, Jacob TA (1982) The metabolism of avermectins B_{1a}, H_2B_{1a} and H_2B_{1b} by liver microsomes. *Drug Metab. & Dispos.* 10:268–274

Pivnichny JV, Shim J-SK, Zimmerman LA (1983) Direct determination of avermectins in plasma at nanogram levels by high-performance liquid chromatography. *J. Pharm. Sci.* 72:1447–1450

Schmid J, Prox A, Baeur E, Koss FW (1980) Abstract No. 434, *7th European Workshop on Drug Metabolism,* Zurich

Stong JD (1987) Determination of ivermectin by fluorescence derivatization. *Anal. Chem.* 59:266–270

Tolan JW, Eskola P, Fink DW, Mrozik H, Zimmerman LA (1980) Determination of avermectin in plasma at nanogram levels using high-performance liquid chromatography with fluorescence detection. *J. Chromatogr.* 190:367–376

Tway PC, Wood Jr JS, Downing GV (1981) Determination of ivermectin in steers and sheep tissues using high-performance liquid chromatography with fluorescence detection. *J. Agric. Food Chem.* 29:1059–1063

Weber NE (1980) Persistent residues: Interface with regulatory decisions. *J. Environ. Path. Toxicol.* 3:35–43

CHAPTER 9

Chemical Assay for Ivermectin in Edible Tissues

George V. Downing

For any animal drug a chemical assay is needed to demonstrate the reduction of drug amounts in edible tissues to negligible levels at appropriate times after the administration of the drug. In the case of ivermectin this was a particular analytical challenge. Because ivermectin is very potent, it is dosed at quite low levels, typically 0.2 mg/kg: hence the residues, even immediately following dosing, are in the parts per billion (ppb) level. Further, the no-effect level (NOEL) of 0.2 mg/kg in animal safety studies results in negligible residues being defined as 10 to 20 ppb for many tissues. Since an acceptable analytical method must provide reliable data at the negligible residue level, the actual analytical method should have a limit of detection approximately tenfold lower than the negligible level.

To develop a method of adequate reliability and sensitivity, it was felt that only a chromatographic method would have the requisite specificity. Ultraviolet detectors available at that time, however, were not sensitive enough to detect the low levels of drug. Fortunately, Tolan and colleagues (1980) descovered an aromatization reaction that resulted in a fluorescent derivative with the desired sensitivity; estimated to be 0.2 ng/ml in plasma. The isolation of the drug from tissue and the subsequent formation of the fluorescent derivative by a modified procedure is the basis of the analytical method that has been successfully applied for determing residue levels in the edible tissues of many species (Tway, Wood, and Downing 1981). The sensitivity of the method is estimated to be about 1 ng/gm.

The fluorescent derivative has been used by other investigators to analyze ivermectin in plasma (Marriner, McKinnon, and Bogan 1987), including the use of the more recently available solid adsorbents to simplify the isolation (Kojima, Yamamoto, and Nakanishi 1987). A modification of the method utilizing solid adsorbents was also developed to determine invermectin levels in human milk as well as in plasma (Chiou, Stubbs, and Bayne 1987). The milk assay has a sensitivity of 0.05 ppb.

With the development of more sensitive ultraviolet detectors, methods for the determination of ivermectin in plasma have been reported using ultraviolet detection with a sensitivity of 2 ng/ml (Pivnichny, Shim, and Zimmerman 1983). A method utilizing normal-phase chromatography and ultraviolet detection with a sensitivity of 4 to 5 ng/ml (Schnitzerling and Nolan 1985) is unique in that the dihydro avermectin B_{1a} and dihydro avermectin B_{1b} components cochromatograph, as contrasted to the reverse-phase chromatographic methods, where the two components are separated. Recently, a method has been published (Alvinerie *et al.* 1987) for the determination in bovine milk using ultraviolet detection and a sensitivity of 2 ng/ml.

Radioactive studies have demonstrated that the parent drug is an adequate marker substance to monitor the depletion of residues in tissues (see Chapter 8.). Even though the drug is metabolized, the parent compound remains a major component of the total residue. In addition, the major component of ivermectin—namely the dihydro avermectin B_{1a} (H_2B_{1a})—is depleted at the same rate as or more slowly than the minor component, dihydro avermectin B_{1b}; since H_2B_{1a} is typically present at concentrations 10 to 20 times higher than H_2B_{1b}, it is used as the marker compound in the assay.

In the method described here (and in detail in Appendix I), the tissue is homogenized with acetone-water and the drug extracted into isooctane. (a modification of the extraction procedure has also been developed to measure levels in bovine milk, in which ammonium hydroxide and ethanol are added to the milk, which is then extracted with ethyl acetate/hexane.). The isooctane extract is evaporated and the residue taken up in methanol and chilled to precipitate fatty material (fat is treated somewhat differently). The extract is further purified by acetonitrile/hexane cleanup to remove hexane-soluble impurities; water is then added to move the drug into a fresh hexane phase. This hexane phase is evaporated and the purified extract taken up in methanol. An aliquot of the methanol is evaporated and the residue derivatized by heating with methyl imidazole/acetic anhydride/dimethyl formamide. The black reaction mixture is cleaned up by adding chloroform and passing the solution over a small silica gel column. The chloroform is evaporated and the sample taken up in methanol for injection onto the HPLC column. Detection is by fluorescence at an excitation wavelength of 364nm and emission at 418nm. Tables 9-1 and 9-2 summarize date for recovering ivermectin from tissues and plasma, using the HPLC/fluorescence determinative residue method.

Confirmation that an observed residue is indeed the drug is an important aspect of the chemical analysis of residues, both from an analytical and regulatory standpoint. Often this is done by a mass spectroscopic method, usually gas chromatography/mass spectroscopy. Ivermectin is particularly unsuited to this type of assay, however; not

TABLE 9.1. Summary of recoveries of ivermectin from tissues by the HPLC/fluorescence method.

Tissue	Added ng/gm	Percent Recovery
Injection Site	9.1	99, 88, 99
	14	93
	18	94, 94
	36	92
Fat	9.1	110, 77
	14	86
	18	83
	27	85
	45	91
Kidney	9.1	88, 88
	18	78
	27	89
Liver	9.1	99
	14	86, 86
	18	83
	27	85, 81
	45	87
	91	88
Muscle	9.1	99, 88
	18	100
	27	96

Range = 77%–110%
Average = 90%
Coefficient of Variation = ± 7%

TABLE 9.2. Summary of recoveries of ivermectin from plasma by the HPLC/fluorescence method.

Added (ng/ml)	Percent Recovery
0.91	110, 110, 110
1.82	110, 110, 110
2.73	73, 73
3.63	83, 83
4.54	88, 88
5.45	92, 73
7.27	96, 83, 83, 96
9.09	77, 88
14.54	83,89

Range = 73% 110%
Average = 91%
Coefficient of Variation = ± 13%

only is it nonvolatile but it is also extremely poorly ionized in the mass spectrometer. While heroic efforts using MS/MS (Tway *et al.* 1984) indicated that the technique had the potential for an identification/confirmation method, it did not seem to be a practical analytical approach. Instead, some unique chemical properties of ivermectin were used to form 2 different derivatives; along with the highly specific fluorescent detection, they serve to confirm the identity of the drug residue. When ivermectin is treated with 1% sulfuric acid in methanol, both of the sugar moieties are removed, resulting in the aglycone; treatment with 1% sulfuric acid in isopropanol, however, removes only one of the sugars, resulting in the formation of the monosaccharide. Both of these compounds form fluorescent derivatives which have retention times different from each other and from the parent drug. Thus, for confirmation the original reaction must result in a fluorescent peak with the proper retention time, and the subsequent acid-treatment products must produce 2 new peaks, each with the appropriate retention times; the original peak, of course, disappears because it is converted to the new product.

The method described in detail in Appendix I has proven to be both versatile and rugged; it has been applied to thousands of samples from many species over the years. In addition to monitoring edible tissues, it has been used to monitor plasma levels in rat, dog, mouse, and human in connection with various studies. It has also been used to determine levels in other tissues from other sources, including those from a snake that had been overdosed with a mouse which had been dosed with ivermectin. The depletion profiles that have been developed using data from this method show considerable variation between species, and between methods of administration. Some of these results are given in Table 9-3, where the time to peak and the half-life of depletion values are given for a number of studies. It should be noted that most injection routes show a prolonged release pattern as compared to oral dosing.

TABLE 9.3. Depletion profiles of ivermectin in various species.

Species	Route	Peak	Plasma t1/2	Liver t1/2
Cattle	SC	27 hrs	2.7 days	4.8
	Oral	24–48	2.6	3.4
Horse	IM	72	4.2, 7.1, 2.1	
	Oral	6	3.5	
Sheep	Oral	6	0.7, 2,5	1.5
Pig	SC	48	4.6	
Human	Oral	1–4	10–12 hrs	

Acknowledgments

The development and application of the ivermectin tissue assay represent the work of many people.

I would like to acknowledge the contributions of the following people: Dr. Patricia C. Tway, Mr. James S. Wood, Jr., Dr. Teresa A. Wehner, Ms. Krystyna T. Czeh, Ms. Eugenia H. Greff, Mr. William E. Tait, and Mr. Richard J. Varsolona.

References

Alvinerie M, Sutra JF, Galtier P, Toutain PL (1987) Determination of ivermectin in milk by high performance liquid chromatography. *Ann. Rech. Vet.* 18:269–274

Chiou R, Stubbs, RJ, Bayne WF (1987) The determination of ivermectin in human plasma and milk by HPLC with Fluorescence detection. *J. Chromatogr.* 416:196–199

Kojima K, Yamamoto K, Nakanishi Y (1987) Determination of 22, 23-dihydroavermectin B_{1a} in dog plasma using solid-phase extraction and high-performance liquid chromatography. *J. Chromatogr.* 413:326–331

Marriner SE, McKinnon I, Bogan JA (1987) The pharmokinetics of ivermectin after oral and subcutaneous administration to sheep and horses. *J. Vet. Pharm. Therap.* 10:175–179

Pivnichny JV, Shim JSK, Zimmerman LA (1983) Direct determination of avermectins in plasma at nanogram levels by high performance liquid chromatography. *J. Pharm. Sci.* 72:1447–1449

Schnitzerling HJ, Nolan J (1985) Normal phase liquid chromatographic determination of nanogram quantities of ivermectin in cattle blood or plasma. *J. Assoc. Office. Anal. Chem.* 68, (1):36–40

Tolan JW, Escola P, Fink DW, Mrozik H, Zimmerman LA (1980) Determination of avermectins in plasma at nanogram levels using high-performance liquid chromatography with fluorescence detection. *J. Chromatogr.* 190:367–376.

Tway PC, Downing GV, Slayback JRB, Rahn GS, Isensee RK (1984) Confirmatory assay for ivermectin in cattle tissue using chemical ionization mass spectrometry/mass spectrometry (MS/MS).*Biomed. Mass Spectrom.* 11,(4):172–176

Tway PC, Wood JS, Downing GV (1981) Determination of ivermectin in cattle and sheep tissues using high performance liquid chromatography with fluorescence detection. *J. Agric. Food Chem.* 29:1059–1063

CHAPTER 10

Safety of Ivermectin in Target Animals

J.D. Pulliam and J.M. Preston

I. Introduction

As part of the overall avermectin development program, target animal safety studies were conducted in many countries by Merck personnel and by independent investigators in universities and other research institutions. In many instances anticipated commercial formulations were studied, but during early development and when excessive dosing demanded, alternative or more concentrated formulations were used. The various test formulations were compared for safety by bridging studies involving assessment of tolerance and bioavailability. Control groups were given vehicle, saline, or left untreated; many studies included both treated and untreated controls.

II. Safety in Horses

Clinical signs of the acute toxic syndrome (toxicity) were first identified when horses were given ivermectin intramuscularly at 12.0 mg/kg (60 times use level). All 4 treated horses showed depression, ataxia, mydriasis, lower lip droop, and depressed respiratory rate, and 1 was euthanized after becoming recumbent. The other 3 recovered gradually over 2 weeks. Some horses in the same trial given 3.0 and 6.0 mg/kg also developed mydriasis (Washko, unpublished; Campbell and Benz 1984).

Biologically significant changes in hematologic or serum biochemical values, with the possible exception of serum iron, have not been observed in samples from ivermectin-treated horses. In the first of 2 experiments, Herd and Kociba (1985) observed small—although statistically significant—changes in 8 serum biochemical constituents, but changes in these same measures were not seen when they repeated the study. They concluded that these minor alterations were biologically insignificant and probably related to feeding, handling, and husbandry. Asquith and Kulwich (1981) also found no untoward hematologic or blood biochemical changes following ivermectin treatment.

Following oral administration of ivermectin paste at 2.0 mg/kg (10 times the use level) for 2 consecutive days, 5 of 11 horses exhibited transient impairment of vision, depression, and ataxia; 2 of the animals were dehydrated during 5 days after initial treatment (Swan, unpublished; Egerton, Seward, and Robin 1983).

Ivermectin oral liquid was given as 3 repeated treatments of 0.6 and 1.0 mg/kg at 2-week intervals to foals aged between 3 weeks and 3 months. After the third dose, 2 of 6 foals given 0.6 mg/kg had transient front limb lameness, which was considered unrelated to treatment, as no such lameness occurred after the first or second administration of 0.6 mg/kg, nor was lameness or any toxic signs seen when ivermectin oral liquid was given at 1.0 mg/kg (DiPietro *et al.* unpublished). Ivermectin in liquid at 0.6 mg/kg and in paste at 1.0 mg/kg was given orally as 3 repeated treatments at 2-week intervals to foals aged 29 to 59 days with no signs of toxicosis (Asquith, unpublished). Ivermectin in paste was also given 3 times at 2-week intervals at 0.6, 1.2, or 1.8 mg/kg to horses in another trial. The repeated doses of 3 or 6 times use level elicited no toxic signs, but 9 times the use level was associated with a slow pupillary light response and a decreased menace reflex after 2 of the 3 treatments (DiPietro, unpublished).

Prior to marketing, ivermectin was given by intramuscular injection at 200 or 300 μg/kg to 824 horses in 30 clinical field trials. Two horses had transient swellings in reaction to the death of *Onchocerca* sp. microfilariae in the skin, and 8 had injection site swellings that lasted less than 14 days and cleared without treatment. Similar field trials with 434 horses aged from 6 weeks to 25 years were conducted at ranches, farms, and stables to assess the field safety of the oral paste formulation. Except for 1 horse that had a transient allergic ventral subcutaneous edema, attributed to activity against *Onchocerca* sp. microfilariae, no adverse effects were seen.

Subcutaneous edema, particularly along the ventral midline, attributed to death of *Onchocerca cervicalis* microfilariae has also been reported by Herd and Donham (1983 a,b), but the swellings generally resolved within 3 to 4 days without additional therapy.

Ivermectin's effect on reproduction and breeding performance in mares and stallions was also investigated. Fifty-eight mares were given oral doses of 0.6 mg/kg during the first 2 weeks following breeding, and at

2-week intervals thereafter, for a total of 6 doses during the period of organogenesis (McKissick *et al.* 1987). Other groups of mares were treated 6 or 7 times with 0.6 mg ivermectin/kg at 2-month intervals beginning at about 90 days of pregnancy (Asquith *et al.* 1988; Godbee, unpublished; Egerton, Seward, and Robin 1983). No anatomical or functional teratogenic defects were discernible in the progeny of either treatment group. Ivermectin administered once at 0.6 mg/kg to 12 stallions had no deleterious effect on libido, seminal characteristics, spermatozoal morphology, testicular measurements or weights, concentrations of testosterone, or the capacity to produce spermatozoa (Squires, unpublished; Egerton, Seward, and Robin 1983).

Due to septic lesions at the injection site and clostridial myositis, which resulted in 2.4 injection site infections and 1.5 deaths reported per 100,000 horse doses sold, the parenteral formulation was withdrawn after 17 months in the U.S. market. The incidence of adverse reaction reports associated with the use of the oral paste formulation, as reported to the manufacturer and based on the sale of tens of millions of doses, has been 0.0003% for reported incidents and 0.0002% for deaths. None of these reported reactions has been confirmed to be caused by ivermectin paste.

III. Safety in Cattle

The acute toxicity of ivermectin given subcutaneously to cattle was investigated at doses of up to 8.0 mg/kg (Washko, unpublished; Leaning, Roncalli, and Brokken 1983). Calves given 8.0 mg/kg developed ataxia and became recumbent within 24 hours after dosing. They had general motor depression, increased respiratory rates, muscular fasiculations, mydriasis, and extensor rigidity of the limbs. One calf died 3 days after treatment, 2 were euthanized, and the fourth recovered. Changes in blood glucose, urea nitrogen, alkaline phosphatase, lactate dehydrogenase, sodium, potassium, hematocrit, and hemoglobin from hemoconcentration reflected the depressed physiologic state and lack of fluid intake in the moribund cattle. Decreased serum iron concentrations within 1 day of treatment were characteristic of the toxic syndrome, but levels returned to normal in 7 to 10 days. No specific gross or histologic changes were associated with ivermectin toxicosis.

Brem and Bulman (1986) examined the hematologic and biochemical values of cattle 1 and 7 days after each of 3 treatments at 200 μg/kg subcutaneously at 30-day intervals. Little or no effect was noted except for improvement of erythrocyte indices, which may have resulted from control of parasites.

Oral and subcutaneous formulations of ivermectin at concentrations equivalent to the marketed products, 4 mg/ml and 10 mg/ml, respectively, or equivalent volume of vehicle were given at 4.0 mg/kg (20 times use level). Affected cattle showed signs of central nervous system depression, including listlessness and ataxia, within the first day following administration; the condition progressed to recumbency and in some instances death. Control cattle given vehicle formulations, all of which included propylene glycol, exhibited similar signs. The contributory effect of the vehicle was further demonstrated by Brokken (unpublished) when he gave single doses as high as 6.0 mg/kg (30 times use level) in a more concentrated formulation (92 mg/ml) without ill effects (Leaning, Roncalli, and Brokken 1983).

Two trials using 208 Jersey and Friesian heifers were conducted to determine the effect of ivermectin at 400 μg/kg (twice use level) on the developing bovine embryo and fetus when administered on 3 occasions during organogenesis. Overall, treatments were administered at 12 time periods between 7 and 56 days after insemination. No effects on pregnancy were detected that could be attributed to ivermectin treatment, nor were any teratogenic effects observed in the calves that were subsequently delivered (Leaning, Roncalli, and Brokken 1983).

To demonstrate the safety of treating cows during the second and third trimesters of pregnancy, 21 cows were allocated to treatments by breed and on the basis of breeding dates. Ivermectin was given at 400 μg/kg (twice use level) monthly, starting as early as the 90th day of pregnancy, for a total of 6 administrations. No adverse effects were observed, and normal calves were born, which indicated that there is no drug-related risk in dosing pregnant cows (Leaning, Roncalli, and Brokken 1983).

A group of 10 bulls was evaluated for breeding performance, including semen quality, before and after treatment at 400 μg ivermectin/kg. Treatment had no deleterious effects on semen concentration, motility, volume, spermatozoal morphology, scrotal and testicular measurements, testicle weights and histomorphology, the capacity to produce spermatozoa, libido, or breeding performance (Galloway, unpublished; Leaning, Roncalli, and Brokken 1983).

Despite a distinct lack of problems during an extensive series of field studies, a low incidence of adverse reactions to death of *Hypoderma* spp. larvae following treatment with ivermectin was observed, primarily in France. Ivermectin is highly effective against *Hypoderma* spp. larvae; the death of migrating (first-instar) *H. bovis* after treatment may be followed by hemorrhage into the spinal canal, which can result in paresis. Cattle with first-instar *H. lineatum* in the esophageal tissues at the time of treatment may experience an eosinophilic, edematous esophagitis; but there have been only a few reports of this reaction. In France, most reactions were reported during an indemnification period. The label warning was revised, and few adverse reactions involving *Hypoderma* spp. have since been reported. Hundreds of millions of doses of the injectable cattle product have been sold as of this writing, with an overall incidence of 0.0001% reported adverse reactions. The other reported adverse reactions were incidental concurrent problems.

The tolerance of cattle to treatment at twice the recommended dose was investigated in 53 field trials comprising 2367 cattle. In the ivermectin- and vehicle-treated cattle, most of the problems related to transient injection site swelling. It was concluded that dosing cattle with ivermectin at twice use level did not result in an increased incidence of health problems compared with animals given vehicle only (Leaning, Roncalli, and Brokken 1983).

In Australia, an injectable formulation of avermectin B_1 (abamectin) is marketed for use in cattle. Although used widely as a pesticide, this is the only abamectin formulation developed for commercial use in animals thus far. Twenty-one trials were conducted with 477 treated and 444 control cattle to evaluate tolerance. Dose levels ranged from 300 μg/kg to 8.0 mg/kg. Safety was examined in 2 acute toxicity studies, 16 field trials at twice use level, 2 breeding cow studies, and in bulls. The acute toxicity trials demonstrated that early signs of toxicosis included depression and ataxia, and that the maximum dose tolerated was about 1.0 mg/kg. In 1 of the field trials, mild signs of toxicity were seen in young calves at 727 μg/kg. In toxicity trials at levels of 2.0 to 8.0 mg/kg or greater, the animals showed more severe signs of toxicity, including ataxia, which progressed to paresis, recumbency, decreased lip and tongue tone, drooling, mydriasis, coma, and death. Abamectin at 300 μg/kg had no effect in the reproduction safety studies in cows and bulls. Following reports of adverse reactions in calves aged 1 week to 3 to 4 months (sometimes associated with overdosing), the label was revised to warn against treating animals under 4 months of age. It has been speculated that this increased susceptibility may have been due to increased permeability of the blood-brain barrier to avermectins in young animals (Button *et al.* 1988). Also in Australia, idiosyncratic toxic reactions were reported in a herd of Murray Grey cattle, which were found to have higher levels of abamectin in the central nervous system than would normally be expected (Seaman *et al.* 1987).

IV. Safety in Sheep and Goats

The acute toxicity syndrome to ivermectin has not been clearly identified in sheep. Sheep given 8.0 mg/kg of ivermectin in propylene glycol were ataxic within 3 hours; they staggered, leaned against the sides of the pen, crossed their legs, were incoordinated, and fell. All were depressed, and 1 became recumbent with reflexes present but delayed. After 24 hours there was marked improvement with only mild incoordination and depression; by 3 days after dosing they appeared clinically normal. Two control sheep given an equivalent volume of propylene glycol vehicle, however, developed comparable signs, and 1 died. No biologically significant or characteristic changes were seen in a series of hematologic and biochemical assays before and after treatment. No gross or histologic changes were found upon necropsy at the termination of the trial (Washko, unpublished; Hotson 1983). Sheep given 4.0 mg/kg ivermectin in propylene glycol in this experiment (and in another in South Africa) also had depression and incoordination. Those in South Africa also had hemoglobinuria, as did the equivalent vehicle-treated controls (Schroder, unpublished; Hotson 1983). These reactions were attributed to the propylene glycol vehicle and are not considered to be a characteristic of ivermectin toxicity in sheep.

A micellar formulation was developed to reduce the incidence of coughing that occurred following drenching with the propylene glycol vehicle. Doses of ivermectin in this currently marketed formulation, up to and including 4.0 mg/kg when given by stomach tube, produced no adverse clinical reactions (Sutherland and Swan, unpublished; Hotson 1983).

A teratology study was conducted in New Zealand wherein 136 ewes were given ivermectin at 400 μg/kg, 138 were given vehicle, and 52 were untreated controls. Groups of ewes were treated twice with a 21-day interval, covering the period from Day 0 to 43 of pregnancy. Records were kept of returns to service, numbers of lambs born, and any incidence of abnormalities. All dead lambs were carefully examined, and a sample of apparently normal lambs was necropsied for thorough examination. No adverse effects resulted from the treatment of ewes in early pregnancy (Hotson 1983). Breeding animal safety was further established in an Australian study with 36 ewes given ivermectin at 400 μg/kg at 14-day intervals from approximately Day 51 of pregnancy until weaning of the lambs at 56 days of age. No adverse effects were seen (Hotson 1983). The injectable ivermectin formulation was given to ewes at 300 μg/kg on 3 occasions at 7-day intervals during the first 3 weeks of pregnancy and to other groups of pregnant ewes at 300 μg/kg during weeks 7, 8, 11, 12, 15, 19, and 20 of gestation. It was concluded that ivermectin administered subcutaneously during the period of organogenesis or the last 14 weeks of gestation had no adverse effect on the ewe or the fetus.

Ivermectin was administered orally 6 times at 400 μg/kg at 21-day intervals to 10 Merino rams. Ten other rams served as untreated controls. A total of 29 semen samples were collected over a 122-day period. Semen was evaluated for volume, density, color, motility, pH, percentage of live sperm, and sperm morphology. One testis was removed from each ram 9 days after the last treatment (Day 114) and histological examinations performed on testicular sections. No adverse effect on semen quality was observed. There were no histological differences between the testicular tissue of treated and control animals 9 days after the sixth treatment. It was concluded that repeated treatment with ivermectin at 400 μg/kg did not impair the reproduction potential of rams (Schröder *et al.* 1986). The injectable ivermectin formulation was also given to rams at 300 μg/kg twice at a 7-day interval. Beginning a week before the first treatment and at weekly intervals until Day 83, each ram was examined and weighed, and semen collected and testicular measurements taken. Semen assessment included evaluation of volume, appearance, wave motion, progressive motility, sperm concentration, percent dead, and cytological examination. The administration of ivermectin subcutaneously to rams at 300 μg/kg twice with a 7-day interval had no adverse effect on breeding performance (Harvey, unpublished).

Extensive field trials were conducted using both the propylene glycol and aqueous micellar formulations at 400 μg/kg (double use dose) in a number of countries, with sheep of different breeds and ages under various conditions of management, nutrition, and climate. More than 12,500 sheep were treated with ivermectin and, in many instances, concomitant treatments such as flukicides or vaccines were given. The only reaction was a low incidence of coughing immediately following dosing. Ivermectin was confirmed to be safe under a variety of conditions encountered in field use (Hotson 1983). In similar studies with the injectable formulation, the only observation was a low incidence of transient pain reaction at the time of injection. Following the sale of hundreds of millions of doses of the oral sheep product, the incidence of adverse reactions, as reported to the manufacturer, has been 0.00002%.

A syndrome of acute toxicity to ivermectin has not been clearly identified in goats, either. Goats injected intramuscularly with ivermectin at levels up to 2.0 mg/kg showed evidence of intense pain during and immediately following injection but no signs of systemic toxicity. It should be noted that this is not a recommended route of administration for ivermectin in any species. Subcutaneous treatment is recommended for cattle, sheep, and swine. Oral doses of 4.0 mg/kg were given to goats in 3 trials. In the first trial, the large volume (5.0 ml/kg—40 times use level) of micellar formulation was given by 30-ml plastic syringe into the goats' mouths, resulting in gagging and most probably aspiration of the formulation, since approximately half of both ivermectin- and vehicle-treated groups died of pneumonia. In 2 subsequent trials, when the formulation was given intraesophageally at 4.0 mg/kg (20 times use level), no signs of toxicity were seen. It was concluded that the effects seen in the first trial (4.0 mg/kg level) resulted from poor dosing technique, as both subsequent, carefully controlled studies found no effects at 4.0 mg/kg in goats. Njanja, Bell, and Wescott (1985) gave groups of goats 0.4, 0.8, and 1.6 mg/kg by subcutaneous injection without eliciting signs of toxicity other than pain reactions that lasted 1 to 2 minutes.

V. Safety in Swine

The signs of acute toxicity to ivermectin in swine were observed in a study where groups of swine were given 1, 10, 50, and 100 times the use level of 300 μg/kg. At 30.0 mg/kg, the pigs were lethargic and ataxic within 24 hours following treatment. Bilateral mydriasis, intermittent tremors, labored breathing, and recumbency occurred. Hematologic and biochemical changes reflected the depressed physiological condition of the animals, which were laterally recumbent and had decreased food and water intake. These effects were noted in values for alkaline phosphatase, cholesterol, triglycerides, glucose, phosphorus, potassium, creatinine, direct bilirubin, and blood urea nitrogen. A posttreatment leukocytosis and neutrophilia observed in some of the pigs given 30.0 mg ivermectin/kg may have been an inflammatory response to the necrosis of connective tissue, fat, and muscle observed at the injection sites following injection of the large-volume dose. Serum iron values were decreased 8 to 14 days following treatment; this transient response has also been associated with the acute toxic syndrome in horses and cattle. Other than the inflammatory reactions at multiple injection sites, no specific gross or histologic changes were attributable to ivermectin. Pigs treated with ivermectin at levels up to 15.0 mg/kg (50 times use level) did not exhibit signs of toxicity (Pulliam, unpublished; Campbell and Benz 1984).

A breeding-animal safety trial was conducted to determine the safety of ivermectin for the developing embryo and fetus during the initial 30 days of pregnancy when implantation and organogenesis occur. Forty-two Yorkshire-cross sows were divided into 6 replicates of 7 treatments. All sows in a replicate were individually mated to the same boar and randomly allocated to treatments. Ivermectin, or an equivalent volume of vehicle only, was administered by subcutaneous injection in the neck at a dose level of 600 μg/kg (twice use level) on 2 occasions (Days 1 and 18, 6 and 24, 12 and 30) during early pregnancy. An unmedicated control group was included in each replicate. The first day after mating that a sow refused to accept the boar was recorded as Day 1 of gestation. Pregnant sows were observed for return to estrus by exposing them daily to a boar for the first 45 days after mating. The sows were observed daily through gestation, farrowing, and weaning of the pigs at 4 weeks of age. All pigs that were dead at birth or that died prior to termination of the trial were necropsied. At least 25% of each sex within each litter were randomly selected for detailed anatomical dissection at about 35 days of age. The clinical and histopathologic data collected during the trial did not reveal significant differences ($p > 0.05$) among the litters from groups of sows treated with vehicle or with ivermectin at 600 μg/kg at various times during the initial 30 days of pregnancy. Nor was there a significant difference ($p > 0.05$) observed between the litters of unmedicated controls and those of the vehicle- and ivermectin-treated groups (Brokken *et al.* 1983).

To demonstrate the safety of treating pregnant sows during the latter two thirds of pregnancy, ivermectin was given at 600 μg/kg (twice use level) at 28-day intervals. In this study, 21 pregnant Yorkshire-cross sows were divided into 7 replicates of 3 sows each following individual hand mating to the same boar. Commencing around 45 days of gestation, each sow within a replicate received either no treatment, ivermectin, or an equivalent volume of vehicle at 28-day intervals, so that 3 treatments were given prior to farrowing. Pigs that were dead at birth and those that died prior to termination of the trial were necropsied. A statistical evaluation of the data did not detect significant differences ($p > 0.05$) between treatment groups with regard to sow weight gain or the weight and number of pigs farrowed. No correlation between the incidence of death or abnormalities of the pigs and the treatments was detected (Brokken *et al.* 1983).

The use of ivermectin in boars was studied in 10 Duroc-cross boars, 9 to 10 months old. During a 7- to 10-week acclimation period, the boars were trained to mount a dummy sow and ejaculate. On Day 0, ivermectin was given at 600 μg/kg, and a comparable volume of vehicle was given to the control boars. Semen was collected on Days -7, 0, 3, and 7 and then weekly until Day 63 following treatment. The semen was evaluated for volume, motility, progressive motility, abnormal sperm, sperm concentration, and pH. No differences were detected between the ivermectin-treated boars and the vehicle-treated controls that would indicate impairment of breeding soundness following dosing with ivermectin (Brokken *et al.* 1983).

Use trials with pigs of various breeds and age, including sows, gilts, barrows, boars, and piglets were conducted in the United States and Europe under field conditions. Ivermectin was given at 300 μg/kg in the U.S. trials and at 600 μg/kg in the European trials. The trials were run under various conditions of management and nutrition; in many instances, concomitant treatments were given. No adverse reactions that could be attributed to treatment were observed in any of the pigs during the observation period of about 2 weeks (Brokken *et al.* 1983). Incidental concurrent adverse reactions following the sale of tens of millions of doses of the swine product have been reported to the manufacturer at a rate of 0.00014%.

VI. Safety in Dogs

The acute toxic syndrome of ivermectin toxicosis in dogs was manifest as mydriasis, depression, tremors, ataxia, stupor, emesis, drooling, and coma, with an LD_{50} for Beagles of approximately 80.0 mg/kg (MacDonald, unpublished). The highest single oral dose without effect was 2.0 mg/kg; for continuous daily dosing for 14 weeks it was 0.5 mg/kg (Norbury, unpublished). Single oral doses of 2.5 mg/kg produced mydriasis. Increasing doses of 5.0 mg/kg elicited mydriasis and tremors, while severe signs—including ataxia—were seen at oral doses of 10.0 mg/kg. One of 4 dogs given 40.0 mg/kg and 2 of 4 dogs given 80.0 mg/kg died (MacDonald, unpublished).

In a 14-week study with daily oral dosing, dogs given 1.0 mg/kg or more developed mydriasis. At 2.0 mg/kg, 4 of 8 dogs additionally lost a small amount of weight and developed tremors, ataxia, anorexia, and dehydration. Euthanasia and necropsy of these 4 dogs revealed agonal gastrointestinal hemorrhage and/or congestion. No other treatment-related gross or histological changes were found (Norbury, unpublished). Subcutaneous injection of ivermectin at 4.7 mg/kg produced mydriasis and salivation, while depression, ataxia, and deaths occurred at 9.4 mg/kg (Seward, Brokken, and Plue 1986).

In assessing the physiologic effects of ivermectin, an intravenous dose of 0.5 mg/kg had no significant effect on blood pressure or heart rate of anesthetized dogs, nor did it modify blood pressure or heart rate responses to autonomic drugs in a standard assay. An intragastric dose of 0.5 mg ivermectin/kg did not affect evoked or basal gastric secretions in dogs with chronic gastric fistula (Clineschmidt, unpublished).

Safety in breeding bitches was evaluated in 2 studies. A dose of 0.5 mg/kg was administered to 14 pregnant bitches on Days 5, 15, 25, and 35 of gestation and to 15 pregnant bitches on Days 10, 20, 30, and 40 of gestation. No teratogenic effects were observed in 48-day fetuses from these bitches treated repeatedly with ivermectin during the first 40 days of gestation. Ivermectin also had no effect on the reproductive status of the pregnant bitches, as measured by the number of implants, resorptions, and live and dead fetuses per pregnant female (Robertson, unpublished).

In the second study, bitches were given repeated oral doses of ivermectin at 600 μg/kg at least twice at monthly intervals before breeding, and then on Days 10, 25, and 45 of gestation, and again monthly after whelping. No adverse effect on reproduction was observed in treated dogs as compared to the controls (Gilman, unpublished).

The effect of ivermectin on spermatogenesis, fertility, and the reproductive performance of 12 Beagle studs was evaluated. Ivermectin was administered orally at 0.6 mg/kg at monthly intervals for 8 months while controls were given water. Semen was collected every 3 days from 28 days before treatment until 83 days after (38 collections/dog). All studs were then bred to 2 nontreated bitches each; litter size, birth weight, and pup abnormalities and mortalities were evaluated. After all pups were whelped, each stud was euthanized and necropsied, and the testes and epididymides were examined microscopically. No adverse effect on reproduction was observed in treated dogs as compared to the controls (Daurio *et al.* 1987).

Following extra-label use of ivermectin products formulated and marketed for horses (EQVALAN®), and for sheep, cattle, and swine (IVOMEC®), it appeared that, within the Collie breed, some dogs were unusually sensitive to the toxic effects of ivermectin (Campbell, Blair, and Seward, 1983; Seward, Blair, Plue, and Brokken, 1983). In a controlled study, 8 Collies affected with Collie eye anomaly (CEA) and 8 Collies clinically free of CEA were studied to determine whether ivermectin was more toxic to members of the Collie breed and if CEA was related. Groups were given 50, 200, or 600 μg ivermectin/kg orally. One dog given 200 μg/kg and 1 given 600 μg/kg developed severe signs of toxicity including ataxia, depression, tremors, recumbency, and mydriasis: 1 died and 1 was euthanized. Two other dogs in these groups had mild transitory signs. Ivermectin tissue assays showed high concentrations of ivermectin in the central nervous system of the 2 Collies that died. Collie eye anomaly was not related to the response to ivermectin (Pulliam, Seward, and Henry 1985). The range of Collie sensitivity to ivermectin was further studied by Paul *et al.* (1987), who found that Collies are sensitive to doses from 100 to 2500 μg/kg, and that the length of time between dosing and onset of clinical signs may indicate the eventual severity of toxicosis and serve as an important prognosticator for the clinician. Physostigmine, 1 mg b.i.d., was found to have limited benefit in treating these dogs, and then only in the more severely depressed and/or comatose stages of ivermectin toxicity. Its use as the sole therapeutic agent or complete antidote for ivermectin toxicosis was not recommended (Tranquilli *et al.* 1987).

The unapproved (extra-label or off-label) use of products designed for large animals continues to result in iatrogenic toxic deaths in dogs (Seward, Brokken, and Plue 1986). Many of these reactions appear to be due to the accidental or erroneous administration of excessive amounts of ivermectin (Preston 1983).

The only currently available formulation for the dog is a tablet to be administered monthly at a dose rate of 6 μg/kg for the prevention of canine heartworm disease. This represents a wide margin of safety, not only in normal dogs—where a single dose of 2.0 mg/kg and daily oral dosing of 0.5 mg/kg for 14 weeks had no effect—but also in ivermectin-sensitive Collies, which tolerate doses of 50 μg/kg without effect (Pulliam, Seward, and Henry 1985; Paul *et al.* 1987).

In dogs with circulating microfilariae, vomiting, excess salivation, blood in feces, soft stool/diarrhea, and depression have been observed after ivermectin treatment (Schlotthauer *et al.* 1986). Although the shocklike reaction in dogs infected with *Dirofilaria immitis* that develops after administration of diethylcarbamazine did not occur following ivermectin treatment (Boreham and Atwell 1983), reactions following ivermectin treatment of microfilaremic dogs may occur, and deaths have been seen (Jackson, Seymour, and Beckett 1986).

The incidence of incidental concurrent adverse reactions, as reported to the manufacturer and based on the sale of tens of millions of doses of ivermectin tablets for use in dogs, is 0.001%. None of these reported reactions has been confirmed to be caused by ivermectin.

References

Asquith RL, Kivipelto J, Harvey JW, Bauer JE (1988) Comparative effects and safety of ivermectin in pregnant mares. *J. Equ. Vet. Sci.* 8:32–35

Asquith RL, Kulwich R (1981) Safety and therapeutic activity of ivermectin as an equine anthelmintic. *J. Equ. Vet. Sci.* 1:18–20

Boreham PFL, Atwell RB (1983) Absence of shock-like reactions to ivermectin in dogs infected with *Dirofilaria immitis*. *J. Helminthol.* 57:279–281

Brem JJ, Bulman GM (1986) An assay of biochemical parameters in cattle medicated at therapeutic level with ivermectin. *Vet. Argent.* 3:365–373

Brokken ES, Barth D, Foster AG, Pulliam JD, Wallace DH (1983) Ivermectin: a new broad-spectrum antiparasitic agent for swine. In *Proceedings of the MSD AGVET Symposium on Recent Developments in the Control of Animal Parasites,* XXII World Veterinary Congress, Perth, Australia, pp 239–258

Button C, Barton R, Honey P, Rickford P (1988) Avermectin toxicity in calves and an evaluation of picrotoxin as an antidote. *Austral. Vet. J.* 65:157–158

Campbell WC, Benz GW (1984) Ivermectin: a review of efficacy and safety. *J. Vet. Pharm. & Ther.* 7:1–16

Campbell WC, Blair LS, Seward RL (1983) Ivermectin vs. heartworm: the present status. Proc. 1983 Heartworm Symp., Orlando, Fla., pp 146–149

Daurio CP, Gilman MR, Pulliam JD, Seward RL (1987) Reproductive evaluation of male Beagles and the safety of ivermectin. *Am. J. Vet. Res.* 48:1755–1760

Egerton JR, Seward RL, Robin B (1983) Ivermectin as an antiparasitic agent for horses. In *Proceedings of the MSD AGVET Symposium on Recent Developments in the Control of Animal Parasites,* XXII World Veterinary Congress, Perth, Australia, pp 49–55

Herd RP, Donham JC (1983a) Efficacy of ivermectin against *Onchocerca cervicalis* microfilarial dermatitis in horses. *Am. J. Vet. Res.* 44:1102–1105

Herd RP, Donham JC (1983b) Control of equine cutaneous nematodiasis by ivermectin. In *Proceedings of the MSD AGVET Symposium on Recent Developments in the Control of Animal Parasites,* XXII World Veterinary Congress, Perth, Australia, pp 286–295

Herd RP, Kociba GJ (1985) Effect of ivermectin on equine blood constituents. *Equ. Vet. J.* 17:142–144

Hotson IK (1983) The development of ivermectin as an antiparasitic agent in sheep. In *Proceedings of the MSD AGVET Symposium on Recent Developments in the Control of Animal Parasites,* XXII World Veterinary Congress, Perth, Australia, pp 42–48

Jackson RF, Seymour WG, Beckett RS (1986) Lower dose of ivermectin as a microfilaricide, 0.05 mg/kg. In Proc. 1986 Heartworm Symp., New Orleans, pp 15–18

Leaning WHD, Roncalli RA, Brokken ES (1983) The efficacy and safety evaluation of ivermectin: A new injectable antiparasitic agent for cattle. In *Proceedings of the MSD AGVET Symposium on Recent Developments in the Control of Animal Parasites,* XXII World Veterinary Congress, Perth, Australia, pp 25–41

McKissick GE, Sutherland IH, Foix J, Olson G (1987) The safety of ivermectin administered orally to pregnant mares. *Equ. Vet. Res.* 7:357–367

Njanja JC, Bell JF, Wescott RB (1985) Apparent lack of toxicity in adult East African goats on parenterally administered ivermectin. *Bull. Anim. Health Prod. Afr.* 33:123–127

Paul AJ, Tranquilli WJ, Seward RL, Todd KS, DiPietro JA (1987) Clinical observations in Collies given ivermectin orally *Am. J. Vet. Res.* 48:684–685

Preston JM (1983) Adverse reactions to unapproved applications (Letters to the Editor) *Vet. Rec.* 112:286

Pulliam JD, Seward RL, Henry RT (1985) Investigating ivermectin toxicity in Collies. *Vet. Med.* 80:33–40

Schlotthauer JC, Stromberg BE, Paul AJ, Todd KS, McCall JW, Dzimianski MT, Blagburn BL, Hendrix CM (1986) Safety and acceptability of ivermectin in dogs with naturally acquired patent infections of *Dirofilaria immitis*. Proc. 1986 Heartworm Symp., New Orleans, pp 29–32

Schröder J, Swan GE, Barrick RA, Pulliam JD (1986) Effect of ivermectin on the reproductive potential of breeding rams. *J. So. Afr. Vet. Assoc.* 57:211–213

Seaman JT, Eagleson JS, Carrigan MJ, Webb RF (1987) Avermectin B_1 toxicity in a herd of Murray Grey cattle. *Austral. Vet. J.* 64:284–285

Seward RL, Blair LS, Plue RE, Brokken ES (1983) The efficacy and safety of ivermectin in dogs. In *Proceedings of the MSD AGVET Symposium on Recent Developments in the Control of Animal Parasites,* XXII World Veterinary Congress, Perth, Australia, pp 259–266

Seward RL, Brokken ES, Plue RE (1986) Ivermectin vs heartworms—A status update. Proc. 1986 Heartworm Symp., New Orleans, pp 1–8

Tranquilli WJ, Paul AJ, Seward RL, Todd Jr. KS, DiPietro JA (1987) Response to physostigmine administration in Collie dogs exhibiting ivermectin toxicosis. *J. Pharm. & Ther.* 10:96–100

CHAPTER 11

Environmental Aspects of Ivermectin Usage in Livestock: General Considerations

B.A. Halley, R.J. Nessel, and A.Y.H. Lu

I. Introduction

A detailed analysis of ivermectin's effect on the environment was an integral component of the overall program to develop ivermectin as an antiparasitic drug for food-producing animals. The analytical studies were designed to determine whether using ivermectin in animals would result in any harmful or undesirable effects on the environment. These studies measured ivermectin's physical properties and its mobility, distribution, and stability in soil and water. Additional studies investigated the drug's effect on a variety of environmentally important organisms. These studies, combined with the clinical use pattern of ivermectin in cattle, sheep, and swine, provided the means to assess ivermectin's environmental impact.

II. Excretion of Ivermectin

When ivermectin is used in food-producing animals, the drug enters the environment as a result of excretion. Radiolabeled drug was used to determine the routes of excretion; the data in Table 11.1 show that most of the radioactivity was excreted in the feces, regardless of animal species or the route of administration (Chiu *et al.*, in preparation). Less than 2% of the radioactivity was found in the urine. (The rat data are included in Table 11.1 for comparison.) Analysis by high-performance liquid chromatography (HPLC) of acetone extracts of feces showed that the major component in feces was the parent drug, and that the remainder of the radioactivity consisted of various ivermectin metabolites (Halley *et al.*, 1989a). Based on both *in vivo* and *in vitro* metabolism studies (Chiu *et al.* 1985; Chiu *et al.* 1986; Miwa *et al.* 1982); and a comparison of retention times on HPLC, the polar metabolites are believed to include the monosaccharides and aglycones of ivermectin, as well as ivermectin's 24-hydroxymethyl derivatives and the corresponding monosaccharides and aglycones. The druglike metabolites would most likely be the 3″-O-desmethyl derivatives (Chiu *et al.* 1984; Chiu *et al.* 1987).

III. Environmental Burden

The amount of ivermectin entering the environment can be predicted from the use pattern of this product in food-producing animals. Accordingly, the environmental burden is determined by the dose, use frequency, excretion pattern, and disposal of the excreted wastes. The approved use level of ivermectin is 0.2 mg/kg body weight for cattle and sheep, and 0.3 mg/kg body weight for swine. The animals may be kept on a pasture, in a small independent feedlot, or in a large commercial feedlot. In general, the animals receive only 1 drug treatment, but up to 3 or 4 treatments per year may be used in year-round parasite-control programs (Halley *et al.*, 1989b).

Manure generated in the feedlot is spread and plowed into the field as fertilizer. Since commercial feedlots produce the largest amounts of manure for farm use, an assessment of this particular use pattern should represent the uppermost environmental burden associated with the use of ivermectin in farm animals. Table 11.2 shows that the calculated amount of ivermectin in soil, based on a U.S. Environmental Protection Agency Publication (U.S. EPA 1974), is in the parts-per-trillion to parts-per-billion range (Halley *et al.*, 1989b). These calculated levels do not take into account the degradation of ivermectin during the period that the animals are kept in the feedlot. The degradation half-life of ivermectin, in

TABLE 11.1. Excretion patterns and composition of radioactive residues in the feces of animals treated with ^{3}H-labeled ivermectin.

Animal species	Dose route in study	Dosage given in study (mg/kg)	Recommended use level (mg/kg)	% of dose excreted[a] in		% of radioactivity excreted in the feces[b] as		
				urine	feces	ivermectin	polars	druglike
Steer	subcutaneous	0.3	0.2	1.5	62	39–45	54	5
Steer	intraruminal	0.3	0.2	0.5	80	[c]	[c]	[c]
Sheep	intraruminal	0.3	0.2	0.5	69	61–69	25	4
Swine	subcutaneous	0.4	0.3	0.4	36	23–43	43	14–34
Rat	oral	0.1	[c]	0.9	83	78	15	6

[a] Excreta were collected 3 days post dose from rats, 7 days post dose from steers, sheep, and swine.
[b] The composition of radioactive residues excreted in the feces was determined by HPLC profiles and reverse isotope dilution assay. Ranges represent values from several determinations. Druglike component refers to the radioactive material eluted from the reverse-phase-HPLC slightly ahead of ivermectin (i.e., slightly more polar).
[c] Not determined.

soil or feces-soil mixtures, has been shown to be in the range of 91 to 217 days in the winter and 7 to 14 days in the summer (Halley *et al.*, 1989a). Furthermore, the calculation assumes that all the drug-related material found in the feces is the parent compound, although Table 11.1 clearly shows that only about half the residue in feces is ivermectin. Other studies have established that metabolites or degradation products are less toxic than ivermectin (Halley *et al.*, 1989a). Thus, in the environment, the ivermectin level present in the soil following the spreading and plowing of manure should be considerably less than the concentrations shown in Table 11.2.

TABLE 11.2. Environmental burden associated with the use of ivermectin in various animal species.

Animal species	Assumptions	Ivermectin in feces[a] (ppb)	Ivermectin in soil[a]
Feedlot cattle	animal weight: 270 kg dose: 54 mg feedlot period: 130 d total waste: 2860 kg manure application: 27 metric tons/ha plowing depth: 15 cm	19	0.2 ppb
Pastured cattle	animal weight: 270 kg dose: 54 mg pasture period: 130 d total waste: 2860 kg animals/ha: 3	19	0.016 mg/m^2
Pastured sheep	animal weight: 36 kg dose: 7.2 mg feedlot period: 120 d total waste: 396 kg animals/ha: 18	18	0.013 mg/m^2
Feedlot swine	animal weight: 25 kg feeder; 150 kg breeder dose: 7.5 mg; 45 mg feedlot period: 168 d total waste: 588 kg; 1949 kg manure application: 27 metric tons/ha plowing depth: 15 cm	18	0.2 ppb
Water-washed swine waste	animal weight: 25 kg feeder; 150 kg breeder dose: 7.5 mg; 45 mg feedlot period: 168 d total waste: 588 kg; 1949 kg spreading rate: 36,600 liter/ha plowing depth: 15 cm	18	0.04 ppb

[a] Ivermectin concentrations expressed as total drug-equivalent without degradation during the feedlot or pasture periods.

IV. Soil Binding and Translocation

The distribution and movement of a chemical in the environment depends on the compound's physical and chemical properties. Table 11.3 shows that ivermectin is rather insoluble in water and has a high octanol-water partition coefficient. These combined properties would indicate that ivermectin should have a high affinity for soil organic matter and a limited movement in the environmental compartments. Soil-binding studies with ^{3}H-labeled ivermectin confirm that it is tightly bound to soils, as evidenced by the high partition coefficient (K_D = 227 to 333) and high organic-carbon binding constant (K_{oc} = 12,600 to 15,700) (Halley *et al.*, 1989a).

A soil column leaching experiment was conducted to study the translocation of ivermectin, its metabolites, and degradation products in soil. In this experiment, steer feces containing radiolabeled ivermectin and metabolites were mixed with four types of soil; each mixture was applied to the top of a 30-cm soil column. Water was allowed to percolate through the soil columns for 7 weeks, and the leachates were collected. The amount of radioactivity recovered in the column leachates was 27% for silt loam, 48% for clay loam, 10% for loam, and 43% for pasture sandy loam (Halley *et al.*, 1989a). HPLC analysis of the leachates showed no detectable levels of ivermectin. At least half of the radioactivity remained in the top 5 cm of the column for each soil type. Thus, only the metabolites or degradants percolated through the columns, whereas ivermectin remained tightly bound to the soils. These studies indicate that ivermectin is rather immobile in soil and will not readily translocate into ground water.

TABLE 11.3. Environmental fate of ivermectin.

Parameter	Experimental data	Possible consequences
Water solubility	very insoluble—5 ppm in saturated solution	rather immobile in the environment
Octanol/water partition coefficient	1651	strong affinity to lipid, soil and organic matter
Vapor pressure[a]	less than 1.5×10^{-9} mm Hg	virtually nonvolatile
UV absorption	maxima at 237, 245, and 253 nm	subject to photodegradation
Soil binding	partition coefficient, K_D = 227–333; organic carbon-binding constant, K_{oc} = 12,600–15,700	very tight soil binding; run-off in surface water and leaching into ground water should be minimal

[a] Vapor pressure of avermectin, which differs from ivermectin only by having a double bond at C-22 and C-23.

V. Stability in Soil and Photodegradation

Strong soil binding and lack of mobility could result in the accumulation of ivermectin in soil. To determine the potential for accumulation, the stability of ivermectin was studied under a variety of experimental conditions. Table 11.4 shows that the degradation half-life of ivermectin varies greatly, depending on the environmental conditions (Halley *et al.*, 1989a). In the laboratory, or outdoors during the winter months, ivermectin in feces/soil mixtures degraded slowly, with half-lives ranging from 90 to 240 days. In contrast, ivermectin degraded very rapidly in the summer, with half-lives of 7 to 14 days. Furthermore, the compound is rapidly decomposed by sunlight: its half-life is only 3 hours when exposed to sunlight as a thin, dry film on glass (Figure 11.1). These results indicate that ivermectin will not accumulate in soil when administered to livestock in the recommended manner.

VI. Toxicity to Soil Microorganisms

The toxicity of ivermectin to soil microbes was determined by studying its effects on soil respiration and nitrification. Feces from treated steers were added to pasture and forest soil so that the mixture contained 30 ppb of ivermectin and metabolites. This concentration is about 150-fold higher than the field concentration shown in Table 11.2. Even at this exaggerated level, ivermectin and its metabolites had no effect on soil respiration (as measured by cumulative CO_2 levels) and soil nitrification (as measured by the rates of conversion of ammonium ion to nitrite and nitrate). Soils containing feces from control or treated steers gave virtually identical results (Halley *et al.*, 1989a). In other studies, ivermectin had no antifungal or antibacterial effects at concentrations as high as 2000 ppm (see Chapter 2).

TABLE 11.4. Degradation half-lives of ivermectin under various experimental conditions.

Condition	$t_{1/2}$
Laboratory, dark, room temperature, in soil/feces mixtures	93–240 days
Outdoors, winter, in soil or in soil/feces mixtures	91–217 days
Outdoors, summer, in soil or in soil/feces mixtures	7–14 days
Outdoors, thin, dry film on glass, sunlight	3 hours

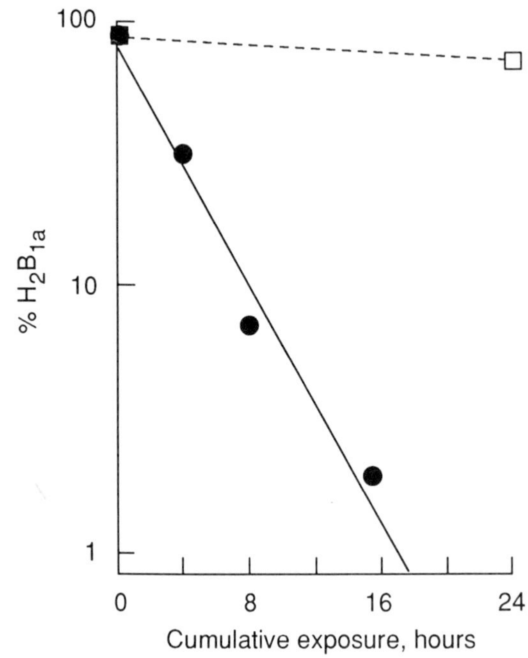

FIGURE 11.1. Photodegradation of H_2B_{1a}. The half-life of tritium-labeled H_2B_{1a}, exposed to sunlight (●) as a thin, dry film on glass in July in Rahway, New Jersey, was about 3 hours. Foil-covered sample (□) was subjected to the same conditions.

VII. Toxicity to Earthworms

Ivermectin's toxicity to the earthworm, *Eisenia foetida,* was studied under controlled laboratory conditions. The compound was added to soil at concentrations of 12 to 200 ppm. Following 28 days of continuous exposure, the LC_{50} was extrapolated to be 315 ppm (Halley *et al.,* 1989a). The no-effect level was 12 ppm.

VIII. Acute Toxicity to Freshwater Organisms

Chlorella pyrenoidosa, a freshwater, unicellular, nonmotile chlorophyte, was used to determine the toxicity of ivermectin toward algae. When *C. pyrenoidosa* was exposed to ivermectin at concentrations of 1 to 10 ppm for 14 days, no effects on overall cell growth, mean specific growth rate, or lag period were observed (Halley *et al.,* 1989a). The only observable effect was on the maximum standing crops (cells/ml). Thus, at these relatively high concentrations, ivermectin had only a moderate effect on the growth characteristics of this alga.

Freshwater organisms such as the water flea *Daphnia magna*, rainbow trout *Salmo gairdneri*, and bluegill sunfish *Lepomis macrochirus* are highly sensitive to ivermectin (Halley *et al.*, 1989a). Table 11.5 shows that the LC_{50} value of ivermectin was approximately 0.025 ppb for *D. magna*, 3.0 ppb for rainbow trout, and 4.8 ppb for bluegill sunfish. Removal of the oleandrose groups of ivermectin to form the monosaccharides and aglycones reduced the compounds' toxicities to Daphnia. Leachates—containing more polar products but no ivermectin—collected from either soil columns or feces/soil columns were much less toxic to Daphnia.

Due to its tight soil binding, the small amount of ivermectin soluble in water should be easily immobilized by suspended soil particles. Table 11.6 clearly shows that the binding of ivermectin to soil reduces the mortality of the daphnids by as much as several orders of magnitude. Thus, the toxicity of ivermectin to freshwater organisms in their natural environment will be greatly reduced because of tight soil binding and rapid photodegradation.

IX. Environmental Safety Assessment

The major route of introducing ivermectin into the soil is via the use of feces from food-producing animals as fertilizer. The ivermectin levels in soils listed in Table 11.2 are therefore valuable in assessing environmental

TABLE 11.5. Toxicity of ivermectin and metabolites to aquatic organisms.

Test species	Length of test (hrs)	Test compound	LC_{50}[a] (ppb)	Approximate nontoxic level (ppb)
Water flea *Daphnia magna*	48	ivermectin	0.025	0.01
		H_2B_{1a} monosaccharide	0.4	0.1
		H_2B_{1a} aglycone	>17[b]	>9
		soil column leachates	[c]	0.48; 3.2
		feces leachates	~6.5	[c]
Rainbow trout *Salmo gairdneri*	96	ivermectin	3.0	0.9
Bluegill sunfish *Lepomis macrochirus*	96	ivermectin	4.8[d]	[e]

[a] Concentration lethal to 50% of exposed population.
[b] LC_{50} could not be accurately determined since the highest concentration of the aglycone used was 17 ppb.
[c] The concentration of ivermectin, its metabolites, and degradation products in the soil column or feces leachates limited the toxicity testing at only 1 or 2 concentrations. Not enough data could be collected to accurately calculate the LC_{50} values or the nontoxic levels.
[d] Extrapolated value.
[e] Not determined. Toxicity observed at all concentrations in definitive test.

TABLE 11.6. Effect of soil on *Daphnia magna* toxicity.[a]

Condition	% DMSO used[b]	No effect level (ppt)	Concentration causing 50% death (ppt)
Ivermectin	0.5	10	15–30
Ivermectin plus			
New Jersey garden soil			
Expt. 1	0.5	>10	100
Expt. 2	0.1	>100	1000
Ivermectin plus			
Iowa clay loam	0.1	>1000	[c]

[a] Dilute solutions of ivermectin were mixed with soil, 2.5 g per 100 ml of solution, and stirred for 1 hour. The soil suspensions were centrifuged and the mortality of daphnids was determined following 48 hours of exposure.

[b] Original trials contained a final concentration of 0.5% DMSO (vehicle). This was reduced to 0.1% in later trials.

[c] Because of the wide range of ivermectin concentrations needed in experiments involving soil, not enough data points were available to calculate the concentration causing 50% death.

safety. These levels are calculated from the ivermectin use pattern and the rate of manure application. Based on the negligible effect at 30 ppb on respiration and nitrification, and the no-effect level of 12 ppm on earthworms, ivermectin would not adversely affect soil microbes and other organisms. Phytotoxicity is also not expected, due to ivermectin's lack of toxicity to freshwater algae over the concentration range of 1 to 10 ppm. Nor has phytotoxicity been observed with abamectin, the related compound now being developed as a pesticide.

Aquatic organisms, such as water fleas and fish, are highly sensitive to ivermectin toxicity. However, due to its low water solubility, high octanol-water partition coefficient, and tight soil binding, ivermectin will be immobile in soil and will not translocate or leach into ground water. Based on the soil-binding data and the Freundlich equation, Halley and colleagues (1989b) have calculated that the ivermectin concentration in runoff and ground water should be below the no-effect level of 0.01 ppb observed for *D. magna* (Table 11.5). Thus, in the environment, the concentration of ivermectin in water should be sufficiently low to cause no adverse effects on freshwater organisms. Other studies have shown that ivermectin (or abamectin) does not appear to be very toxic to birds (Kelso 1984), chickens (Mousa *et al.* 1986; Zeman 1987), ducks (see Chapter 13), and mammals (Nessel, Jacob, and Robertson 1983). The effect of ivermectin on manure-dwelling or -feeding insects is discussed in Chapter 12.

X. Cattle Feedlot Environmental Safety Study

A cattle feedlot environmental fate study was also carried out to evaluate ivermectin's potential ecological impact (Nessel *et al.*, 1989). Five cattle were housed in each of 2 identical, unpaved, dirt feedlot pens at a density of approximately one animal per 200 square feet. Animals in the treated group were given a single dose (0.2 mg/kg) of ivermectin. Control animals received no treatment. Surface runoff and percolated water collected during a 28-day trial period contained no significant amounts (< 0.01 ppb) of ivermectin. The collected water also showed no ivermectin-related toxicity to *D. magna* (no-effect level, 0.01 ppb). Furthermore, none of the subsurface (8–30 cm depth) core soil samples collected after 28 days contained any detectable amounts of ivermectin (detection limit = 1 ppb). This field trial supports our laboratory data and indicates that ivermectin in feces is unlikely to cause adverse environmental effects in surface or subsurface waters.

Our studies on environmental safety have been based on the currently approved uses of ivermectin. As new programs or treatment methods are developed, their potential environmental impact will need to be assessed.

Acknowledgements

We would like to thank Drs. Peter Wislocki, William VandenHeuvel and S.H.L. Chiu for their constructive comments on this manuscript.

References

Chiu SHL, Buhs RP, Sestokas E, Taub R, Jacob TA (1985) Determination of ivermectin residue in animal tissues by high-performance liquid chromatography-reverse isotope dilution assay. *J. Agric. Food Chem.* 33:99–102

Chiu SHL, Sestokas E, Taub R, Buhs RP, Green M, Sestokas R, VandenHeuvel WJA, Arison BH, Jacob TA (1986) Metabolic disposition of ivermectin in tissues of cattle, sheep, and rats. *Drug Metab. & Dispos.* 14:590–600

Chiu SHL, Sestokas E, Taub R, Smith JL, Arison B, Lu AYH (1984) The metabolism of avermectin-H_2B_{1a} and -H_2B_{1b} by pig liver microsomes. *Drug Metab. & Dispos.* 12:464–469

Chiu SHL, Taub R, Sestokas E, Lu AYH, Jacob TA (1987) Comparative in vivo and in vitro metabolism of ivermectin in steers, sheep, swine, and rat. *Drug Metab. Rev.* 18:289–302

Halley BA, Jacob TA, Lu AYH (1989a) The environmental impact of the use of ivermectin: Environmental effects and fate. *Chemosphere*, in press.

Halley BA, Nessel RJ, Lu AYH, Roncalli RA (1989b) The environmental safety of ivermectin: An overview. *Chemosphere*, in press.

Kelso PC (1984) Ivermectin cures scaly mite infestation. *Vet. Med.* 79:446

Miwa GT, Walsh JS, VandenHeuvel WJA, Arison B, Sestokas E, Buhs R, Rosegay A, Avermitilis S, Lu AYH, Walsh MAR, Walker RW, Taub R, Jacob

TA (1982) The metabolism of avermectins B_{1a}, H_2B_{1a}, and H_2B_{1b} by liver microsomes. *Drug Metab. & Dispos.* 10:268–274

Mousa S, Grad N, Sokkar I, Raheem MA (1986) Investigations on the efficacy of ivermectin for ectoparasites and nematodes in chickens. I. Testing for drug safety to chickens. II. Anthelmintic efficacy of ivermectin for experimental ascaridiasis in chickens. *Assiut Vet. Med. J.* 17(33):223, 225–233

Nessel RJ, Jacob TA, Robertson RT (1983) The human and environmental safety aspects of ivermectin. In Leaning WHD, Siegmund OH, Fraser CM (eds) *Recent Developments in the Control of Animal Parasites,* MSD-AGVET, Rahway, NJ, pp 98–100

Nessel RJ, Wallace DH, Wehner T, Tait W, Gomez L (1989) Environmental fate of ivermectin in a cattle feedlot. *Chemosphere,* in press.

US EPA (1974) Development document for effluent limitations guidelines and new source performance standards for the feedlots-points source category. Washington, DC; EPA-440/1-74-004-a

Zeman P (1987) Systemic efficacy of ivermectin against *Dermanyssus gallinae* (de Geer, 1778) in fowls. *Vet. Parasitol.* 23:141–146

CHAPTER 12

Environmental Aspects of Use of Ivermectin and Abamectin in Livestock: Effects on Cattle Dung Fauna

R.A. Roncalli

I. Role of Animal Droppings in the Ecosystem

Animal droppings have played an important role in our ecosystem for millions of years. In fact, they help preserve it by returning valuable nutrients to the soil as they decompose.

Dung fauna encompass a range of inhabitants, including insects, nematodes, bacteria, yeast, and fungi. The number of invertebrates and micro-organisms involved in the decomposition of dung can be very high. Putnam (1983), for instance, reported that there may be "as many as 10^{11} bacteria per ml of sheep dung and 10^6 fungal mycelia and 10^{10} actinomycetals per ml." In cattle dung there may be as many as 2,000,000 yeast cells per gram. It has been suggested that in 10 grams (dry weight) of decaying cow dung, there can be as many as 500 nematodes, 100 collembolans, 15 mites, 5 enchytraids, and several hundred insect larvae (chiefly beetle and dung-fly). The assemblage of inhabitants and their role in the disintegration of dung varies, however, as may their cumulative effects. This depends on many factors, including seasonality, microclimate, ecosystem, and artificial control of the dung community. Physical factors such as rain, snow, and frost (White 1960; Bastiman 1970), trampling or disturbance by animals—especially birds—are of great importance in the breakdown of dung.

The role played by the different members of the dung community in the degradation process will vary according to the habitat. In fact, while dung-burying beetles play a major role in the dispersal of dung in pasture in some tropical areas, this does not appear to be the case in temperate areas, where the number of dung-burying beetles is much lower. The degradation of fecal material in temperate areas appears to be primarily a decomposition process. Earthworms have also been reported as major organisms responsible for dung degradation (White 1960).

Early in the 1960s, the Commonwealth Scientific and Industrial Research Organization (CSIRO) in Australia and the United States Department of Agriculture (USDA) encouraged the introduction of Afro-Asian dung-burying beetles into each country's ecosystem. One of the main purposes of this plan was to reduce the prevalence of dung-breeding flies—such as Australia's bush fly and the horn fly—by the use of the beetles to degrade the dung. Over the last 20 years, 41 dung beetle species have been released in Australia; of these, 21 are known to have become established (Ridsdill-Smith in press). Six species of dung beetles were released in the United States (Fincher 1986), and most of these species are now established. It appears that in both Australia (Doube 1986) and the United States (Legner and Warkentin 1983) the results of the projects to control buffalo and horn flies were disappointing. As a result, the official USDA program was terminated in October 1987.

II. Effect of Ivermectin on Larvae of Dung-Breeding Diptera

A number of Muscidae, such as the horn fly, the face fly, and the stable fly, are often associated with the dung of herbivorous mammals. The horn fly, *Haematobia irritans*, and its subspecies, *H. irritans exigua* (buffalo fly) and *H. thirouxi potans*, are biting species that annoy cattle and cause considerable losses (i.e., reduction in average daily gain). Drummond (1987) estimated that in the United States alone the horn fly causes annual losses to the cattle industry of $679 million. Roberts (1952) has postulated that cattle having to contend with large numbers of buffalo flies—one of Australia's major pests—will be less productive (i.e., decreased weight gain and milk production). Moreover, Drummond (1987) reported that the face fly (*Musca autumnalis*) generates annual losses of $59 million to the U.S. cattle industry (feedlot and range cattle); those losses appear to be the result of an increase in the incidence of pinkeye, with a resulting effect on weaning and yearling weight. According to the same author the annual loss in feedlot cattle and dairy cows caused by the stable fly (*Stomoxys calcitrans*) in the United States is $418 million.

During the past 9 years a number of trials have been conducted to assess the effect of ivermectin and abamectin on larvae of cattle dung-breeding Diptera. In laboratory tests, Schmidt and Kunz (1980) determined the effect of ivermectin on stable flies (*S. calcitrans*) and horn flies (*H. irritans*). Ivermectin prevented the flies' development from larvae to adults. The effective dose of ivermectin was 0.048 ppm (LC_{50}) and 0.186 ppm (LC_{90}) for stable flies, and 0.003 ppm (LC_{50}) and 0.006 ppm (LC_{90}) for horn flies.

Meyer, Simco, and Lancaster (1980) reported that ivermectin given to cattle subcutaneously at 200 μg/kg had an effect on larvae of the face fly (*M. autumnalis*) for 14 days after treatment. Miller and colleagues (1981) showed that a single injection to cattle of 200 μg ivermectin/kg controlled larvae of horn flies (*H. irritans*) for up to 4 weeks after treatment. When ivermectin was given daily at a dose of 1 μg/kg orally, it killed all horn fly larvae in the manure. An oral dose level of 5 μg/kg killed all of the face flies, about 60% of the stable flies (*S. calcitrans*), and 90% of the house flies (*M. domestica*) in the manure. Ivermectin, given by subcutaneous injection at a dose of 5 μg/kg/day, prevented development of horn flies in the manure. On the other hand, injections of 10 μg/kg daily did not control stable fly larvae.

The results of a trial conducted by Schmidt (1983) at the USDA Livestock Laboratory (Kerrville, TX) showed that intramuscular treatment of cattle with ivermectin at a dose rate of 200 μg/kg prevented emergence of adult horn flies (*H. irritans*) from manure for up to 28 days after treatment. Some *H. irritans* developed into adults from manure collected at 35 days after treatment and then aged for 14 days. According to Ridsdill-Smith (1988), a single subcutaneous injection of abamectin at a dose rate of 200 μg/kg killed bush fly (*M. vetustissima*) larvae for 2 weeks after injection.

In a trial carried out in Australia (Burrows and Picton, unpublished results), *H. irritans exigua* (buffalo fly) were cultured from feces collected from 5 cattle injected subcutaneously with 200 μg abamectin/kg body weight. No flies emerged from the feces of the treated cattle for up to 21 days following treatment.

The results of 2 trials conducted in South Africa (D'Assonville and Soll, unpublished results; D'Assonville, unpublished results) showed that larval stages of the face fly *M. xanthomelas*, one of the vectors for *Parafilaria bovicola*, and *H. thirouxi potans*, the horn fly of central, east, and southern Africa, were killed in feces of cattle treated with sustained-release boluses delivering 40 μg ivermectin/kg/day.

III. Effect of Ivermectin and Abamectin on Afro-Asian Dung Beetles (*Onthophagus gazella* and *Onthophagus binodis*)

A. Onthophagus gazella

A series of trials (see Tables 12.1 and 12.2) was conducted in Australia to examine the effects of ivermectin and abamectin fecal residues on larval and adult stages of *Onthophagus gazella*. Cattle were treated once, subcutaneously, at 200 or 300 μg/kg body weight. The trials were carried out in sequential order, to assess the effect of the drugs' residues in feces at different time intervals following the placement of the beetles.

In these trials feces from treated and untreated animals were placed in buckets, along with pairs of *O. gazella,* and observed for the beetles' viability, production of brood balls, and emergence of new beetle populations for up to 35 days after treatment. The feces were not exposed to sunlight, eliminating any effects resulting from degradation of ivermectin and abamectin (which may occur under field conditions). The results of these trials indicate that neither ivermectin nor abamectin at the above doses had any effect on adult *O. gazella*. Both compounds did, however, prevent larval development: for ivermectin, up to 21 days following treatment, for abamectin, up to 28 days.

TABLE 12.1. Ivermectin vs dung beetles (*Onthophagus gazella*): ivermectin in cattle trials (Australia).

Investigator(s)	Drug	Route	Dose (μg/kg)	Results: Adults	Results: Larvae
J. Picton (1980) unpublished	ivermectin	S.C.[a]	300	No effect	Failed to develop 44–52 hours after treatment
J. Picton & R. W. Butler unpublished	ivermectin	S.C.	300	No effect	Failed to develop 1, 3, and 5 days after treatment
J. Picton & R. W. Butler unpublished	ivermectin	S.C.	300	No effect	Failed to develop 7 and 14 days after treatment No effect at 21, 28 and 35 days after treatment

[a] S.C. = subcutaneous.

TABLE 12.2. Ivermectin vs dung beetles (*Onthophagus gazella*): ivermectin and abamectin in cattle trials (Australia).

Investigator(s)	Drug	Route	Dose (μg/kg)	Results: Adults	Results: Larvae
J. Picton & R. O. Burrows	ivermectin	S.C.[a]	200	Not determined	Failed to develop 7 and 10 days after treatment
	abamectin	S.C.	200	Not determined	Failed to develop 7, 10 and 14 days after treatment
R. O. Burrows & J. Picton	abamectin	S.C.	200	No effect	Failed to develop 21 days after treatment Unaffected 28 days after treatment

[a] S.C. = subcutaneous.

In Texas, *O. gazella* are active in the early fall. During September–October 1980, Schmidt (1983) observed that the presence and burrows of adult beetles were approximately the same in manure from untreated cattle as in manure of cattle treated with ivermectin.

B. *Onthophagus binodis*

Ridsdill-Smith (1988) conducted a trial in southwestern Australia to assess the effect of abamectin, given to cattle subcutaneously at the prescribed dose, on the development of *Onthophagus binodis* in manure. Dung was collected 1, 2, 4, 8, and 11 weeks after treatment with abamectin and transferred to plastic boxes. Pairs of *O. binodis* were placed in dung of untreated cattle and abamectin-treated cattle. While the survival of adult dung beetles was not influenced by the treatment, the production of brood balls was decreased for 2 weeks in dung from cattle treated with abamectin. The survival of immature dung beetles was affected for 4 weeks. In the same trial, levamisole given orally did not seem to influence the beetles. Ridsdill-Smith suggested replacing the treatment with abamectin with another anthelmintic from September to November, which is the main breeding period of beetles in southwestern Australia. The use of abamectin in other months should not influence dung beetle breeding.

The abamectins are not the only compounds to affect the larval stages of the dung beetle. A number of published reports have indicated that various anthelmintics and insecticides (phenothiazine, dichlorvos, coumaphos, etc.) affect dung beetles, while thiabendazole and levamisole have little effect. Also of interest is the fact that superphosphate, which is used in many sites to improve pastures, decreased brood ball production and survival of the dung beetle *O. granulatus* (Holm and Wallace 1987).

IV. Effect of Ivermectin on Other Dung Insects

Schmidt (1983), in his trial conducted in Texas, also evaluated the effect of ivermectin (200 μg/kg intramuscularly) on native insects. Emergence of some insects—such as sphaerocerids, sepsids, and 2 species of Gymnodia—from feces of treated animals was severely reduced. In addition, more parasitic wasps were present in the control manure. On the other hand, about the same number of gnats and of staphylinids emerged from both treated and untreated feces. Mites were plentiful in both types of feces.

Wall and Strong (1987), in a trial conducted at Bristol University (U.K.), collected dung from cattle treated with an experimental sustained-release bolus delivering 40 μg/kg/day as well as from untreated cattle and observed the dung for 100 days. In this trial the dung from treated animals contained "few, or in some cases no Coleoptera or Diptera." *Aphodius* spp. was the most abundant (89.4%) of the Coleoptera found in the untreated dung. The authors expressed concern about the potential adverse impact of ivermectin usage on the condition of pastures.

In their study on the effect of treating cattle with a sustained-release ivermectin device (above), Wall and Strong recorded the number of earthworms appearing in dung pats, and underlying soil, at various intervals after the initiation of treatment. The resulting data did not show any clear-cut effect of ivermectin on the number or time of appearance of earthworms.

V. Effect of Different Ivermectin Formulations on Degradation of Cattle Fecal Pats

Schmidt (1983) observed the aging of manure from animals treated with an intramuscular injection of ivermectin at a dose of 200 μg/kg. Several pats of manure collected from the pens of treated and untreated cattle were molded in pans and placed on the surface of a stony-shaped area inside a wire enclosure. At the end of the 29-day test, the consistency and form of the manure from the treated and untreated groups appeared to be the same. Schmidt stated that "since manure from treated cattle also appeared to disintegrate at the same rate as manure of untreated animals, on the basis of the results reported here, the manure of treated animals should pose no greater threat of pollution than untreated manure in grazing areas."

Wall and Strong (1987) reported that feces of untreated cattle were well decomposed 40 days after deposition, and for the most part had disappeared after 100 days. On the other hand, feces of cattle treated with the ivermectin bolus releasing 40 μg/kg/day were solid and intact after 100 days. Strong and Brown (1987) inferred that this was due to the fact that Coleoptera were almost absent from treated feces of any age. In this trial, feces were collected from housed cattle, mixed, and placed into a circular mold of corrugated cardboard and transferred to a 5m x 10m enclosure in a pasture.

McKeand, Bairden, and Ibarra-Silva (1988) reported on the effect of ivermectin given as a pour-on formulation at a rate of 500 μg/kg to calves at 3, 8, and 13 weeks after turnout to pasture in western Scotland. One week after the third treatment fecal pats were selected, labeled, and left *in situ*. After 9 weeks there was no marked difference in the rates of breakdown of the feces between the dung pats of the ivermectin-treated calves and those of the untreated controls. Although the fauna present in the cattle dung were not monitored, these authors suggest that if the fauna involved in the decay of dung were adversely affected by the ivermectin, these species would have rapidly repopulated the pats.

The results of the 3 trials described appear to indicate that there is a difference with regard to ivermectin formulations and degradation of cattle fecal pats. No difference was, in fact, detected between the injectable and the pour-on formulations versus the untreated controls. There was a difference, however, when an experimental formulation (sustained-release bolus) was used. Two of the trials were conducted under conditions which may not have been an accurate representation of a true field situation. Future trials should be run under field conditions as was done in the study by McKeand and colleagues (1988), i.e., evaluation of dung pats left *in situ*. In fact, there are several factors to consider in running these trials. Under natural circumstances, dung beetles (which are mostly flying insects) regularly migrate to and from dung pats. Also, disintegration of fecal pats will be accelerated by trampling by animals, the weathering effects of wind and rain, or other environmental factors.

VI. Conclusions

Ivermectin and abamectin have an effect on some important dung fauna, such as the larval stages of Diptera and of some dung beetles. The effect on biting flies (i.e., the horn fly) could be considered beneficial, but its practical impact under field conditions remains to be determined. Ivermectin and abamectin appear to affect dung beetles mainly in the larval stages, and this could be considered harmful. The importance of these findings to those situations in which beetles play a major role in dung degradation is still under evaluation.

Although the population dynamics of coprophagous insects is not well known and varies greatly from area to area, the use of ivermectin and abamectin is not expected to pose a threat to dung beetle populations. Localized use of the abamectins on particular herds of cattle at infrequent intervals is unlikely to significantly affect overall beetle population sizes. In fact, only a portion of a single generation of dung beetles will be affected, as suppression of larval development will occur for a limited period of time after treatment of cattle. Not all cattle will be treated in the same herd or in neighboring herds at the same time, and feces from untreated cattle will always be available to sustain beetle populations. Another factor to consider is the effect of ivermectin on earthworms, which play an important role in the degradation of dung in numerous countries (e.g., the United Kingdom, New Zealand). The estimated LC_{50} of ivermectin for earthworms under controlled laboratory conditions was 300 mg/kg (ppm) of soil, a value which is much more than can be encountered in the environment; the no-effect level of ivermectin was 12 ppm (Halley, Nessel, and Lu (1988). The final word on these issues will be obtained only through a series of controlled field studies in different areas of the world. A number of these trials have already been initiated, and the results will provide valuable information on this area of research, which is still not well understood.

References

Bastiman B (1970) Problems of pasture contamination and herbage rejection under intensive grazing. In *11th Progress Report of Experimental Husbandry and Experimental Horticultural Stations,* NAAS, pp 62–69

Doube BM (1986) Biological control of the buffalo fly in Australia: the potential of the Southern Africa dung fauna. *Misc. Pubs. Entomol. Soc. of Amer.* (No. 61):16–34

Drummond RO (1987) Economic aspects of ectoparasites of cattle in North America. In *The Economic Impact of Parasitism in Cattle,* MSD AGVET Symposium, Montreal, Quebec, Canada, pp 9–24

Fincher GT (1986) Importation, colonization, and release of dung-burying scarabs. *Misc. Pubs. Entomol. Soc. of Amer.* (No 61):69–76

Halley BA, Nessel RJ, Lu AYH (1988) Environmental aspects of ivermectin usage in livestock: general considerations. (Chapter 11)

Holm E, Wallace MMH (1987) The influence of superphosphate on the establishment of introduced dung beetles in south-eastern Australia. *J. Aust. Inst. Agric. Sci.* 5:202–203

Legner EF, Warkentin RW (1983) Questions concerning the dynamics of *Onthophagus gazella* (Coleoptera:Scarabaeidae) with symbovine flies in the lower Colorado desert of California. *Proc. 51st Ann. Conf. Calif. Mosquito & Vector Contr. Assoc.* pp 99–101

McKeand J, Bairden K, Ibarra-Silva AM (1988) The degradation of bovine fecal pats containing ivermectin. *Vet. Rec.* 122:587–588

Meyer JA, Simco JS, Lancaster JL (1980) Control of face fly larval development with ivermectin, MK-933. *Southwest. Entomol.* 5:207–209

Miller JA, Kunz SE, Oehler DD, Miller RW (1981) Larvicidal activity of Merck MK-933, an avermectin, against the horn fly, stable fly, face fly and house fly. *J. Econ. Entomol.* 74:608–611

Putnam RJ (1983) Carrion and dung: The decomposition of animal wastes. In *The Institute of Biology's Studies in Biology* No. 156, Edward Arnold Publishers, London, pp 1–62

Ridsdill-Smith TJ (in press) Some effects of ivermectin on non-target organisms in cattle dung. *Proc. 5th Austral. Conf. Grassland Invert. Ecol.*

Ridsdill-Smith TJ (1988) Survival and reproduction of *Musca vetustissima* Walker (Diptera:Muscidae) and a scarabaeine dung beetle in dung of cattle treated with avermectin B1. *J. Aust. Entomol. Soc.* 27:175–178

Roberts FHS (1952) *Insects Affecting Livestock.* Angus and Robertson, Sydney, Australia, pp 117–124

Schmidt CD (1983) Activity of an avermectin against selected insects in aging manure. *Envir. Entomol.* 12:455–457

Schmidt CD, Kunz SE (1980) Testing immature laboratory-reared stable flies and horn flies for susceptibility to insecticides. *J. Econ. Entomol.* 73:702–703

Strong L, Brown TA (1987) Avermectins in insect control and biology: a review. *Bull. Entomol. Res.* 77:357–389

Wall R, Strong L (1987) Environmental consequences of treating cattle with the antiparasitic drug ivermectin. *Nature* 327:418–421

White E (1960) The distribution and subsequent disappearance of sheep dung on Pennine moorland. *J. Anim. Ecol.* 29:243–250

CHAPTER 13

Environmental Aspects of Abamectin Use in Crop Protection

P.G. Wislocki, L.S. Grosso, and R.A. Dybas

I. Introduction

The use of any chemical as a pesticide results in the exposure of the environment to the chemical. The extent of this exposure depends on the way the chemical is applied—pattern, rate, and frequency—as well as its persistence in the environment. Humans can control all these parameters save the last. A chemical's persistence is determined by its physico-chemical properties: half-life in soil and water, photolytic stability, and soil-binding ability. These same factors also affect the chemical's bio-availability to living organisms.

In Chapter 20 Dr. Dybas discusses the agricultural uses of abamectin. It will be used at a maximum rate of 0.025 lb active ingredient/acre (28 g/hectare) 3 times/season, or at a maximum rate of 0.02 lb active ingredient/acre (22 g/hectare) up to 10 times/season. Abamectin is also being used by homeowners to control fire ants at a use rate of only 0.00011 lb active ingredient/acre (123 mg/hectare). The compound is formulated in a bait used at a rate of more than a million particles/acre. The bait particles are rapidly scavenged by foraging fire ants. This use will not lead to significant exposure to the environment and therefore is not a topic of discussion in this chapter.

The risk to nontarget organisms associated with the use of a pesticide depends upon both its toxicity to nontarget organisms and their exposure to the pesticide. As a pesticide, abamectin is very toxic to target pests. It is also toxic to certain nontarget organisms; however, the pesticide's properties and use patterns reduce the exposure of nontarget organisms. In this regard abamectin has many positive attributes. It degrades rapidly and its physiocochemical properties prevent it from bioconcentrating or bioaccumulating in the environment. An analysis of abamectin's physio-chemical properties and their effect on its environmental fate per se, as well as the chemical's toxicity and risk to nontarget organisms, follows.

The nomenclature used in this chapter should be clarified. The product that is being developed for agricultural use is designated *abamectin*. It refers to a mixture of not less than 80% avermectin B_{1a} and not more than 20% avermectin B_{1b}. (Figure 13.1). Certain studies presented here used radioactively labeled avermectin B_{1a}; they are designated accordingly.

II. Environmental Fate of Abamectin

The studies on the environmental fate of a compound describe not only how a compound is degraded in the environment but also the extent to which it is available to biological organisms. This section addresses abamectin's rate of degradation, its bioavailability, and its uptake into biological systems.

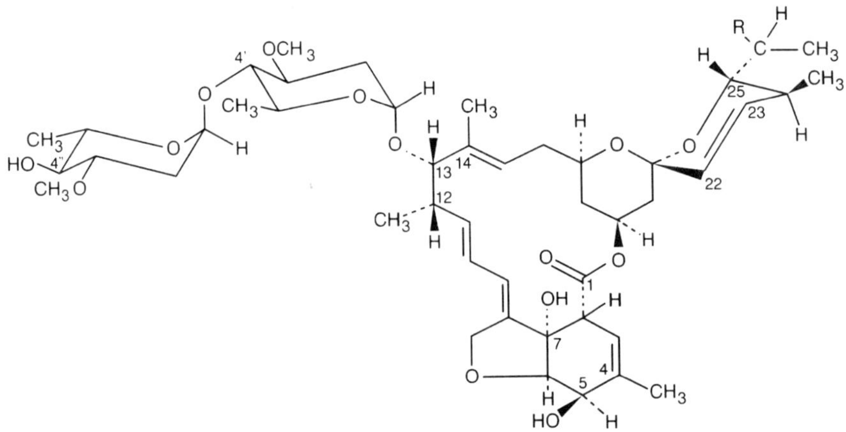

a-Component R = $C_2H_5 \geq 80\%$
b-Component R = $CH_3 \leq 20\%$

ABAMECTIN = AVERMECTIN B_1

FIGURE 13.1. The structure of abamectin.

A. PHOTOLYSIS

Abamectin undergoes rapid photolysis under a number of different conditions. Photolysis occurs when abamectin is exposed to light in water, on soil particles, or as a thin film on either inert (glass) or biological surfaces, such as leaves. The degradation occurs by oxidative and photooxidative mechanisms.

1. Water

In a water photolysis experiment avermectin B_{1a} was exposed to sunlight and its degradation was followed by HPLC. Under these conditions avermectin B_{1a} degraded with a half-life of less than 12 hours. Products formed during the course of photolysis included a less polar degradate identified as a photo isomer, the delta-8,9 Z isomer of avermectin B_{1a}, and 2 fractions more polar than avermectin B_{1a}, designated the moderately polar and polar fractions. During the course of this degradation the characteristic UV absorption at 245 nm is lost. (Absorption is due to the presence of a diene moiety at carbons 8 through 11 in the molecule.) This loss of absorbance also occurs when abamectin is photolyzed in organic solvents (Mrozik *et al.* 1988). The terminal degradation products of water photolysis were contained in the polar fraction. Its toxicity and that of the other fractions are discussed later.

2. Soil

When soil containing avermectin B_{1a} was exposed to sunlight on glass plates, it degraded to multiple products rapidly, with a half-life of 21 hours.

3. Thin Film

Abamectin is exceptionally susceptible to degradation when it is present on a surface as a thin film. Such degradation occurs even in the absence of light; however, it is greatly accelerated in the presence of light. Both under laboratory light and in simulated sunlight, a thin film of abamectin degrades with an initial half-life of 4 to 6 hours. Both avermectin B_{1a} and avermectin B_{1b} degrade at the same rate (J. MacConnell and R. Demchak, personal communication). The degradation products include the delta-8,9 isomer of avermectin B_{1a} and a polar and moderately polar fraction. HPLC profiles of the polar degradates generated on plants and on glass demonstrated that these degradates were similar. The degradates on glass contained a multitude of components, some of which had from 1 to 6 additional oxygens compared to the parent compound. Other components had lost the features of the macrocyclic ring, including the loss of UV absorbance at 245 nm; only the sugar portion of the molecule was recognizable by NMR or mass spectroscopy. These data indicate that extensive degradation occurs when abamectin is exposed to light.

B. Hydrolysis

The facility with which avermectin B_{1a} undergoes hydrolysis was determined at pH 5, 7, and 9 (the pH range normally found in surface and ground water). After 28 days at 25°C, avermectin B_{1a} remained unchanged, indicating that it was not readily hydrolyzed under these conditions.

C. Soil Metabolism

In collaboration with Donald Bull (Bull *et al.* 1984), soil metabolism studies were performed at concentrations of 0.1, 1.0, or 50 ppm in 3 soil types: Lufkin fine sandy loam, Houston clay, and construction-grade sand. Avermectin B_{1a} had half-lives ranging from 20 to 47 days. It degraded to at least 13 products. The major product was identified by NMR and mass spectroscopy as the 8a-hydroxy derivative of avermectin B_{1a}. This compound appears to be the result of microbial metabolism, since sterilized soil did not metabolize abamectin. Under anaerobic conditions the rate of metabolism decreased significantly.

D. Solubility

A major factor which determines the behavior of a chemical in the environment is its solubility. Because abamectin is quite insoluble in water, determining its actual solubility was very difficult. For this reason the method of May and Wasik (1978) was used. By this dynamic method it was determined that the solubility of avermectin B_{1a} was 7.8 ppb in water.

E. Soil Binding

The bioavailability of a compound to biological systems in the environment is strongly influenced by its ability to bind to soil. A compound that binds tightly and is not mobile will result in a much lower level of exposure than one which does not bind tightly. The ability of abamectin to bind to soil was examined by 3 different methods: soil thin-layer chromatography (TLC), batch equilibrium binding studies, and soil column leaching studies. In all 3 systems it was determined that avermectin B_{1a} is an immobile pesticide. When its mobility was determined by soil TLC using 6 different soils—including Lakeland sand, which contained only 0.1% organic matter—avermectin B_{1a} did not move from the origin; when compared with standards, it was classified as an immobile pesticide. To determine the binding constant of abamectin to soil, batch equilibrium studies were performed. The results of these studies indicated that avermectin B_{1a} binds very tightly to soil particles in relation to the organic matter content of the soil. The binding constant, Koc, based on the organic content of the soils, was approximately 4000 or greater, demonstrating the immobile nature of abamectin. In a soil column leaching study, avermectin B_{1a} was applied to 38-cm-high columns of soil. Water equivalent to 22 to 23 inches of rainfall was applied to the columns over a 28-day period beginning immediately or after 29 days of aging. Approximately 80% to 99% of the radioactivity, which included avermectin B_{1a} and polar degradates, remained in the top 6 cm of the column. Some radioactivity, including a small amount of avermectin B_{1a} and polar degradates, did pass through the column, apparently due to channeling effects in the column. There was no significant difference between the aged and unaged columns, indicating that any degradation products formed during the aging period are not more mobile than the parent compound. These studies further demonstrate the immobile nature of abamectin and indicate its lack of bioavailability in the environment.

F. Plant Uptake

The ability of plants to take up abamectin residue from the soil is a measure of these residues bioavailability. This is a pragmatic issue because crops are often rotated into fields where pesticides have been used to treat previous crops. A rotational crop study (Moye *et al.* 1987) was performed using 3 different soil types that had organic matter contents from 0.14% to 38.3%. Although total applications of up to 0.36 lbs active ingredient per acre were used, there was no bioconcentration of residues. Indeed, the highest average level of total radioactive residues of avermectin B_{1a} found in any plant part was only 11.6 ppb. This level is quite low compared to total radioactive residues in soil of 1070 ppb. Examination of the properties of the plant residues by extraction indicated that 95% of the residues were not avermectin B_{1a}-related: they could not be extracted with acetone, which removes avermectin B_{1a} and its degradates. Plant metabolism studies have shown that radioactive fragments from avermectin B_{1a} can be incorporated into the natural products of plants. Therefore, the radioactive residue in the plants is due to their uptake of small fragments of the avermectin B_{1a} molecule and the incorporation of 1- and 2-carbon fragments into natural plant constituents.

G. Bioconcentration in Fish

The fact that chlorinated pesticides concentrate and accumulate in fish and organisms higher on the food chain led to a general concern about the ability of pesticides to bioconcentrate and bioaccumulate in the environment. Not only are the possible ecological effects of concern, but so also is the possible hazard to humans from consuming high levels of bioconcentrated residues. Because abamectin is very insoluble in water and has an octanol water partition coefficient of 9900, it seemed possible that it could bioconcentrate. When its bioconcentration factor in bluegill sunfish was determined, however, abamectin was shown not to bioconcentrate. The study was performed under dynamic (flow-through) conditions by ABC Laboratories (Columbia, MO). Bluegill sunfish were exposed to avermectin B_{1a} at a concentration of 0.099 ppb for 28 days. The residues in the fish reached a steady-state concentration at 10 days. From days 28 to 42 the fish were kept in water without avermectin B_{1a} for the depuration phase of the experiment. The concentration of residues in the whole fish was 6.8 ppb on day 28, but this decreased rapidly to only 0.32 ppb on day 42. Using the uptake and depuration rates, it was calculated that abamectin has a steady-state bioconcentration factor of only 52. Therefore, abamectin neither accumulates nor persists in fish. This is probably due to the large size of the molecule. Avermectin B_{1a} has a molecular weight of 872. Its size prevents it from being a truly lipophilic compound. Brooke, Dobbs, and Williams (1986) have reported this phenomenon with other high molecular-weight compounds. These results are consistent with animal metabolism studies that have shown that the compound neither accumulates nor persists in rats or goats (Maynard *et al.*, unpublished data). Therefore, abamectin will neither bioconcentrate in individual organisms nor bioaccumulate in the food chain.

H. Fate in the Aquatic Environment

To assess abamectin's fate in the aquatic environment a simulated field study was performed in collaboration with Wildlife International (Easton, MD). Abamectin was applied by 1 of 2 methods to tanks of water 2 feet deep containing a 3-inch layer of pond sediment. The water was either sprayed directly with the diluted emulsifiable concentrate (EC) formulation to simulate the drift route of exposure, or soil was sprayed directly with the diluted formulation and added to the water immediately or 4 days later to simulate runoff. Samples of water and sediment were taken at various times for up to 52 days after treatment and analyzed for abamectin.

The abamectin in tanks treated directly with spray (drift simulation) was rapidly distributed between the sediment and the water. Between the zero-time sampling and the 19-hour sampling, the levels of abamectin in the water decreased 4- to 15-fold. After the initial distribution and rapid degradation the level of abamectin decreased with a half-life of about 4 days. The half-life of abamectin in sediment was approximately 2 to 4 weeks. If one assumes an application rate of 0.025 lb active ingredient/acre (the highest maximum application rate for any use) and that 5% of the use rate impacts on nearby surface water, then the level of abamectin in the water the day after the application was only 26 ppt. By 2 days the level decreased to 8 ppt. This decreased to less than 1.25 ppt (the limit of detection) by 15 days after treatment. The levels of abamectin in the water over time are shown graphically in Figure 13.2.

In the simulated runoff study, soil was added to the water immediately after treatment with abamectin or after 4 days of exposure to the elements. Water and sediment from tanks treated with pre-aged soil did not contain detectable levels of abamectin. Sediment and water from the tanks to which soil was added immediately did contain abamectin residues. Since abamectin binds very strongly to soil, one can assume a runoff of 0.1% of the applied abamectin. Also, in common agricultural practice an area tenfold greater than the pond size is needed to sustain a viable farm pond. Using these assumptions, the levels of residues in the water were calculated to be in the range of 1 to 3 ppt for 15 days after the addition of soil. The residues in the water dropped to 0.28 ppt by day 31 and to less than 0.03 ppt by day 51. Residues of abamectin in the sediment trended downward during the 51-day period and fell within the range of 100 to 300 ppt. The levels of abamectin in the water over time are shown graphically in Figure 13.3.

This study also examined loss of abamectin on the soil surface. A layer

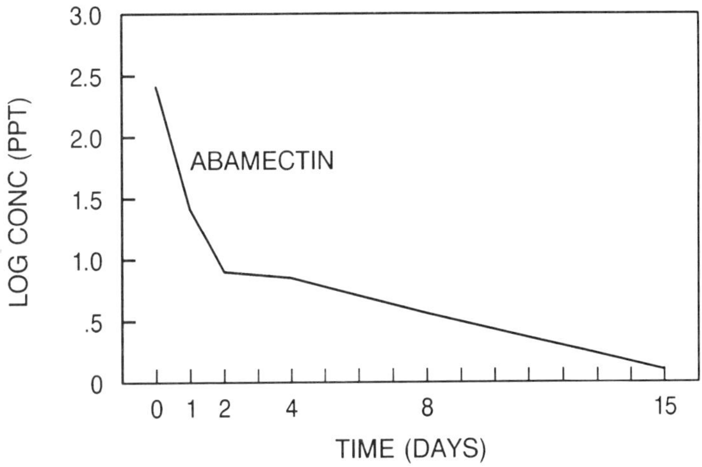

FIGURE 13.2. Decrease in the concentration of abamectin (ppt) over time in the water of tanks subjected to drift simulation.

of soil that had been sprayed with abamectin was analyzed at 0, 1, 2, and 4 days. Abamectin degraded rapidly, with a half-life of 8 hours (Figure 13.4).

This simulated field study demonstrates that abamectin degrades readily both on soil and in the aquatic environment.

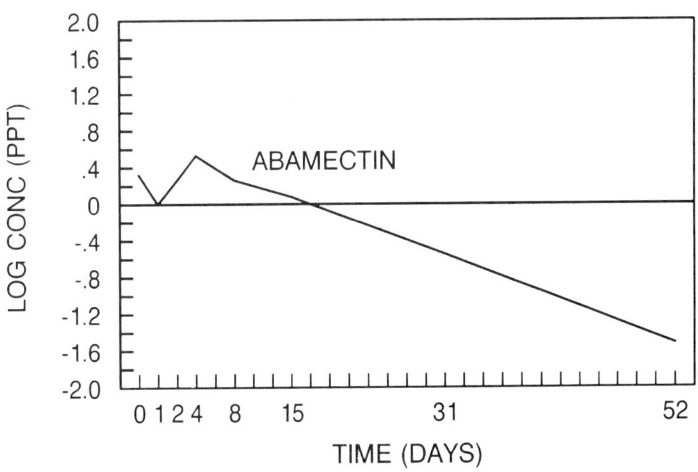

FIGURE 13.3. Decrease in the concentration of abamectin (ppt) over time in the water of tanks subjected to runoff simulation.

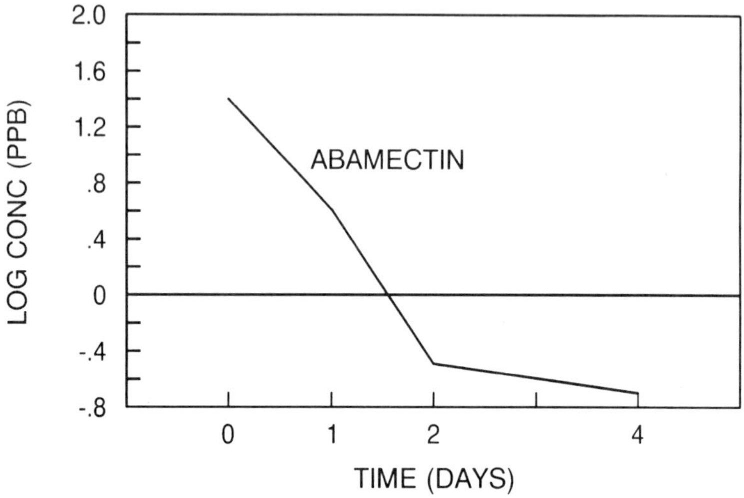

FIGURE 13.4. Decrease in the concentration of abamectin (ppt) over time in soil sprayed directly with abamectin.

I. Fate in the Terrestrial Environment

Soil dissipation studies and crop residue trials were performed to determine the residues of abamectin on soil and crops (Tway *et al.*, unpublished data). Because these studies are actual field studies, they most accurately depict the residue levels to which terrestrial organisms will actually be exposed. In the soil dissipation studies the initial levels of abamectin in the top 2 inches of soil were from 10 to 20 ppb. This is ¼ to ½ of the theoretical level of 42 ppb expected to be found at zero time when 0.025 lb active ingredient/acre is applied to soil. Minimal residues were found at the 2-to-4-inch level, and no residues were found at a soil depth of 4 to 6 inches. Residues depleted rapidly and did not accumulate, even after 12 weekly applications.

Residue data on crops were determined to establish tolerances in raw agricultural commodities and food and feed additives. These residue values can also be used to estimate the exposure of terrestrial organisms to abamectin. Residue data are available for 4 crops: cotton foliage, celery plants, citrus fruits, and tomatoes. The cotton foliage trials were performed in South Africa at application rates different from those in the United States when calculated at the U.S. rate of 0.02 lb active ingredient/acre, the initial residue values were approximately 1 ppm. Within 3 days the residue values were approximately 5% of the initial values. In 20 residue trials on celery plants, the plants were treated at 10 weekly intervals at a rate of 0.02 lb active ingredient/acre. At zero time after the last of 10 weekly applications the average residue value in the whole celery plants was 170 ppb. By 7 days after the application the residues had declined to 9.5 ppb, which is less than 6% of the initial residue levels. These data demonstrate that even repeated applications of abamectin do not result in accumulated residues—they deplete rapidly. Residue results from cotton foliage and celery plants can be used as surrogate data for grasses and leaves and leafy crops, respectively, in risk assessments. Due to their small surface-to-mass ratios, citrus fruits and tomatoes have lower initial residues of abamectin. The zero-time residue levels in citrus fruits treated with 0.025 lb active ingredient/acre average from 14 to 45 ppb. The residues declined to approximately 20% of initial values by 7 days. The initial residue level of abamectin on tomatoes was less than 17 ppb. By 3 days after the application the residue levels were less than 5 ppb and usually less than 2 ppb, the limit of detection of the analytical method. These data on citrus fruits and tomatoes can be used as surrogate data for other fruits. Metabolism studies on citrus fruits (Iwata *et al.* 1985; Maynard *et al.* 1989), cotton (Bull *et al.* 1984), and celery (Moye *et al.*, unpublished data) have also demonstrated the rapid degradation of avermectin B_{1a} on plants. These studies have shown that the degradation products formed are the delta 8,9 isomer of avermectin B_{1a}, the moderately polar fraction, and the polar fraction. These fractions are made up of multiple components. Because the polar fraction is the major degradate, and because it is similar to the polar fraction generated on glass, the glass-derived material was used for toxicology studies. The results of these studies is discussed below. The delta 8,9 isomer is present on plants at 10% to 20% of the total residue of it and its parent compound. It also degrades at the same rate as its parent compound. Because the delta 8,9 isomer is closely related to its parent, it was also tested for toxicity in mice.

The soil dissipation and residue data indicate that, under field use conditions, the residue levels of abamectin do not accumulate, even when multiple applications are made; moreover, the residue levels deplete rapidly, greatly limiting exposure.

J. Conclusions

The environmental fate data demonstrate that abamectin photodegrades rapidly in the environment and is metabolized in the soil. Its solubility in water is limited, and it binds to soil very tightly. It does not bioconcentrate in fish and is not taken up from soil into plants. Both aquatic and terrestrial studies confirm the rapid degradation of abamectin in the environment, and its concomitant lack of accumulation and persistence.

III. Effects of Abamectin on Nontarget Organisms

Because it is impossible to target a chemical pesticide solely to the pest causing crop damage, it is necessary to determine the effects of pesticide use on nontarget organisms. The safety of pesticides to nontarget organisms can be assessed by a comparison of the information derived from a series of tests in various indicator organisms and actual residue data. The toxicity data presented here are unpublished (Wislocki *et al.*).

A. Aquatic Organisms

Although abamectin will not be applied directly to surface water, some exposure could occur either via drift during the course of application or through runoff from treated fields. Therefore, it is important to assess abamectin's toxicity to aquatic organisms that may inhabit waters adjacent to treated areas.

1. Invertebrates: Acute Toxicity

Invertebrates vary widely in their sensitivity to abamectin. (Studies were performed by Springborn Life Sciences, Wareham, MA.) As seen in Table 13.1, mysid shrimp are the most sensitive invertebrate. The 96-hour LC_{50} for mysid shrimp, an estuarine organism, was 0.022 ppb. Pink shrimp, however, had a 96-hour LC_{50} of 1.6 ppb, 2 orders of magnitude higher than for the mysid shrimp. Daphnia, a freshwater invertebrate, had a 48-hour LC_{50} of 340 ppt. Both blue crabs and Eastern oysters were much less sensitive to the toxic effects of abamectin. They had 96-hour LC_{50} values of 153 and 430 ppb, respectively. The water photolysis products of avermectin B_{1a} and the major soil metabolite. 8a-hydroxyavermectin B_{1a} were also tested for their acute toxicity to Daphnia by ABC Laboratories (Columbia, MO). These degradation products were much less toxic than the parent compound (Table 13.2). The polar fraction—which is the terminal degradation product of the photolysis of abamectin in water—had an LC_{50} of greater than 100 ppb, more than 160 times that of avermectin B_{1a}, which had an LC_{50} of 0.63 ppb. The moderately polar fraction (which is formed transiently) was 10 times less toxic than its parent compound. The delta-8,9 isomer and the

TABLE 13.1. Acute toxicity of abamectin to aquatic invertebrates.

Invertebrate	LC_{50} (ppb)[a]
Daphnia *(Daphnia magna)*	0.34
Pink Shrimp *(Panaeus duorarum)*	1.6
Mysid shrimp *(Mysidopsis bahia)*	0.022
Eastern oysters *(Crassostrea virginica)*[b]	430
Blue crab *(Callinectes sapidus)*	153

[a] The LC_{50} values are after 96 hours of exposure, except for Daphnia, which represents 48 hours of exposure.
[b] Exposure occurred at the embryo-larval stage of the life cycle

TABLE 13.2. Acute toxicity of avermectin B_{1a} degradates to Daphnia.

Degradates[a]	LC_{50} at 48 hours (ppb)
Polar	>100
Moderately polar	6.8
delta 8,9-isomer of avermectin B_{1a}	27.2
8a-hydroxyavermectin B_{1a}	26

[a] All degradates were isolated from a water photolysis reaction, except 8a-hydroxyavermectin B_{1a}, which was made synthetically.

8a-hydroxy derivative were 40 times less toxic than avermectin B_{1a}. Therefore, abamectin degrades to less toxic metabolites.

2. Fish: Acute Toxicity

The acute toxicity of abamectin has been determined in 5 different species of fish (Table 13.3). Their response to abamectin is much more uniform than that observed for invertebrates. The LC_{50} for rainbow trout is 3.2 ppb, while that for bluegill sunfish is 9.6 ppb. (Studies were performed by Springborn Life Sciences, Wareham, MA.) The sheepshead minnow, an estuarine fish tested for toxicity, had an LC_{50} of 15 ppb. The channel catfish and carp had higher LC_{50} values, of 24 and 42 ppb, respectively, when determined by ABC Laboratories (Columbia, MO). There was only a 1 order of magnitude difference among the fish species examined, while there were 4 orders of magnitude difference among the invertebrate species examined.

3. Chronic Toxicity

The results of the environmental fate studies indicate that chronic exposure to abamectin should be minimal and without effects. Its rapid photolytic degradation and strong binding to sediment preclude its being bioavailable to aquatic organisms in a chronic manner. Nonetheless, 3 chronic exposure studies have been performed (Table 13.4). Full life-cycle studies have been done with daphnia and mysid shrimp. (Studies were performed by Springborn Life Sciences, Wareham, MA.) An early

TABLE 13.3. Acute toxicity of abamectin to fish.

Fish	LC_{50} at 96 hours of exposure (ppb)
Rainbow trout	3.2
Bluegill sunfish	9.6
Sheepshead minnow	15
Channel catfish	24
Carp	42

TABLE 13.4. Chronic toxicity of abamectin to aquatic organisms.

Organism	MATC (ppb)[a]	ACR[b]
Daphnia *(Daphnia magna)*, life cycle	0.03–0.09	6.5
Mysid *(Mysidopsis bahia)*, life cycle	0.0035–0.0093	3.8
Rainbow trout, early life stage	0.52–0.95	4.6

[a] The maximum acceptable toxicant concentration (MATC) is expressed as a value between the highest no-effect level (NOEL) and the lowest effect level (LEL).

[b] The acute-to-chronic ratio (ACR) is obtained by dividing the LC_{50} by the MATC. The MATC for this calculation was determined by calculating the geometric mean of the NOEL and LEL.

life-stage study was performed with rainbow trout by ABC Laboratories (Columbia, MO). In all 3 cases abamectin had no chronic effects. The difference between the LC_{50} determined in each species and the no-effect level (NOEL) observed in the chronic study was less than tenfold. The NOELs observed were 30, 3.5, and 520 ppt for Daphnia, mysid shrimp, and rainbow trout, respectively. A common way of expressing the no-effect level in a chronic study is to determine the maximum acceptable toxicant concentration (MATC). This value is the geometric mean of the NOEL and the lowest effect level (LEL). When the acute-to-chronic ratio (ACR), the ratio of the LC_{50} to the MATC, was determined, it was found that the ACRs were in the range of 4 to 7. This indicates that abamectin would not have chronic effects on these test organisms but could exhibit acute effects.

4. Plants

Abamectin is essentially nonphytotoxic, permitting its use even on sensitive ornamental plants. Its phytotoxicity to nontarget terrestrial plants will be discussed in Chapter 20. However, 2 studies were performed to assess its phytotoxicity to aquatic plants. (Studies were performed by Springborn Life Sciences, Wareham, MA.) These studies indicated that abamectin was relatively nontoxic to duckweed *(Lemna gibba)* and to freshwater algae *(Selenastrum capricornatum)*. The concentration of abamectin calculated to decrease frond production in duckweed by 50% was 3.9 ppm. A concentration greater than 100 ppm would be required to reduce the algae cell proliferation by 50%.

5. Conclusions

Aquatic organisms vary greatly in their sensitivity to abamectin. Aquatic plants are only minimally affected by high concentrations of abamectin. Certain invertebrates, however, are quite sensitive, with LC_{50} values in the ppt range, while other invertebrates are much less sensitive. Fish are fairly uniform in their response to abamectin and are 2 to 3 orders of magnitude less sensitive than mysid shrimp. Degradation products of abamectin are 1 to 3 orders of magnitude less toxic than abamectin itself.

B. Terrestrial Organisms

Despite the diversity of terrestrial organisms, only a limited number can be tested for the effects of pesticides. Certain organisms are chosen because of their importance to the environment. These include nitrogen-fixing bacteria, earthworms, bees, and birds. The effects of pesticides on mammalian species are determined during the assessment of the toxicity of the pesticide to humans when rodents and other mammalian species are used for extensive testing. The results of these tests on mammalian species are presented in Chapter 6.

1. Soil Micro- and Macroorganisms

The effect of abamectin on the bacteria, which convert ammonium ion to nitrate, was studied in humic sandy soil and loam soil by TNO (The Netherlands). Forty and 400 ppb abamectin had no effect on either the decrease in the level of ammonium ion or on the increase of nitrate. At a use rate of 0.025 lb active ingredient/acre, the maximum theoretical concentration of abamectin in the top inch of soil immediately following application would be approximately 85 ppb within the range of the experimental concentrations. Therefore, abamectin should not affect nitrogen-fixing bacteria.

Eisenia foetida was used to study the effects of abamectin on earthworms (Biospherics, MD). The 28-day LC_{50} was determined to be 38 ppm, indicating that the use of abamectin should not have an effect on earthworms.

2. Bees

The toxicity of abamectin to bees was assessed in laboratory studies by applying it directly to the bees, by putting it in their food, and by exposing the bees to foliage that had been treated at various times prior to harvesting (Atkins, personal communications). Abamectin was found to be quite toxic to the bees. In 2 studies it had contact LC_{50} values of 0.002 and 0.017 μg/bee at 24 and 48 hours, respectively. When abamectin was fed to bees, it had an LD_{50} of 0.009 μg/bee. However, citrus or alfalfa foliage that had been treated with abamectin 24 to 48 hours earlier was not toxic. Abamectin rapidly loses its toxicity to bees upon exposure to the environment.

3. Birds

The bobwhite quail and mallard duck are the species normally chosen for avian toxicity tests. In Table 13.5 the results of a number of studies with

TABLE 13.5. Toxicity of abamectin to birds.

Bird	LD_{50} (mg/kg)[a]	LC_{50} (ppm)[b]	Reproductive effects, NOEL (ppm)[c]
Mallard duck	[d]	383	12
Bobwhite quail	2000	3102	[d]

[a] Single oral dose.
[b] Birds were fed abamectin in the diet for 5 days and then fed regular diet for 3 days.
[c] Birds were fed abamectin for 18 weeks from prior to mating through egg laying.
[d] Not determined.

these two species are presented. The studies were performed by Wildlife International (Easton, MD). Abamectin was not very toxic to the bobwhite quail. The LD_{50} was greater than 2 g/kg. When quail were fed abamectin in their diet for 5 days, followed by 3 days on untreated feed, the LC_{50} was 3102 ppm. Mallard ducks were somewhat more sensitive: the LC_{50} after 5 days of dietary exposure was determined to be 383 ppm.

An avian reproduction study was performed in the mallard duck. When ducks were fed 3, 6, or 12 ppm abamectin in their diet for 18 weeks, there was no statistically significant effect on any parameter of reproduction. These dietary levels are greater than those which would occur in the environment.

4. Mammals

Mammalian toxicity data (discussed in detail in Chapter 6) indicate that abamectin has an LD_{50} of approximately 10.0 mg/kg in mice. Studies were also performed on the two degradation products, the delta 8,9 isomer of avermectin B_{1a} and the polar fraction. The delta 8,9 isomer is at least eightfold less acutely toxic than its parent compound, but it possesses the same level of subchronic toxicity. For this reason residue data now include the level of this isomer. The polar fraction isolated from the degradation of abamectin on glass is more than 500 times less acutely toxic than abamectin and is greater than 20 times less toxic in the most sensitive subchronic test.

5. Conclusions

Abamectin does not affect nitrogen-fixing bacteria, even at levels higher than those which would be present in the environment. At high concentrations abamectin can have a toxic effect on earthworms and birds. However, these effects occur at concentrations which are higher than those found in the environment. The toxicity of abamectin to bees is mitigated by its rapid degradation, such that residues of abamectin present on foliage 24 to 48 hours after treatment are not toxic. Abamectin's polar degradation fraction—the major degradation fraction—is much less toxic than abamectin itself.

IV. Risk Assessment

In order to assess the risk of a pesticide to the environment one must compare the exposure levels that cause a toxic effect with the exposure levels expected from using the compound. Environmental fate data yield an estimate of the environmental concentration, while toxicity studies indicate the concentration at which toxic effects can occur.

A. Aquatic Organisms

The rapid photolytic degradation of abamectin in water to much less toxic degradation products and its strong binding to soil indicate that levels of abamectin in water should be low. This was shown to be the case in the simulated field study, which should give the worst-case scenario for drift and runoff. To simulate drift, the water was sprayed directly with the diluted formulation. Under these conditions, some mixing occurred: this would decrease the amount of surface degradation. Also, both the runoff and drift tanks were covered with tarpaulins to prevent cross-contamination; since the treatments were applied in the afternoon, the tanks were not uncovered until the next morning, permitting mixing to occur prior to environmental exposure. Water analyses also included abamectin bound to particles suspended in the water. Therefore, the residue values obtained represented a worst-case situation—and even then they were very low.

The levels of abamectin in water resulting from runoff were in the range of only 1 to 3 ppt during the 15-day period after treatment, and lower thereafter. This level is below the lowest NOEL determined, which was in the mysid shrimp chronic life-cycle study (Table 13.4). The mysid shrimp is the most sensitive organism to the toxic effects of abamectin. The levels of abamectin resulting from drift are initially high, assuming that 5% of the applied pesticide impacted on the surface water. This level of abamectin is greater than would be expected, given the rapid photolysis abamectin would undergo as it drifted to the water and settled on the surface rather than being sprayed directly into the surface. Initial residue levels of 266 ppt are below the LC_{50} levels for even Daphnia, the freshwater organisms most sensitive to abamectin. These levels are also below the NOEL for rainbow trout determined in the early life-stage study. By 2 days the residues have decreased to 8 ppt, below the LC_{50} for mysid shrimp and below the NOEL for Daphnia. At 2 days the concentration of abamectin in water is at levels that may affect shrimp (8 ppt vs an

MATC of approximately 5 ppt). However, these are exaggerated residue levels derived from the tank study. A stagnant 2-foot-deep body of water is not representative of an estuary, which undergoes mixing from the influx of fresh water and the action of tides. Therefore, the use of abamectin should not have an acute or chronic effect on aquatic organisms.

B. Terrestrial Organisms

As indicated previously, the use of abamectin results in soil residue levels of 10 to 20 ppb in the top 2 inches of soil immediately after application. This level is not sufficient to have an effect on earthworms (LD_{50} of 28 ppm) or nitrogen-fixing bacteria (NOEL greater than 400 ppb). In fact, abamectin levels as high as 2000 ppm do not have antifungal or antibacterial activity (see Chapter 2). Abamectin foliar residues aged for 24 to 48 hours are not toxic to bees. Moreover, abamectin is not significantly toxic to nontarget beneficial insects (see Chapter 20). All these facts suggest that abamectin is a good candidate for use in integrated pest-management programs.

The concern over the impact of pesticides on terrestrial organisms centers on their effects on birds and mammals. It is also assumed that protecting these animals protects other animals, such as amphibians and reptiles. Abamectin is acutely toxic to birds. However, birds are much less sensitive to abamectin than are other species. The lowest LC_{50} observed, 383 ppm, was in the mallard duck (Table 13.5). The NOEL for reproductive effects in the mallard duck was 12 ppm. Therefore, if residue levels of abamectin on avian feedstuffs are below 12 ppm, no adverse acute or chronic effects on birds would be expected. One method used to determine the levels of residues of pesticides on foodstuffs for terrestrial animals is to use the data accumulated by Hoerger and Kenaga (1972) and Kenaga (1973). Those data—from residue trials and tolerances for a number of pesticides—were used to predict levels of residues in various foodstuffs (Table 13.6). Based on a use rate of 0.025 lb active ingredient/acre, theoretical residue levels greater than 12 ppm would not be expected. Therefore, the use of abamectin should not pose a risk to avian species.

By comparing the theoretical levels from Kenaga with those derived from the actual use of the compound, it can be seen that abamectin does not give the high initial levels predicted by Kenaga's calculations and it depletes very rapidly. This is due to its rapid photodegradation on surfaces (initial half-life of 4 to 6 hours). In the 20 celery trials performed in the United States, in which repeated applications were made, the average residue level was only 0.17 ppm, which is ¼ that proposed by Kenaga. Again, the residues deplete rapidly, to less than 0.01 ppm by 7 days. Mammalian species vary greatly in their sensitivity to abamectin.

TABLE 13.6. The theoretical maximum and typical concentrations of abamectin expected on terrestrial food items immediately after application of abamectin at 0.025 lb active ingredient (ai)/acre (citrus) and 0.02 lb ai/acre (cotton, vegetables) (Kenaga 1973).

	0.025 lb ai/acre		0.02 lb ai/acre	
Food items	Maximum (ppm)	Typical (ppm)	Maximum (ppm)	Typical (ppm)
Short grass	6.0	3.1	4.8	2.5
Long grass	2.7	2.3	2.2	1.8
Leafy crops, leaves	3.0	0.9	2.5	0.7
Forage, insects	1.5	0.8	1.2	0.7
Seed pods	0.3	0.12	0.2	0.1
Fruit	0.15	0.04	0.1	0.03

The lowest acute toxicity value, obtained in the weanling rat, was an LD_{50} of 1.5 mg/kg. If one assumes that a wild mammal will consume 20% of its body weight in food/day, it would have to ingest residue levels of 7.5 ppm, 44 times higher than the average found on celery, to reach the LD_{50} level. Several other factors should be mentioned. The exposure levels assume that all mammalian foodstuffs have the same residue level as the target crop. In actuality, this is not the case. Animals would also consume foodstuffs outside the direct application area, where residue levels would be lower. Also, laboratory animals were dosed by gavage, which has been shown to yield a twofold greater toxicity to abamectin than in feed administration. Thus an additional twofold safety factor exists for wild mammalian species.

The lowest subchronic toxicity value was obtained in the materno-toxicity-teratogenicity study in the CF-1 mouse. The NOEL was 0.05 mg/kg by gavage and 0.1 mg/kg in the diet. In this study multiple doses of abamectin were given. Using the dietary NOEL, a mammal which ingests 20% of its body weight in food/day would have to consume greater than 0.50 ppm of abamectin in the diet for several days. The low initial residue levels—which are 3 times lower than this amount—and the rapid degradation eliminate the possiblility of continuous exposure: no maternotoxic or teratogenic effects should occur.

Residues in fruit are much lower than those in celery, and, therefore, no effects from fruit consumption should occur. Insects are a major food source for certain mammals. Given the low residue levels on plants and the rapid degradation of abamectin, insects will not have high residues of abamectin. Insects will not bioconcentrate residues of abamectin. A study by Bull (1986) demonstrated that the half-life of abamectin in insects is less than a half a day. Insects should not contain abamectin residues at levels sufficient to be toxic to those animals consuming them.

V. Conclusions

Abamectin neither persists nor accumulates in the environment. It rapidly photolyzes in water, on soil, and as a thin film on both inert and biological surfaces. Soil metabolizes abamectin at a moderate rate. Its strong binding to soil prevents it from entering the aquatic environment, reduces its concentration in water, and limits its bioavailability. These characteristics reduce the environmental exposure to abamectin to a level below that which would cause effects on aquatic or terrestrial organisms. Therefore, when label directions are followed, abamectin can be used in an environmentally safe manner.

References

Brooke DN, Dobbs AJ, Williams N (1986) Octanol water partition coefficients (P): measurement, estimation and interpretation, particularly for chemicals with P 10^5. *Ecotox. & Envir. Safety* 11:251–260

Bull DL (1986) Toxicity and pharmacodynamics of avermectin in the tobacco budworm, corn earworm and fall armyworm *(Noctuidae lepidoptera). J. Agric. Food Chem.* 34:74–78

Bull DL, Ivie GW, MacConnell JG, Gruber VF, Ku CC, Arison BH, Stevenson JM, VandenHeuval WJA (1984) Fate of avermectin B1a in soil and plants. *J. Agric. Food Chem.* 32:94–102

Hoerger FD, Kenaga EE (1972) Pesticide residues in plants. Correlation of representative data as a basis for estimation of their magnitude in the environment. In F. Coulston and F. Korte (eds) *Environmental Quality,* Vol 1, Academic Press, New York, pp 9–28

Iwata I, MacConnell JG, Flor JE, Putter I, Dinhoff TM (1985) Residues of avermectin B_{1a} on and in citrus fruits and foliage. *J. Agric. Food Chem.* 33:467–471

Kenaga EE (1973) Factors to be considered in the evaluation of the toxicity of pesticides to birds in their environment. In F. Coulston and F. Korte (eds) *Environmental Quality and Safety,* Vol 2, Academic Press, New York, pp 161–181

May WE, Wasik SP (1978) Determination of the aqueous solubility of the polynuclear aromatic hydrocarbons by a coupled liquid chromatography technique. *Anal. Chem. 50:175–182*

Maynard MS, Iwata Y, Wislocki PG, Ku CC, Jacob TA, (1989) The fate of avermectin B_{1a} on citrus fruits: 1. Distribution and magnitude of the ^{14}C residue and avermectin B_{1a} on citrus fruits from a field study. *J. Agric. Food Chem.* 37:178–183

Moye HA, Malagodi MH, Yoh J, Leibee GL, Ku CC, Wislocki PG (1987) Residues of avermectin B_{1a} in rotational crops and soils following soil treatment with [^{14}C] avermectin B_{1a}. *J. Agric. Food Chem.* 35:859–864

Mrozik H, Eskola P, Reynolds GF, Arison BH, Smith GM, Fisher MH (1988) Photoisomers of avermectins. *J. Org. Chem.* 53:1820–1823

CHAPTER 14

Worker Safety Aspects of Abamectin Use in Crop Protection

L.S. Grosso, R.A. Dybas, and S.F. Rickard

I. Introduction

Abamectin is the avermectin selected for agricultural use. Its various formulations, and the uses that have been developed, are described in Chapter 20.

Although abamectin is applied to ornamental plants, crops, and trees at extremely low rates, its high oral mammalian toxicity (Chapter 6) initially raised concern regarding the safety of workers mixing, loading, and applying the product, as well as those harvesting treated crops. An established quantitative exposure model developed for registered pesticides indicated a significant correlation between dermal exposure and application rate (Reinert and Severn 1985). The exposure model was based on data generated from exposure monitoring of workers in orchards during ground application of pesticides using high-pressure or airblast equipment. A linear regression analysis of the data failed to intercept the origin, thus predicting substantial exposure to such products used at low rates of application. The reported values are normalized to 3000 cm^2 of exposed skin, the amount for an applicator wearing long pants, a short-sleeved open-necked shirt, and no gloves or facial protection. The authors argue that the correlation ($r=0.7$) permits an estimate of exposure during airblast application of any pesticide with a certain level of confidence. It should be pointed out that the model does not consider the bioavailability of individual products (such as dermal penetration), and thereby again overestimates exposure.

The studies on which the exposure model was based were conducted with pesticide products used at conventional rates of application (0.25 to

8.0 lbs active ingredient/acre). Obviously, the model greatly overestimates exposures for lower application rates. To demonstrate actual exposure data for abamectin when applied with similar equipment, a worker-exposure study was conducted using conventional airblast equipment in typical California citrus groves, under typical working conditions. Airblast equipment was chosen because this application method has been reported to result in the highest levels of exposure. Moreover, the results could be used as a "worst-case" approximation for other application methods.

The safety to agricultural workers reentering and harvesting crops treated with abamectin was also a concern during the early phases of product development. It is widely accepted that reentry into pesticide-treated sites can present a significant hazard to workers/harvesters. This has been especially true with the acutely toxic organophosphates and carbamates. Worker exposure is mainly by dermal contact with residues sorbed to particulate matter. Measurement of dislodgeable residues is therefore a means of estimating worker exposure to a pesticide during routine harvesting practices (Gunther *et al.* 1977).

Workers can be exposed to foliar pesticide residues via dermal contact and inhalation. Most evidence from field studies now indicates that greater than 99% of total exposure to pesticides occurs by dermal contact (hands and forearms) with residues bound to particulate matter on foliage (Zweig *et al.* 1984). Transfer of pesticide residues to humans during reentry activities is governed more by the physical nature of the residues than by their chemical properties. Inhalation exposure to vapor phase and particulate residue also occurs, but it is minor—1% of the dermal exposure. Inhalation exposure of workers to abamectin residues is considered to be negligible due to the extremely low vapor pressure of the compound ($<1.5\times10^{-9}$ torr), coupled with its low application rate.

Pesticide residues sorbed to particulate matter adhering to foliar or fruit surfaces are measured as dislodgeable foliar residues (DFR) by techniques developed by Iwata and colleagues (1977). Zweig and colleagues (1984) have summarized the results of 35 field studies on human dermal exposure and dislodgeable foliar residues (DFR) from harvesting operations on a number of crops with a variety of pesticides. Table 14.1 lists the ratios of dermal exposure to dislodgeable foliar residues obtained. Considering the variety of pesticides and crops studied, the calculated ratios are very similar, and thus there appears to be a good correlation between dermal exposure and dislodgeable pesticide residues. Therefore, Zweig and colleagues (1984) have proposed that it should be possible to calculate daily dermal exposure of workers/harvesters, as a first approximation, by multiplying the dislodgeable foliar residue concentration (DFR: $\mu g/cm^2$) obtained experimentally by the empirical factor 5000. The resulting Zweig-Popendorf Factor is 5000 cm^2/hour.

To utilize the Zweig-Popendorf Factor, dislodgeable foliar residue

TABLE 14.1. Ratios of dermal exposure to dislodgeable foliar residues.

Pesticide	Crop	Activity	$R \times 10^{-3}$
Carbaryl (day 1)	Strawberries	Harvesting	4.34
Carbaryl (day 2)	Strawberries	Harvesting	2.82
Carbaryl (day 3)	Strawberries	Harvesting	6.17
Captan	Strawberries	Harvesting	6.17
Captan	Strawberries	Harvesting	8.57
Captan	Strawberries	Harvesting	2.90
Captan	Strawberries	Harvesting	8.00
Captan	Strawberries	Harvesting	2.62
Captan	Strawberries	Harvesting	5.97
Captan	Strawberries	Harvesting	4.73
Benomyl	Strawberries	Harvesting	7.19
Benomyl	Apples	Thinning	0.5
Chlorobenzilate	Citrus	Harvesting	5.33[a]
OP Compounds	Citrus	Harvesting	5.1[b]
OP Compounds	Peaches	Harvesting	1.9[c]
Empirical Factor = 5×10^3			

[a] Corrected for one side of the leaf surface.
[b] Geometric mean from 14 observations.
[c] Geometric mean from 9 observations.
(From Zweig *et al.*, (1984) *J. Agric. Food Chem.* 32:1232.)

studies with abamectin were conducted on the labor-intensive crop, ornamental chrysanthemums. Abamectin residues on chrysanthemum were obtained from leaf-punch samples from greenhouse-grown cultivars. To prove the correlation factor as proposed by Zweig and colleagues (1984), an actual worker reentry study was conducted using greenhouse grown chrysanthemums in Holland under conditions and practices typical of that country.

The data developed for the tasks of mixing/loading and application of abamectin to citrus trees, as well as for harvesting citrus and ornamental crops, can be used in conjunction with the toxicology data as presented in Chapter 6 to calculate the margins of safety (MOS) of the product to the workers.

II. Worker Exposure to Abamectin during Airblast Treatment of Citrus Groves

Abamectin is formulated as a 0.15 lb/gallon emulsifiable concentrate (0.15 EC) for use on a variety of crops. Because exposure during airblast application is generally considered to be a "worst case," typical conditions of mixing/loading and application of the product in citrus groves were tested. The study involved a total of 4 applications: 3 consisted of 3 tankloads and 1 of 4 tankloads, for a total of 13 monitorings during 4 work periods of 4 hours each. Rates of exposure were calculated for workers wearing long-sleeved chambray shirts, long denim pants, and shoes. Test conditions also included the wearing of gloves, and the effectiveness of minimal hygiene. Measured residues were corrected for recoveries from field-fortified (spiked) controls. For residue values less than the sensitivity of the detection method, 50% of the method's sensitivity was used as the magnitude of the residue. For example, with a sensitivity of 0.5 $\mu g/cm^2$, nondetectable residues were reported as 0.25 $\mu g/cm^2$ for the purposes of quantitation.

With the exception of exposure of the hands, dermal exposure was measured with multilayer dosimeters affixed to full-body protective suits. The dosimeters were placed at conventional locations to represent body areas for which surface areas have been estimated: back of neck, front and "V" of neck, shoulders/upper arms, forearms and wrists, thighs, and ankles/lower legs. Three types of dosimeters were used for each worker. These were:

- Conventional clothing I: 100% lightweight cotton shirt material on the upper body; 65/35% polyester/cotton pants material on the lower body.
- Conventional clothing II: 65/35% lightweight polyester/cotton chambray shirt material on the upper body; 100% cotton work-weight denim material on the lower body.
- Protective clothing I: 100% cotton coverall material on upper and lower body dosimeters.

A total of 42 dosimeters were tested on each person. Exposure of the face was estimated by swabbing 4 areas of 20 cm^2 each: forehead, left cheek, right cheek, and throat. Because the workers wore goggles and respirators, the swabs were taken from areas not covered by protective gear. Exposure of hands was measured from total residue in hand rinses. Exposure by inhalation was measured by sampling the air in the worker's breathing zone with an MSA Fixt-Flo personal air pump, and charcoal tube traps. For each type of measurement, samples spiked in the field were used as concurrent recovery and stability controls.

There were no detectable residues in charcoal air-monitoring tubes; therefore, inhalation exposures were not calculated. Using the industrial hygiene convention, a lognormal distribution was chosen to represent the data. This convention is based on the understanding that the conditions conducive to (but not all necessary for) the occurrence of lognormal distributions are found in occupational environmental data (Leidel, Busch, and Lynch 1977).

Table 14.2 presents the geometric means and geometric standard deviations calculated from the adjusted measured values. For risk-assessment purposes, unprotected whole-body exposure was compared to dermal exposure calculated from residues when wearing conventional clothing II (chambray shirt and denim pants) and gloves over washed hands.

As shown in Table 14.2, the exposure/minute was greater for mixer/

TABLE 14.2. Worker exposure to abamectin.

Unprotected whole body exposure		Adjusted ng ai/minute	Adjusted ng ai/g ai/handled
Mixer/loader	Geometric mean	24,915	14,111
	GSD[a]	4.74	4.60
Sprayer	Geometric mean	7547	7989
	GSD	4.88	4.32
Wearing long pants long sleeve shirt, impermeable gloves, and washing hands			
Mixer/loader	Geometric mean	604	342
	GSD	1.51	1.29
Sprayer	Geometric mean	414	439
	GSD	1.79	1.60

[a] As an estimator of the variance of the data, the geometric mean is multiplied and divided by the geometric standard deviation (GSD).

loaders than for sprayers. This is consistent with previously published field studies (Reinert and Severn 1985). When gloves were not worn, the exposure/g ai handled for mixers was also greater than for sprayers. Also, most of the reduction in exposure was due to the wearing of gloves. However, when gloves were worn, the exposure/g ai handled was essentially similar for mixers and sprayers.

Table 14.2 also shows that wearing denim long pants and chambray long-sleeved shirt can reduce total bodily exposure irrespective of facial washings by more than 94% compared to unprotected whole-body exposure (regardless of rate function): this is consistent with popular assumptions of 80% to 100% protection by clothing (Reinert *et al.* 1987). Also, most of the reduction in exposure was due to wearing gloves. However, almost all of the exposure calculated for clothed skin resulted from the fact that more than 50% of the totals were contributed by using 50% of the method's sensitivity in the calculations for these residues on dosimeters that were below the sensitivity of the method (5ng/cm^2). Actual exposure would be considerably lower than calculated exposure. Cloth was highly effective in trapping abamectin residues. This was not unexpected, as abamectin is known to bind to cellulosic and other substrates very well.

To conclude, the actual rates of exposure for workers in this study would be less than 50% of the calculated rates; the estimates are extremely conservative, as 50% of the limit of sensitivity of the analytical method was added in each case where there were no detectable residues. Due to the low expected exposure to abamectin, workers were monitored for a 4-hour period (1/2 workday) while applying 3 tankloads of spray

(1 replicate included 4 tankloads) rather than single tankloads (as is the convention for these studies).

Calculations of margins of safety (MOS) to the exposure conditions described may be computed utilizing the toxicology data from Chapter 6 as follows:

- Lowest no-effect level of abamectin technical based on maternotoxicity in the CF-1 mouse—0.05 mg/kg/day by oral gavage.
- Monkey dermal penetration is less than 1% using ^{3}H—abamectin technical; ^{3}H—abamectin in the 0.15 EC undiluted; or ^{3}H—abamectin 0.15 EC diluted in water

The CF-1 mouse is extremely sensitive to abamectin and provides a very conservative model for predicting the safety of abamectin to humans. Data discussed in Chapter 6 demonstrate that primates (rhesus monkeys) are far less sensitive to abamectin than the CF-1 muose or any of the other mammalian species tested. Also, human data available on ivermectin, the human and animal health drug analog of abamectin, further support the safety of abamectin in humans. In fact, the clinical dosages of ivermectin in animals and humans range from 0.15 to 0.3 mg/kg, and even the lowest of these is lethal to the CF-1 mouse.

The dermal penetration of abamectin is extremely low: less than 1% when applied either as the technical material or in the 0.15 EC formulation, diluted or undiluted. The following analysis compares the MOS for workers who are unprotected with those who use typical protective clothing and personal hygiene during airblast application of abamectin at 0.025 lb ai/acre to citrus. The exposure data for each of these test conditions are presented in 2 different ways. The traditional expression of pesticide exposure to applicators is an amount of active ingredient per unit of time. The first set of MOS calculations, therefore, presents the geometric mean exposures in ng/minute. These values are then adjusted for the length of time the particular task is performed during a typical workday; i.e., 1 hour for mixers/loaders and 8 hours for sprayers.

The second set of MOS calculations presents the geometric mean exposures in ng of active ingredient per gram of active ingredient handled. These values are then adjusted for the total amount of active ingredient handled by each worker type during a typical workday in which a maximum of 20 acres of citrus would be treated by airblast sprayer. Therefore, mixers/loaders and sprayers would handle the following amount of abamectin active ingredient per day

$$20 \text{ acres/day} \times 11.34 \text{ grams ai/acre} = 226.8 \text{ grams ai/day}$$
$$(0.025 \text{ lb ai/acre} = 11.34 \text{ g ai/acre})$$

Margins of safety for the methods of exposure expression are calculated as follows:

Exposure expressed as active ingredient per time
Exposure = ng/min × 10^{-6} mg/ng × 60 min/hr × 1/60 kg
Exposure = mg ai/kg body weight hour
Factoring for dermal penetration (dfp)—1%
Exposure = mg/kg/hr × 100^{-1}
MOS = *NOEL (mg/kg)* ÷ Exposure (mg/kg/hr) × 1/100
Exposure for mixer/loader = mg/kg/hr
Exposure for sprayers = mg/kg/8hr
Exposure expressed as active ingredient per gram active ingredient handled
Exposure = ng/g ai × 10^{-6} mg/ng × 0.5 lbs ai/day × 454 gr/lb × 1/60 kg
Factoring for dermal penetration (dfp)—1%
Exposure = mg/kg/day × 1/100
MOS for mixers/loaders/applicators = NOEL (mg/kg/day) ÷ Exposure (mg/kg/day) × 1/100

Table 14.3 compares the Margins of Safety based on time of exposure and amount of active ingredient handled between mixers/loaders and applicators for whole body unprotected and when wearing conventional clothing (chambray shirt and denim pants) and using personal hygiene.

Margins of Safety (MOS) have been presented for agricultural workers who handle the product during mixing, loading, and application functions. Actual human-exposure values have been measured for these tasks under typical conditions reflective of product labels approved by regulatory agencies in various countries. The exposure data developed for abamectin

TABLE 14.3. Abamectin margins of safety (MOS) based on maternotoxicity for pesticide applicators-mixers/loaders and sprayers.

MOS based on time of exposure/per day[a]	Mixers/loaders	Sprayers
Unprotected whole body exposure	200	83
Protected whole body exposure	8333	1562
MOS based on amount ai handled per day[b]	Mixers/Loaders	Sprayers
Unprotected whole body exposure	94	166
Protected whole body exposure	3846	3030

[a] Mixers/Loaders handle pesticides for a maximum of 1 hour per day to prepare sufficient material for sprayers to work for a maximum of 8 hours.
[b] The quantity of active ingredient handled is based on a maximum of 20 acres treated per day.

clearly show that the existing model available for applicators grossly overestimates exposure. Based on the available safety data on the avermectins in the most sensitive model (CF-1 mouse), in addition to human data and exposure data, we believe that there are adequate margins of safety for workers who mix/load or spray abamectin using airblast equipment with or without the use of conventional clothing.

III. Worker Exposure to Abamectin during Reentry

To estimate the safety of abamectin to workers harvesting ornamental plants by utilizing the Zweig-Popendorf Correlation, a dislodgeable foliar residue study was conducted in a commercial chrysanthemum propagation greenhouse at DeLier, Netherlands. Abamectin was applied in 3 weekly applications of 27 g ai/hectare (0.024 lb ai/acre) as 1.5 l formulation of the 1.8EC (18 g/l EC) in 1500 l of water per hectare.

Surface extracts from the abamectin-treated chrysanthemum foliage were prepared for assay by the method of Gunther and colleagues (1977) to determine dislodgeable foliar residues to which workers might be exposed while harvesting cuttings from the treated plants. Of the various production tasks, harvesting of chrysanthemum propagation cuttings is believed to represent the most labor-intensive and "worst case" for worker exposure to pesticide residues in greenhouse operations. Because DFR data are commonly used to estimate exposure for workers entering treated crop areas to perform cultural tasks, they are used in making a risk assessment to determine margins of safety (MOS) for the worker (Adams 1984). In this procedure, the empirically derived Zweig-Popendorf Factor of 5000 cm^2/hour (based on one surface of the leaf, as were these data) is applied to the DFR data to estimate exposure. The Zweig-Popendorf Factor provides a very conservative estimate of worker safety, since exposure values are derived from harvesters wearing cotton gloves (which are known to significantly overestimate residues on the hands).

Leaf-punch samples for residue analysis were collected directly into separate glass jars from each of 2 untreated and 4 treated plots before and at 2, 4, 8, 16, and 24 to 30 hours, and at 3 and 7 days after the third application. Immediately after collection, surface residues of abamectin were removed from the leaf discs, and the aqueous solutions were frozen until analyzed by an HPLC-fluorescence method for residues of abamectin (avermectin B_{1a} and avermectin B_{1b}) and its corresponding Δ8, 9-isomer. Residues were reported on a leaf surface area and used to predict dermal exposure and margins of safety for workers. Extra leaf punches from the control plots were collected to be used as control and field fortification samples; these samples measured the abamectin stability and recovery through sample preparation, storage, and assay.

The results of the study are summarized in Table 14.4. The dissipa-

TABLE 14.4. Dislodgeable foliar residues of abamectin and its 8,9-isomer on chrysanthemum (average of 4 replicates).

Sampling time	Total residues (ng/cm^2) with standard deviation deviation
Before 3rd Spray	1.30 ± 0.52
2-hr. post spray	22.04 ± 1.74
4-hr. post spray	19.85 ± 1.68
8-hr. post spray	21.50 ± 3.95
16-hr. post spray	21.92 ± 2.33
24–30 hr. post spray	11.59 ± 1.06
3 days	5.16 ± 0.62
7 days	2.16 ± 0.89

tion curve for both residue species is similar (Figure 14.1). The "prior to last application" samples for all 4 treated plots had average avermectin $B_{1a}/\Delta 8,9$-isomer residues of 1.2 ng/cm^2 and 0.14 ng/cm^2 avermectin B_{1b}. The residues at 2 hours following the last application averaged 19.2 ng/cm^2 for the combined residues of $B_{1a}/\Delta 8.9$ isomer and 2.9 ng/cm^2 avermectin B_{1b}. Abamectin is unstable in the presence of sunlight, but these residues did not decay through Hour 16, as the treated chrysanthemums were protected from light in the late afternoon by drawing close the greenhouse thermal shades. Between Hours 16 and 30, after the thermal shades were opened, the residues decayed, with average residues at 30 hours of 10.1 ng/cm^2 avermectin B_{1a} and 1.5 ng/cm^2 avermectin B_{1b}. At 7 days after the last application, residues averaged 1.9 ng/cm^2 avermectin B_{1a} and 0.23 ng/cm^2 avermectin B_{1b}, essentially identical to the residues found at 7 days following the second of 3 applications. No buildup or accumulation of residues was observed following multiple applications in greenhouse conditions. No difference was found in the recoveries from leaf disc samples spiked in the field and those spiked in the laboratory. Application of the Zweig-Popendorf Factor to the DFR data from this study results in the following estimate of worker exposure to abamectin residues. The average for total DFR residues of abamectin and its $\Delta 8,9$-isomer was 22 ng/cm^2 at 16 hours after the third of 3 weekly sprays at the recommended rate of 27 g abamectin/hectare, immediately prior to the reentry phase.

DFR = 22 ng/cm^2 or 0.022 μg/cm^2
Zweig-Popendorf Factor = 5,000 cm^2/hr
Assume 8-hour workday and 60-kg person

$$\textit{Exposure} = 0.022\ \mu g/cm^2 \times 5000\ cm^2/hr \times 8\ hrs$$
$$= 880\ \mu g/person/day$$

OR

$$\textit{Exposure} = 880\mu g/person/day = 14.7\ \mu g/kg/day \text{ for a 60 kg person}$$

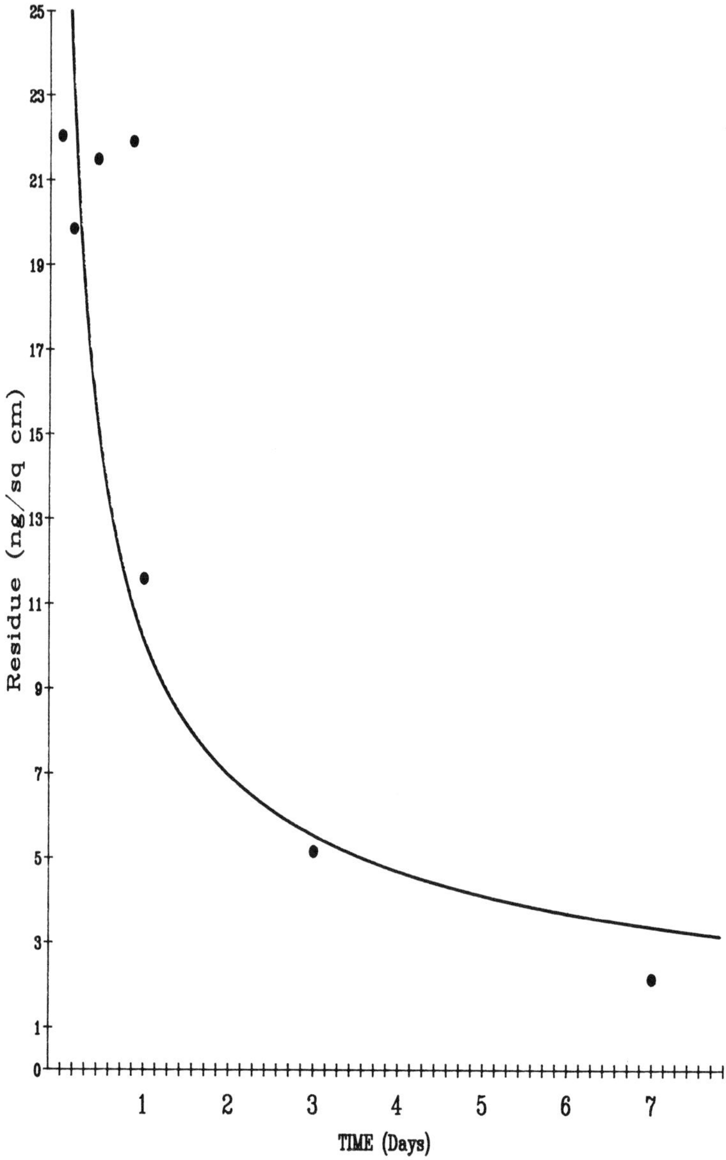

FIGURE 14.1. Abamectin 8,9 isomer dislodgeable residue dissipation.

The margins of safety (MOS) for exposure of harvesters to abamectin dislodgeable foliar residues are calculated as a ratio of exposure to the lowest NOEL for toxicological effects. For abamectin, the lowest NOEL is 0.05 mg/kg/day for maternotoxicity in CF-1 mice. The dermal penetration factor as developed in monkeys is less than 1%.

$$\begin{aligned} \text{NOEL} &= 50\ \mu g/kg/day \\ \text{Exposure} &= 14.7\ \mu g/kg/day \\ \text{MOS} &= \text{NOEL/exposure} \times 100\ \text{(dpf)} \\ &= \frac{50}{14.7} \times 100 = 340 \\ \text{MOS} &= 340 \text{ for maternotoxicity} \end{aligned}$$

It was believed that this worker exposure of 14.7 μg/kg/day from foliar residues of abamectin estimated via the Zweig-Popendorf Factor was an overestimate of exposure, resulting in a very conservative MOS.

To confirm the accuracy of the Zweig-Popendorf Factor with abamectin under the same greenhouse conditions, an actual worker reentry study was conducted in the Netherlands. This study measures the dermal exposure of workers to foliar residues of abamectin during harvest of propagation cuttings from greenhouse-grown chrysanthemums that had been treated with abamectin (0.15 EC) at its maximum recommended use rate. Residues from coveralls, hats, gloves, and hand rinses of harvesters were used to estimate exposure, which was then used in a risk assessment to determine margins of safety for workers involved in the culture and production of greenhouse ornamentals.

The study was conducted in the same commercial chrysanthemum propagation greenhouse at DeLier, Netherlands as that used for the DFR study. Each of 4 workers was dressed in a disposable Tyvek spun-olefin coverall and baseball hat with prepared dosimeters attached to the front and the back of the hat, the chest, back, upper and lower arms, and upper and lower legs. The workers wore cotton gloves. Each worker was assigned to a separate treated plot for harvesting. At the end of each of four 1-hour work periods, the dosimeters and gloves were removed into separate numbered bags. After the gloves were removed, each worker's hands were rinsed 3 times. Control and fortified (spiked) samples from the field, along with the experimental samples, were immediately frozen following their collection for subsequent analysis using an HPLC-fluorescence method which determines abamectin (avermectin B_{1a} and avermectin B_{1b}) and the Δ8,9-isomer.

Abamectin residues were found only on the gloves, lower-leg dosimeters, and in the hand-rinse solutions; in 1 case low-level residues were found on the chest dosimeter. The data are presented in Table 14.5.

Average exposure was 70,863 ng/hr with a coefficient of variation (CV) of 5.4%. Approximately 97% of the total exposure was on the hands, 3% on the clothing, and less than 1% on the face and clothed body. Because 50% of the limit of quantitation was used when no residues were measured on a given dosimeter, calculated exposures of the face and neck (except in 1 case) and the clothed body were calculational artifacts that were insignificant in estimating exposure. Body protection by long pants

TABLE 14.5. Individual worker exposure data.

Worker body no.	Total (ng/hr)	Hands	Face & neck	Clothes	Body
.101	76,546	74,184	80	2054	227
.102	70,069	66,088	132	3284	566
.103	68,299	66,212	80	1780	227
.104	68,537	66,488	80	1742	227
Average:	70,863	68,243	93	2215	312
S.D.	3869	3964	26	726	169

and long-sleeved shirt was minimal since 97% of exposure occurred on the hands. When body exposure occurred, it was usually only the lower leg dosimeters that had been in contact with treated foliage.

Residue concentration in cotton gloves is believed to grossly overestimate exposure from actual residues present and available for dermal penetration of the workers' hands (Reinert *et al.* 1987). This is supported by previously reported studies in which cotton gloves were clearly shown to represent a "worst case" for estimating potential exposure of the hands to dislodgeable residues. Because of its almost irreversible binding to cellulosic and other fibers in the gloves, abamectin would not be dislodged from gloves or penetrate through to the hand. This was shown by finding 99.7% of hand exposure in the glove extracts and less than 0.3% of the total residue in the solvent hand rinse. Average residues in gloves from other studies reported in the literature are usually 3 to 10 times those in solvent rinses.

From the exposure data presented above, MOS may be determined for the greenhouse harvester of abamectin-treated chrysanthemums. The following calculations assume an 8-hour workday, 1% dermal penetration for abamectin, and a 60-kg person:

$$
\begin{aligned}
\textit{Exposure} &= 70.86\ \mu\text{g/worker/hour} = 567\ \mu\text{g/worker/8-hr workday} \\
&= 9.45\ \mu\text{g/kg/day dermal exposure for a 60-kg person} \\
&= 9.45\ \mu\text{g/kg/day} \times 1\%\ \text{dermal penetration} \\
&= 0.0945\ \mu\text{g/kg/day systemic exposure} \\
\textit{NOEL} &= \text{Maternotoxicity in CF-1 mouse } 0.05\ \text{mg/kg/day} \\
\textit{MOS} &= \frac{\text{NOEL}}{\text{Systemic exposure}} \\
&= \frac{50\ \mu\text{g/kg/day}}{0.0945\ \mu\text{g/kg/day}} \\
&= 529
\end{aligned}
$$

The actual exposure value of 9.45 μg/kg/day developed in this study agrees well with the calculated value of 14.7 μg/kg/day based on measured foliar dislodgeable residues and using the Zweig-Popendorf Factor. A similar DFR study was also conducted by Merck Sharp &

TABLE 14.6. Harvester exposure.

Study site	Basis	Worker Exposure	MOS Maternotoxicity
Netherlands	Actual worker exposure	9.45 μg/kg/day	529
Netherlands	Predicted exposure from DFR	14.7 μg/kg/day	340
California	Predicted exposure from DFR	10.7 μg/kg/day	467

Dohme Research Laboratories in California (Jenkins *et al.* 1987). In this study AVID 0.15 EC was applied to greenhouse-grown chrysanthemums twice, 5 days apart, at 28 g abamectin per hectare (0.025 lb ai/acre) in 2338 l of water. At 2 hours after the second spray, total DFRs of abamectin and its 8.9 isomer were present at 16 ng/cm^2, which compares favorably to the 22 ng/cm^2 found in the Holland DFR study.

Using the California data and the Zweig-Popendorf Factor, daily harvester exposure is estimated to be 10.67 μg/kg/day (0.016 μg/kg/day $\times$ 5000 cm^2 $\times$ 8 hours = 640 μg/day = 10.67 μg/kg/day). The MOS may then be calculated accordingly [MOS = NOEL / exposure = 50 μg/kg/day/10.67μg/kg/day $\times$ 100 (dermal penetration)] as 467.

The worker-exposure data from the 3 greenhouse studies are summarized in Table 14.6.

These MOS determinations in Table 14.6 are remarkably consistent, whether calculated from actual worker-exposure data or from worker-exposure estimates derived from measured foliar residues. The MOS from the DFR studies are slightly more conservative than the MOS from the worker reentry actual exposure study, which represented "worst-case" exposure data. The MOS calculated from the worker reentry study was based upon direct measurement of abamectin residues on harvesters of cuttings from greenhouse chrysanthemums treated with the maximum recommended rate of abamectin, and used in combination with the lowest NOEL for toxic effects in the most sensitive species of test animal, the CF-1 mouse. The data show the model used for predicting harvester exposure to pesticide dislodgeable foliar residues is reasonably accurate, and further prove this work task may be performed safely with abamectin.

References

Adams, JD (1984) Pesticide Assessment Guidelines, Subdivision K. Exposure: Reentry Protection. US EPA Office of Pesticide Programs.

Gunther FA, Iwata Y, Carmen GE, Smith CA (1977) The citrus reentry problem: research on its causes and effects and approaches to its minimization. *Resid. Rev.* 67:1–139.

Iwata Y, Spear RC, Knaak JB, Foster RJ (1977) Worker reentry into pesticide-treated crops. Procedure for the determination of dislodgeable pesticide residues on foliage. *Bull. Envir. Contam. Toxicol.* 18(6):649–655.

Jenkins JJ, Rosenthal HS, Mollet J, Brown RD, Norton J, Dybas RA (1987) Dislodgeable residues of avermectin B_{1a} and its delta 8,9-isomer following application of AVID 0.15 EC to greenhouse grown chrysanthemums. ACS Services. 193rd National Meeting, AGROCHEMICALS No. 3.

Leidel NA, Busch KA, Lynch JR (1977) Occupational Exposure Sampling Strategy Manual. National Institute for Occupational Safety and Health p 131.

Reinert JC, Nielsen AP, Davis JE, Hickey KD, Nigg HN, Ware GW, Lunchick C (1987) Pesticide Assessment Guidelines, Subdivision U. Applicator Exposure Monitoring, US EPA Office of Pesticide Programs, p 163.

Reinert JC, Severn DJ (1985) Dermal exposure to pesticides, the Environmental Protection Agency's viewpoint in Honeycutt. In ACS Symposium Series 273, American Chemical Society, Washington, DC, pp 257–268.

Zweig G, Gao R, Witt J, Popendorf W, Bogen K (1984) Dermal exposure to carbaryl by strawberry harvesters. *J. Agric. Food Chem.* 32:1232–1276.

CHAPTER 15

Use of Ivermectin in Cattle, Sheep, Goats, and Swine

G.W. Benz, R.A. Roncalli, and S.J. Gross

I. Introduction

This chapter presents a summary of the efficacy data that form the basis for the clinical use of ivermectin in cattle, sheep, goats, and swine. At least 2 adequate and well-controlled trials investigated each ivermectin formulation's effect on each parasite species. Most of the trials were conducted by MSDRL investigators, though investigators at other laboratories also contributed. The efficacy percentages presented here are those upon which the regulatory approvals were based. Animal health applications of ivermectin have been reviewed (Campbell *et al.* 1983; Campbell and Benz 1984; Benz 1985; Campbell 1985; Bennett 1986; Barragry 1987). Clinical usages have also been summarized concerning cattle (Leaning, Roncalli, and Brokken 1983), sheep (Hotson 1983), and swine (Brokken *et al.* 1983). Recent reports that expand the basis of the label claims are included.

I. Use in Cattle

A. Injectable Formulation

IVOMEC Injection is a sterile solution containing 1.0% w/v ivermectin. The product is indicated for the treatment and control of gastrointestinal nematodes (including hypobiotic *Ostertagia* fourth-stage larvae), lungworms, and certain other nematodes; grubs; sucking lice; psoroptic and sarcoptic mange mites; sand tampans; and larvae of the Old World screwworm fly. It is to be administered subcutaneously in front of or behind the shoulder at 1.0 ml/50 kg body weight.

Endoparasite Activity

The recommended dose of 200 μg ivermectin/kg was selected upon completion of numerous dose-titration trials. Adult *Cooperia oncophora, C. punctata, Trichostrongylus colubriformis,* and *Nematodirus helvetianus* each required a dose between 100 μg/kg and 200 μg/kg; fourth-stage larvae of *Haemonchus placei, C. oncophora, N. helvetianus,* and *T. colubriformis* required a dose of 200 μg/kg.

Trial data used for registration of label efficacy claims are summarized in Table 15.1. In work performed subsequent to the original registrations, hemorrhagic dermal lesions caused by *Parafilaria bovicola* were observed to require at least 70 days for regression (Swan *et al.* 1983). Efficacy of more than 99% was found for *Thelazia* spp. adults (Carmichael, Soll, and Scherer 1985).

Infections with *Ostertagia* and *Cooperia* acquired up to at least 7 days after an ivermectin injection, as well as with *Dictyocaulus viviparus* acquired up to at least 14 days later, are controlled (Barth 1983; Armour *et al.* 1985), presumably because the drug persists following injection. Based on this persistent effect, control programs utilizing ivermectin injections at 3, 8, and 13 weeks after turnout onto spring pasture have been effective in controlling gastrointestinal parasites as well as lungworms (Ryan *et al.* 1986; Taylor, Mallon, and Kenny 1985; Jacobs, Fox, and Ryan 1987). In such programs, cattle on pastures contaminated with *D. viviparus* infective larvae have been found to be resistant to lungworm disease in the next grazing season, probably because infective larvae ingested between treatments induced immunity; gastrointestinal nematodes in the second season were not apparent but inhibited *Ostertagia* larvae did accumulate (Armour et al. 1988).

Ectoparasite Activity

The dose rate confirmed as optimal against nematode parasites was also found to be highly effective against several economically important ectoparasites.

TABLE 15.1. Efficacy in registration trials of ivermectin given subcutaneously at 200 μg/kg against adult and fourth-stage nematode parasites of cattle.

Parasite	% Reduction	
	Adults	Larvae[a]
Gastrointestinal nematodes		
Haemonchus placei	98	96
Mecistocirrus digitatus	100	ND[b]
Ostertagia ostertagi	>99	98
O. ostertagi hypobiotic larvae		>99
O. lyrata	99	ND[b]
Trichostrongylus axei	>99	98
T. colubriformis	93	97
Cooperia spp.	97	97
C. oncophora	95	99
C. punctata	98	95
C. pectinata	>99	ND[b]
Nematodirus helvetianus	84	ND[b]
N. spathiger	99	ND[b]
Strongyloides papillosus	>99	ND[b]
Toxocara vitulorum	100	ND[b]
Bunostomum phlebotomum	>99	>99
Oesophagostomum radiatum	98	>99
Lungworms		
Dictyocaulus viviparus	100	>99
D. viviparus hypobiotic larvae		100[c]
Other nematodes		
Parafilaria bovicola	[d]	ND[b]
Thelazia spp.	>99	ND[b]

[a] Developing fourth-stage larvae.
[b] No data are available.
[c] Includes fourth- and/or fifth-stage larvae.
[d] Subcutaneous lesions require 70 days for regression.

Grubs

The common cattle grubs in the Northern Hemisphere, *Hypoderma bovis* and *H. lineatum*, are highly susceptible to ivermectin. All 3 larval stages are killed following treatment. Efficacy in confirmation trials was 100% in most instances, although a few third instars (larvae), which were near to emergence from their host at the time of treatment, were expelled even though they had been grossly affected and were probably dead. Killing *Hypoderma* first instars during their normal migratory route may cause adverse host–parasite reactions—such as eosinophilic esophagitis leading to bloat (*H. lineatum*) or hemorrhage, (*H. bovis*) which affects the spinal cord and most often leads to hindquarter paralysis. These reactions can be avoided by not treating cattle with ivermectin during this migratory season (as determined by local epidemiologic patterns).

The tropical cattle grub affecting cattle in Latin America, *Dermatobia hominis*, is also controlled effectively (Roncalli 1984b).

Lice

Lice that ingest blood or body fluids from their host (i.e., sucking lice), including *Haematopinus eurysternus, Linognathus vituli,* and *Solenopotes capillatus,* are highly susceptible to therapeutic treatment. Ivermectin given subcutaneously at 200 μg/kg kills adult sucking lice as they feed upon blood or its constituents; the drug persists sufficiently long so that newly emerged larvae as well as nymphs are also killed as they begin to feed. In the registration trials, viable lice were recovered from cattle 1 week after treatment but none thereafter (up to 8 weeks). Lice surviving on ivermectin-treated cattle during the first week after treatment should be considered infective to nonmedicated cattle. To avoid reinfestation, ivermectin-medicated cattle should not be mingled with those untreated during the balance of the winter season, when these parasites are still active on their host.

Biting lice (*Damalinia bovis*) are not eliminated consistently from cattle given a therapeutic injection of ivermectin. This may be related to their superficial feeding pattern. A claim stated as "aid in the control" of *D. bovis* is registered in Europe and some Southern Hemisphere countries. In the United States, treatment of infested cattle was ineffectual; whether there are susceptibility differences among *D. bovis* populations from various geographic localities has not been determined.

Mites

Among mange mites, *Sarcoptes scabiei* var. *bovis* is the most sensitive to ivermectin. This species burrows more deeply into the dermis than do other species and evidently consumes blood or body fluids directly. In registration trials, live sarcoptic mites from medicated animals were recovered at 1 week following injection with ivermectin, but not thereafter (up to 8 weeks).

Psoroptes ovis does not burrow into the skin as deeply as *Sarcoptes*. Nonetheless, no live psoroptic mites were recovered during confirmation trials after 2 weeks following treatment although, in subsequent trials, a few *P. ovis* have been found on cattle treated 20 days previously (Wright and Guillot 1984). An isolation period of at least 14 days following treatment is adequate for use in control programs (Strickland and Gerrish 1987). Very few live mites can be recovered subsequent to treatment; the persistence of ivermectin following injection presumably accounts for the few recovered mites not being able to reestablish viable populations (Guillot, Wright, and Oehler 1986).

Chorioptes bovis, living on the superficial dermal surface, is the least responsive of the cattle mites studied; only an "aid in control" claim is registered in certain countries.

Ticks

Ticks also are affected by ivermectin. *Boophilus microplus* and *B. decoloratus,* which are single-host species, are more sensitive than multihost ticks. Ingestion of blood by adult females is interfered with; eventually they fall off, usually only partially engorged, and few eggs are produced. The efficacy of therapeutic doses against *Boophilus* spp. is sufficient for the registration of "aid in control" claims in several countries. *Boophilus* strains resistant to organophosphates, DDT, synthetic pyrethroids, and amidine were sensitive to ivermectin (Roncalli *et al.* 1984).

Effects against most multihost ticks are too transient for meaningful efficacy claims; however, a claim has been registered for the sand tampan (*Ornithodoros savignyi*) present in South Africa (Soll *et al.* 1984).

Screwworms

Among fly larvae (screwworms) that develop in the wounds of cattle, a therapeutic injection of ivermectin effectively controls Old World screwworm fly (*Chrysomya bezziana*) larvae for 14 days following treatment. Established infestations are less effectively controlled and may require additional measures. Screwworms of *Cochliomyia hominivorax* are not controlled by such ivermectin treatment.

Oral Formulations

IVOMEC oral solution for cattle contains 0.4% w/v ivermectin and should be administered at 2.5 ml/50 kg body weight using standard dosing equipment. IVOMEC cattle paste contains 0.153% w/v ivermectin and is administered orally by depressing the handle of the Medigun applicator completely to deliver 23 mg ivermectin per 113.5 kg (250 lb) body weight. These formulations are indicated for the treatment and control of gastrointestinal nematodes, lungworms, grubs, and sucking lice.

Endoparasite Activity

Efficacy data used for registration of nematode efficacy claims for both oral formulations are listed in Table 15.2.

Ectoparasite Activity

Complete efficacy is lacking against mange mites following oral administration of ivermectin to cattle, presumably because less ivermectin is absorbed systemically and it persists for a shorter duration compared to the subcutaneous route.

The common cattle grubs in the Northern Hemisphere, *Hypoderma*

TABLE 15.2. Efficacy in registration trials of ivermectin given orally at 200 μg/kg against nematode parasites of cattle.

Parasite	% Reduction	
	Adults	Larvae[a]
Gastrointestinal nematodes		
Haemonchus placei	>99	100
Ostertagia ostertagi	>99	99
O. ostertagi hypobiotic larvae		>99
O. lyrata	>99	>99
Trichostrongylus axei	>99	>99
T. colubriformis	100	>99
Cooperia oncophora	>99	100
C. punctata	>99	>99
Nematodirus helvetianus	97	98
Strongyloides papillosus	>99	ND[b]
Bunostomum phlebotomum	>99	100
Oesophagostomum radiatum	100	100
Trichuris ovis	>99	ND[b]
Lungworms		
Dictyocaulus viviparus	100	>99

[a] Developing fourth-stage larvae.
[b] No data are available.

bovis and *H. lineatum*, were killed with 100% efficiency in development trials and the same precautions observed with the injectable formulation regarding potential adverse host–parasite reactions during the autumn migratory season should be observed. Infestations of sucking lice (*Haematopinus eurysternus* and *Linognathus vituli*) present on cattle in the development program were eliminated after 1 week following oral treatment.

TOPICAL FORMULATION

IVOMEC Pour On for cattle contains 0.5% w/v ivermectin and is applied along the topline in a narrow strip extending from the withers to the tailhead. The volume of application is 1 ml/10 kg body weight. This formulation is for the treatment and control of gastrointestinal nematodes, lungworms, grubs, sucking and biting lice, chorioptic and sarcoptic mange mites, and as an "aid in control" of ticks (*Boophilus microplus*).

Endoparasite Activity

The recommended dose rate of 500 μg/kg was selected following a series of dose-titration trials. Dose-confirmation data against gastrointestinal nematodes and lungworms (Hotson *et al.* 1985; Alva-Valdes *et al.* 1986; Yazwinski *et al.* 1986) are summarized in Table 15.3. The formulation has

TABLE 15.3. Efficacy in registration trials of ivermectin applied topically at 500 μg/kg against nematode parasites of cattle.

Parasite	% Reduction	
	Adults	Larvae[a]
Gastrointestinal nematodes		
Haemonchus placei	>99	93
Ostertagia ostertagi	>99	96
O. ostertagi hypobiotic larvae		>99
Trichostrongylus axei	96	99
T. colubriformis	80	84
Cooperia spp.	95	96
C. oncophora	96	ND[b]
C. punctata	100	ND[b]
Strongyloides papillosus	97	ND[b]
Oesophagostomum radiatum	>99	100
O. venulosum	100	ND[b]
Trichuris spp.	87	ND[b]
Lungworms		
Dictyocaulus viviparus	100	>99

[a] Developing fourth-stage larvae.
[b] No data are available.

sufficient persistence of activity to control *Ostertagia* spp. infections acquired up to 14 days after treatment and *Dictyocaulus viviparus* acquired up to 28 days after treatment.

Ectoparasite Activity

Ivermectin applied topically to cattle effectively controls several ectoparasites (Barth *et al.* 1986; Alva-Valdes *et al.* 1986; Hotson *et al.* 1985). Infestations of *Chorioptes bovis* as well as *Sarcoptes scabiei* var. *bovis* are controlled. However, the formulation does not completely eliminate *Psoroptes ovis* and, in such cases, the use of IVOMEC Injection should be considered. Sucking lice (*Haematopinus eurysternus, Linognathus vituli,* and *Solenopotes capillatus*) as well as biting lice (*Damalinia bovis*) are effectively controlled. Horn flies (*Haematobia irritans*) are controlled for up to 35 days following product application. Northern Hemisphere grubs (larvae of *Hypoderma bovis* and *H. lineatum*) and tropical grubs (*Dermatobia hominis*) are controlled. The topical formulation "aids in the control" of *Boophilus microplus* (Cramer *et al.* 1985).

Sustained-Release Bolus

Development of a sustained-release bolus is in progress. Initial trials utilizing an osmotic pump to deliver ivermectin at steady-state rate (Pope *et al.* 1985) over 28 days demonstrated that prophylaxis against newly ingested larvae (Egerton, Suhayda, and Eary 1986), as well as therapy against established infections could be accomplished with a dose of 40 μg/kg/day (Baggott, Batty, and Ross 1986). The same dose prevented the engorgement by adult female multihost ticks (Soll, Carmichael, and Gross 1987).

Prototype boluses (Eckenhoff *et al.* 1987; Wilkinson *et al.* 1987) for commercial use (Soll, Carmichael, and Harvey 1988) are envisaged to deliver ivermectin at steady-state rate over 120 days. There are 2 boluses in development that are identical in all respects except that 1 bolus will delivery 8 mg ivermectin daily for cattle expected to weigh 200 kg after the end of the delivery period, whereas the other will deliver 12 mg daily for cattle to attain 300 kg. Each bolus will be delivered orally into the distal pharynx or anterior esophagus so as to preclude damage during administration. After 120 days, the bolus is expected to promptly cease delivery.

Use in Sheep

Oral Formulation

IVOMEC or ORAMEC Liquid for sheep is a 0.08% w/v solution of ivermectin to be given orally to sheep at 2.5 ml/10 kg body weight using standard drenching equipment. Dose rates and equipment should be checked before drenching commences to ensure proper volumes are delivered. The oral formulation is for the treatment and control of gastrointestinal nematodes, lungworms, nasal bots, and itch mites.

Endoparasite Activity

The recommended dose rate of 200 μg/kg for sheep was selected following a series of dose-titration trials. Dose-confirmation data against gastrointestinal nematodes and lungworms, used for registration, are summarized in Table 15.4. Strains of *Haemonchus contortus, Ostertagia circumcincta,* and *Trichostrongylus colubriformis* tolerant to benzimidazoles, levamisole, and morantel (and an *H. contortus* strain tolerant to rafoxanide) were fully susceptible to ivermectin. *Haemonchus* resistance to ivermectin has been reported following repeated treatments in laboratory (Egerton, Suhayda, and Eary 1988) and, at short intervals, field situations (Carmichael *et al.* 1987; van Wyk and Malan 1988; van Wyk *et al.* 1987; Echevarria and Trindade, 1989). *Trichostrongylus colubriformis* resistance under laboratory conditions also has been reported (Giordano, Tritschler, and Coles 1987).

Ectoparasite Activity

Efficacy also was demonstrated against all three instars (larvae) of nasal bots, *Oestrus ovis* (Roncalli 1984a), and against itch mites, *Psorergates*

TABLE 15.4. Efficacy in registration trials of ivermectin given orally at 200 μg/kg against nematode parasites of sheep.

Parasite	% Reduction	
	Adults	Larvae[a]
Gastrointestinal nematodes		
Haemonchus contortus	99	98
H. contortus hypobiotic larvae		100
H. placei	>99	ND[b]
Ostertagia circumcincta	>99	99
O. circumcincta		99
Trichostrongylus axei	99	99
T. colubriformis	>99	>99
T. vitrinus	>99	96
Cooperia curticei	>99	93
C. oncophora	97	96
Gaigeria pachyscelis	>99	99
Nematodirus battus	>99	>99
N. filicollis	99	98
N. spathiger	98	99
Strongyloides papillosus	>99	>99
Chabertia ovina	>99	97
Trichuris ovis	97	94
Oesophagostomum columbianum	100	97
O. venulosum	100	97
Lungworms		
Dictyocaulus filaria	>99	96

[a] Developing fourth-stage larvae.
[b] No data are available.

ovis (Hotson 1983). Ivermectin delivered orally to sheep does not control other mange infestations.

INJECTABLE FORMULATION

IVOMEC Injection, the same 1.0% w/v solution used in cattle, is also employed for sheep. The product is administered subcutaneously at 0.5 ml/25 kg body weight, using care to ensure that the skin has been penetrated before attempting delivery of the dose. It is indicated for the treatment and control of gastrointestinal nematodes, lungworms, nasal bots, mange mites, and itch mites.

Endoparasite Activity

The dose of 200 μg ivermectin/kg utilized orally in sheep was selected for this formulation based on other usages. Registration trials subsequently confirmed high efficacy against gastrointestinal nematodes and lungworms (Table 15.5). Efficacy against *Protostrongylus rufescens* has also been demonstrated (Dakkak *et al.* 1986).

TABLE 15.5. Efficacy in registration trials of ivermectin given subcutaneously at 200 μg/kg against nematode parasites of sheep.

Parasite	% Reduction	
	Adults	Larvae[a]
Gastrointestinal nematodes		
Haemonchus contortus	99	>99
Ostertagia circumcincta	>99	>99
O. trifurcata	100	98
Trichostrongylus axei	100	ND[b]
T. colubriformis	98	>99
T. vitrinus	100	93
Nematodirus filicollis	92	93
N. spathiger	ND[b]	95
Cooperia curticei	99	>99
Oesophagostomum columbianum	>99	>99
O. venulosum	100	ND[b]
Chabertia ovina	100	98
Trichuris ovis	87	ND[b]
Strongyloides papillosus	ND[b]	>99
Gaigeria pachyscelis	100	>99
Lungworms		
Dictyocaulus filaria	>99	>99
Protostrongylus rufescens	100	ND[b]

[a] Developing fourth-stage larvae.
[b] No data are available.

Ectoparasite Activity

Efficacy was confirmed in registration trials against the parasitic larval stages of the nasal bot, *Oestrus ovis*.

Infestations caused by mange mites, *Sarcoptes scabiei,* and itch mites, *Psorergates ovis,* also are controlled by ivermectin given subcutaneously. In contrast to the oral formulation, which does not control *Psoroptes ovis,* sheep given the injectable formulation do experience marked reductions in *Psoroptes* numbers and clinical signs. A second injection 7 days later may be required to eliminate all the living mites (Roncalli and Sutherland 1986). These reductions in psoroptic mites on sheep are presumably related to the longer persistence of ivermectin following subcutaneous administration, compared to oral administration, as well as to the feeding patterns of *Psoroptes* on sheep (Kirkwood 1985).

Use in Goats

ORAL FORMULATION

IVOMEC or ORAMEC Liquid for goats is the same 0.08% w/v solution of ivermectin as used in sheep, and is to be given at 2.5 ml/10 kg body weight. Standard drenching equipment can be utilized provided proper volumes are delivered. The product is indicated for the treatment and control of gastrointestinal nematodes and lungworms.

The same dose rate of 200 μg/kg, demonstrated to be efficacious in sheep, is used in goats. Data from dose-titration (Swan and Gross 1985) and dose-confirmation trials used for registration of efficacy claims are summarized in Table 15.6. Ectoparasites affecting goats were not sufficiently responsive to be included on the list of efficacy claims.

Injectable Formulation

In goats, there is insufficient efficacy against nematodes to justify use of the injectable formulation (IVOMEC Injection) otherwise recommended in cattle and sheep.

Use in Swine

Injectable Formulation

IVOMEC Injection containing 1.0% w/v ivermectin, the same formulation recommended for use in cattle and sheep, also is utilized in swine for the treatment and control of gastrointestinal roundworms, lungworms, kidney worms, lice, and mites. A dilute formulation containing 0.27% w/v ivermectin is recommended for young pigs.

The recommended dose of the 1.0% formulation is 1 ml/33 kg body weight (300 μg ivermectin/kg) adminstered subcutaneously. In young pigs, especially those below 16 kg for which less than 0.5 ml 1.0% IVOMEC Injection is indicated, dosing accuracy is important; the use of a

Table 15.6. Efficacy in registration trials of ivermectin given orally at 200 μg/kg against nematode parasites of goats.

Parasite	% Reduction	
	Adults	Larvae[a]
Gastrointestinal Nematodes		
Haemonchus contortus	>99	>99
Ostertagia circumcincta	>99	100
Trichostrongylus colubriformis	>99	>99
Nematodirus spathiger	100	100
Chabertia ovina	100	ND[b]
Strongyloides papillosus	>99	100
Oesophagostomum columbianum	100	100
Lungworm		
Dictyocaulus filaria	100	ND[b]

[a] Developing fourth-stage larvae.
[b] No data are available.

syringe that can deliver accurately as little as 0.1 ml is recommended. Alternatively, young pigs should be given 1 ml of the 0.27% formulation per 9 kg (20 lb) body weight.

Endoparasite Activity

Efficacy data used for the registration of nematode efficacy claims are summarized in Table 15.7. Kidney worms, *Stephanurus dentatus,* are controlled (Plue *et al.* 1986). Further, ivermectin given to sows 7 to 14 days before farrowing effectively controls transmission of *Strongyloides ransomi* larvae to newborn pigs.

Ectoparasite Activity

Infestations of lice (*Haematopinus suis*) and mange mites (*Sarcoptes scabiei* var. *suis*) were effectively controlled during registration trials. In mange control programs, all animals in a herd must be treated and a consistent program of retreatment adhered to (Hogg 1984). Sows preferably should be treated prior to breeding and 7 to 14 days prior to farrowing (Courtney, Ingalls, and Stitzlein 1983). Boars should be treated at least twice annually, although frequency of and need for treatments depend on exposure. All feeder pigs received for finishing should be treated before placement in clean quarters; pigs exposed to contaminated soil, premises, or other pigs may need retreatment if reinfestation occurs.

IVOMEC Injection in swine has a persistent drug level sufficient to control sarcoptic mite infestations throughout the life cycle, from egg to adult. Because the ivermectin effect is not immediate, however, care must be taken to prevent reinfestation from exposure to untreated animals or contaminated facilities. Generally, pigs should not be moved to clean

TABLE 15.7. Efficacy in registration trials of ivermectin given subcutaneously at 300 μg/kg against nematode parasites of swine.

Parasite	% Reduction	
	Adults	Larvae[a]
Gastrointestinal nematodes		
Ascaris suum	100	>99
Hyostrongylus rubidus	98	99
Oesophagostomum spp.	96	95
Strongyloides ransomi	99	ND[b]
Trichuris suis	80	ND[b]
Lungworms		
Metastrongylus spp.	100	ND[b]
Kidney Worms		
Stephanurus dentatus	>99	>99

[a] Developing fourth-stage larvae.
[b] No data are available.

quarters or exposed to uninfested pigs for approximately 1 week after treatment. Sows should be treated at least 1 week before farrowing to minimize transfer of mites to newborn pigs. Louse eggs are unaffected by IVOMEC Injection and may require up to 3 weeks to hatch; louse infestations developing from hatching eggs may require retreatment.

References

Alva-Valdes R, Wallace DH, Holste JE, Egerton JR, Cox JL, Wooden JW, Barrick RA (1986) Efficacy of ivermectin in a topical formulation against induced gastrointestinal and pulmonary nematode infections, and naturally acquired grubs and lice in cattle. *Am. J. Vet. Res.* 47:2389–2392.

Armour J, Bairden K, Batty AF, Davison CC, Ross D (1985) Persistent anthelmintic activity of ivermectin in cattle. *Vet. Rec.* 116:151–153.

Armour J, Bairden K, Ryan WG (1988) Immunity of ivermectin treated cattle to challenge from helminth parasites in the following season. *Vet. Rec.* 122:223–225.

Baggott DG, Batty AF, Ross DB (1986) The control of mature nematode infections in cattle by sustained delivery of ivermectin. Proceedings of the 14th World Congress on Diseases of Cattle, Vol. 1, Dublin, Ireland, pp 160–165.

Barragry TB (1987) A review of the pharmacology and clinical uses of ivermectin. *Can. Vet. J.* 28:512–517.

Barth D (1983) Persistent anthelmintic effect of ivermectin in cattle. *Vet. Rec.* 113:300.

Barth D, Batty AF, Robin B, Preston JM (1986) Efficacy of a topical formulation of ivermectin against cattle ectoparasites. Proceedings 14th World Congress of Diseases of Cattle, Vol 1, Dublin, Ireland, pp 157–159.

Barth D, Preston JM (1985) Efficacy against somatic *Strongyloides ransomi* larvae. *Vet. Rec.* 116:366–367.

Bennett DG (1986) Clinical pharmacology of ivermectin. *J. Am. Vet. Med. Assoc.* 189:100–104.

Benz GW (1985) Animal health applications of ivermectin. *Southwest. Entomol.* (*Suppl.*) 7:43–50.

Brokken ES, Barth D, Foster AG, Pulliam JD, Wallace DH (1983) Ivermectin, a new broad-spectrum antiparasitic agent for swine. In Proceedings of the MSD AGVET Symposium "Recent Developments in the Control of Animal Parasites," in association with the XXII World Veterinary Congress, Perth, Australia, pp 239–258.

Campbell WC (1985) Ivermectin: An update. *Parasitol. Today* 1:10–16.

Campbell WC, Benz GW (1984) Ivermectin: A review of efficacy and safety. *J. Vet. Pharm. Therap.* 7:1–16.

Campbell WC, Fisher MH, Stapley EO, Albers-Schonberg G, Jacobs TA (1983) Ivermectin: A potent new antiparasitic agent. *Science* 221:823–828.

Carmichael IH, Soll MD, Scherer H (1985) The use of ivermectin in the control of bovine thelaziosis. 11th Conference World Association for the Advancement of Veterinary Parasitology, Rio de Janeiro, Abstract 106.

Carmichael IH, Visser R, Schneider D, Soll MD (1987) *Haemonchus contortus* resistance to ivermectin (Letter to Editor). *J. S. Afr. Vet. Assoc.* 58:93.

Courtney CH, Ingalls WL, Stitzlein SL (1983) Ivermectin for the control of swine scabies: Relative values of prefarrowing treatment of sows and weaning treatment of pigs. *Am. J. Vet. Res.* 44:1220–1223.

Cramer LG, Carvalho LAF, Bridl AA, Amaral NK, Barrick RA (1985) Topically applied ivermectin: Efficacy against *Boophilus microplus* in cattle. 11th Conference World Association for Advancement of Veterinary Parasitology, Rio de Janeiro, Abstract 126.

Dakkak A, Robin B, Kachani M (1986) Efficacy of ivermectin in the ewe. *Rev. Med. Vet.* (Toulouse) 137:781–787 (in French).

Echevarria FAM, Trindade GNP (1989) Anthelmintic resistance by *Haemonchus contortus* to ivermectin in Brazil: A preliminary report. *Vet. Rec.* 124:147–148.

Eckenhoff B, Cortese R, Wright JC, Wilkinson PK, Zingerman JR, Pope DG (1987) Osmotically-driven ruminal delivery system for long term rate controlled delivery of ivermectin. *Pharm. Res.* (*Suppl.*) 4:46.

Egerton JR, Suhayda D, Eary CH (1986) Prophylaxis of nematode infections in cattle with an indwelling rumino-reticular ivermectin sustained release bolus. *Vet. Parasit.* 22:67–75.

Egerton JR, Suhayda D, Eary CH (1988) Laboratory selection of *Haemonchus contortus* for resistance to ivermectin. *J. Parasit.* 74:614–617.

Giordano DJ, Tritschler JP, Coles GC (1987) Selection of ivermectin resistant *Trichostrongylus colubriformis* in lambs. Proceedings 12th Conference World Association for Advancement of Veterinary Parasitology, Montreal, Abstract No. 8A-5.

Guillot FS, Wright FC, Oehler D (1986) Concentration of ivermectin in bovine serum and its effect on the fecundity of psoroptic mange mites. *Am. J. Vet. Res.* 47:525–527.

Hogg A (1984) Eradication of sarcoptic mange in swine with ivermectin. Proceedings 8th International Pig Veterinary Society Congress, Ghent, Belgium, p 206.

Hotson IK (1983) The development of ivermectin as an antiparasitic agent in sheep. In Proceedings of the MSD AGVET Symposium "Recent Developments in the Control of Animal Parasites," in association with the XXII World Veterinary Congress, Perth, Australia, pp 42–55.

Hotson IK, Bliss WJ, Cox JL, Roncalli RA, Sutherland IH (1985) Efficacy of topically administered ivermectin against cattle parasites. 11th Conference World Association for Advancement of Veterinary Parasitology, Rio de Janeirio, Abstract 112.

Jacobs DE, Fox MT, Ryan WG (1987) Early season parasitic gastroenteritis in calves and its prevention with ivermectin. *Vet. Rec.* 120:29–31.

Kirkwood AC (1985) Some observations on the biology and control of the sheep scab mite *Psoroptes ovis* (Herring) in Britain. *Vet. Parasitol.* 18:269–279.

Leaning WHD, Roncalli RA, Brokken ES (1983) The efficacy and safety evaluation of ivermectin: A new injectable antiparasitic agent for cattle. In Proceedings of the MSD AGVET Symposium "Recent Developments in the Control of Animal Parasites," in association with the XXII World Veterinary Congress, Perth, Australia, pp 25–41.

Plue RE, Brokken ES, Ericsson GF, Foster AG, Wallace DH (1986) A review of ivermectin efficacy against adult and immature *Stephanurus dentatus*. Proceedings 9th International Pig Veterinary Society Congress, p 375.

Pope DG, Wilkinson PK, Egerton JR, Conroy J (1985) Oral controlled-release delivery of ivermectin in cattle via an osmotic pump. *J. Pharm. Sci.* 74:1108–1110.

Roncalli RA (1984a) Efficacy of ivermectin against *Oestrus ovis* in sheep. *Vet. Med. Small Ani. Clinic.* 79:1095–1097.

Roncalli RA (1984b) The biology and the control of *Dermatobia hominis,* the tropical warble-fly of Latin America. *Prevent. Vet. Med.* 2:569–578.

Roncalli RA, Hotson IK, Benitez-Usher C, Bridi AA (1984c) Efficacy of ivermectin against *Boophilus* spp. in cattle. Proceedings of 29th Annual Meeting of American Association of Veterinary Parasitologists, New Orleans, Abstract 12.

Roncalli RA, Sutherland IH (1986) The use of ivermectin injectable against *Psoroptes ovis* (Acarina: Psoroptidae) in sheep. Proceedings 31st Annual Meeting American Association of Veterinary Parasitologists, No. 10.

Ryan WG, Armour J, Bairden K, Fox MT, Jacobs DE (1986) Early season use of ivermectin to control parasitic gastroenteritis and bronchitis in calves. Proceedings of the 14th World Congress of Diseases of Cattle, Dublin, Ireland, Vol. 1, pp 185–190.

Soll MD, Carmichael IH, Gross SJ (1987) Control of induced infestations of adult *Amblyomma hebraeum* with sustained release ivermectin. *Onderstepoort J. Vet. Res.* 54:17–20.

Soll MD, Carmichael IH, Harvey RG (1988) Prophylactic efficacy of sustained-release ivermectin against induced nematode infestations in cattle. *J. S. Afr. Vet. Assoc.* 59:9–11.

Soll MD, Swan GE, Schroder J, Bezuidenhout JD (1984) Efficacy of ivermectin against the sand tampan (*Ornithodoros savignyi*). *Vet. Rec.* 114:70.

Strickland RK, Gerrish RR (1987) Infestivity of *Psoroptes ovis* on ivermectin-treated cattle. *Am. J. Vet. Res.* 48:342–344.

Swan GE, Gross SJ (1985) Efficacy of ivermectin against induced gastrointestinal nematode infections in goats. *Vet. Rec.* 117:147–149.

Swan GE, Soll MD, Carmichael IH, Schroder J (1983) Efficacy of ivermectin against *Parafilaria bovicola*. *Vet. Rec.* 113:260.

Taylor SM, Mallon TR, Kenny J (1985) Comparison of early season suppressive anthelmintic prophylactic methods for parasitic gastroenteritis and bronchitis in calves. *Vet. Rec.* 117:521–524.

van Wyk JA, Malan FS (1988) Resistance of field strains of *Haemonchus contortus* to ivermectin, closantel, rafoxanide and the benzimidazoles in South Africa. *Vet. Rec.* 123:226–228.

van Wyk JA, Malan FS, Gerber HM, Alva RMR (1987) Two field strains of *Haemonchus contortus* resistant to rafoxanide. *Onderstepoort J. Vet. Res.* 54:143–146.

Wilkinson PK, Baggott DG, Zingerman JR, Pope DG, Eckenhoff B (1987) *In-vivo* performance of a new osmotically driven, long term rate controlled delivery system for ivermectin in cattle. *Pharm. Res.* (Supplement) 4:46.

Wright FC, Guillot FS (1984) Effect of ivermectin in heifers on mortality and egg production of *Psoroptes ovis*. *Am. J. Vet. Res.* 45:2132–2134.

Yazwinski TA, Wood N, Holtzen HM, Presson BL, Kilgore RL (1986) Measuring the anthelmintic efficacy of a new formulation of ivermectin. *Vet. Med. Small Ani. Clinic.* 81:1175–1177.

CHAPTER 16

Use of Abamectin in Cattle

G.W. Benz and J.L. Cox

I. Introduction

This chapter presents a summary of the efficacy data that form the basis for the clinical use of abamectin (avermectin B_1) in cattle. The product is formulated in the same vehicle as used for IVOMEC (ivermectin) Injection. At the present time, AVOMEC (abamectin) Injection is registered only in Australia.

At least 2 adequate and well-controlled trials investigated the effect on each parasite species. Most of the trials were conducted by MSDRL researchers, though investigators at other laboratories also contributed. The efficacy percentages presented here are those upon which regulatory approval was based. Other efficacy data obtained with abamectin but formulated in a different vehicle, and not relied upon for registration, have been presented (Benz and Ernst 1979; Egerton *et al.* 1979; Wescott *et al.* 1980).

II. Efficacy

AVOMEC Injection is a sterile solution containing 1.0% w/v abamectin. The product is indicated for the treatment and control of gastrointestinal nematodes (including inhibited immature *Ostertagia ostertagi*), lungworms (*Dictyocaulus viviparus*), and sucking lice (*Linognathus vituli*) (Scott *et al.* 1985). It is to be administered subcutaneously in front of or behind the shoulder at 1 ml/50 kg body weight.

A. Endoparasite Activity

The recommended dose of 200 μg abamectin/kg was selected upon completion of dose-titration trials involving nematodes primarily, but also taking into account data against sucking lice (*Linognathus vituli*) and tropical cattle ticks (*Boophilus microplus*).

Trial data based on subcutaneous injection of abamectin and used for registration of label-efficacy claims are summarized in Table 16.1. Claims registered in Australia include the following:

Haemonchus placei (adults and fourth-stage larvae)
Ostertagia ostertagi (adults, fourth-stage larvae, and hypobiotic larvae)
Trichostrongylus axei (adults)
Cooperia spp. (adults and fourth-stage larvae)
Chabertia ovina (adults)
Oesophagostomum radiatum (adults and fourth-stage larvae)
Dictyocaulus viviparus (adults and fourth-stage larvae)

Several of the trials involved comparisons of the efficacy of abamectin and ivermectin (Table 16.2). Ivermectin and abamectin differ only by reduction of one double bond, each product utilizes the same vehicle, and each is administered subcutaneously at the same dose rate. Based on comparable efficacies, the following additional nematode efficacy claims based on ivermectin data have been registered in Australia:

Table 16.1. Efficacy in registration trials of abamectin given subcutaneously at 200 μg/kg against adult and fourth-stage nematode parasites of cattle.

	% Reduction	
Parasite	Adults	Immatures[a]
Gastrointestinal Nematodes		
Haemonchus placei	100	100
Ostertagia ostertagia	>99	>99
O. ostertagi hypobiotic larvae		>99
Trichostrongylus axei	>99	ND[b]
Cooperia spp.	>99	100
Chabertia ovina	100	ND[b]
Oesophagostomum radiatum	>99	100
Lungworms		
Dictyocaulus viviparus	100	100

[a] Developing fourth-stage larvae.
[b] No data are available.

TABLE 16.2. Comparative efficacy in registration trials of abamectin and ivermectin, each given subcutaneously at 200 μg/kg, against adult and fourth-stage nematode parasites of cattle.

	Abamectin % Reduction		Ivermectin % Reduction	
Parasite	Adults	Immatures[a]	Adults	Immatures
Gastrointestinal Nematodes				
Haemonchus placei	100	100	>99	100
Ostertagia ostertagi	100	>99	>99	>99
O. ostertagi hypobiotic larvae		>99		>99
Trichostrongylus axei	100	ND[b]	>99	ND[b]
Cooperia spp.	>99	100	>99	>99
Chabertia ovina	100	ND[b]	100	ND[b]
Oesophagostomum radiatum	100	100	100	>99

[a] Developing fourth-stage larvae.
[b] No data are available.

Ostertagia lyrata (adults and fourth-stage larvae)
Trichostrongylus axei (fourth-stage larvae)
Trichostrongylus colubriformis (adults and fourth-stage larvae)
Strongyloides papillosus (adults)
Bunostomum phlebotomum (adults and fourth-stage larvae)

AVOMEC Injection effectively controls infections with *Haemonchus placei, Ostertagia* spp., *Cooperia* spp., and *Oesophagostomum radiatum* acquired up to at least 7 days after treatment, and *Dictyocaulus viviparus* acquired up to at least 14 days after treatment. Data to substantiate these claims were obtained using ivermectin (Bremner *et al.* 1983; Barth 1983; Armour *et al.* 1985) as well as abamectin.

Since registration, the uses of abamectin for nematode control have been reported (Tahir, Holroyd, and Copeman 1986; De Chaneet *et al.* 1988). The high efficacy of abamectin against oxfendazole-resistant *Trichostrongylus axei* in cattle also has been reported (Eagleson and Bowie 1986).

B. Ectoparasite Activity

The abamectin dose rate confirmed as optimal against nematode parasites was also found to be highly effective against sucking lice, *Linognathus vituli*. Among treated cattle, no live lice were found on Day 14 after treatment until observations were terminated on Day 56.

Abamectin is sufficiently efficacious against tropical cattle ticks, *Boophilus microplus*, to justify an "aid-in-control" label claim. A single subcutaneous injection at 200 μg/kg significantly reduces the numbers of engorged female ticks dropped from treated cattle for at least 21 days, and the reproductive potential among surviving female ticks is reduced by interference with egg production.

References

Armour J, Bairden K, Batty AF, Davison CC, Ross D (1985) Persistent anthelmintic activity of ivermectin in cattle. *Vet. Rec.* 116:151–153.

Barth D (1983) Persistent anthelmintic effect of ivermectin in cattle. *Vet. Rec.* 113:300.

Benz GW and Ernst JV (1979) Anthelmintic activities of the B_1a fraction of avermectin against gastrointestinal nematodes in calves. *Am. J. Vet. Res.* 40:1187–1188.

Bremner KC, Berrie DA, Hotson IK (1983) Persistence of the anthelmintic activity of ivermectin in calves. *Vet. Rec.* 113:569.

De Chaneet GC, Casey R, Dixon FF, Besier RB, Mitchell RK (1988) Effect of avermectin B_1 and benzimidazole anthelmintics on worm egg output of treated cattle. *Austral. Vet. J.* 65:85–86.

Eagleson JS, Bowie JY (1986) Oxfendazole resistance in *Trichostrongylus axei* in cattle in Australia. *Vet. Rec.* 119:604.

Egerton JR, Ostlind DA, Blair LS, Eary CH, Suhayda D, Cifelli S, Riek RF, Campbell WC (1979) Avermectins, a new family of potent anthelmintic agents: efficacy of the B_1a component. *Antimic. Agents Chemother.* 15:372–378.

Scott PG, Burrows RO, Hotson IK, Cox JL (1985) Avermectin B_1 as an anti-parasitic agent for cattle. 11th Conference World Association for Advancement of Veterinary Parasitology, Rio de Janeiro, Abstract 83.

Tahir MS, Holroyd RG, Copeman DB (1986) Treatment of beef calves with ivermectin and avermectin B_1 in dry tropical Australia. 6th International Congress of Parasitology, Brisbane, Australia, Abstract 651.

Wescott RB, Farrell CJ, Gallina AM, Foreyt WJ (1980) Efficacy of avermectin B_1a for treatment of experimentally induced nematode infections in cattle. *Am. J. Vet. Res.* 41:1326–1328.

CHAPTER 17

Use of Ivermectin in Horses

W.C. Campbell, W.H.D. Leaning, and R.L. Seward

I. Products

A. Eqvalan Paste™; Zimecterin Paste™

This is a paste, for oral use, containing 1.87% w/w ivermectin. In the United States, it is available in a prefilled syringe, calibrated so that each increment represents the amount of drug needed for 250 lb (114 kg) of body weight at the rate of 200 μg/kg. Each syringe contains enough paste to treat one mature horse. The syringe sold in international markets is calibrated to deliver the amount of drug needed for 100 kg (220 lb) of body weight at 200 μg/kg.

B. Eqvalan Liquid™

This product is a clear, ready-to-use liquid for professional administration by stomach tube (nasogastric intubation) or as an oral drench. It contains

1% ivermectin and various excipients. The recommended dosage is 200 μg/kg, and each ml contains enough ivermectin to treat 110 lb (50 kg) of body weight.

C. Eqvalan Injectable™

Eqvalan injectable™ is a micellar formulation containing 20 mg of ivermectin per milliliter of sterile aqueous solution (2.0% w/v) intended for intramuscular injection. Manufacture and distribution of this product were suspended in 1984. Adverse reactions have included some that were severe or even fatal. In most instances contamination of the injection site with bacteria (*Clostridium* sp.) appears to have been involved, while in others the reaction appears to have been of the anaphylactoid type and was associated with inadvertent intravenous injection or the presence of polysorbate 80 in the micellar formulation.

II. Antiparasitic Efficacy

A. General

Most of the early studies on the efficacy of ivermectin in horses involved intramuscular injection of the drug. Because the injectable product is no longer commercially available its efficacy will not be discussed in detail here, and readers are referred to reviews by Campbell and Benz (1983); Egerton, Seward, and Robin (1984); Leaning (1984); Madigan (1984); Weiss (1984); Slocombe and colleagues (1984); Klei and colleagues (1984); and Campbell (1985).

The efficacy of parenterally and orally administered ivermectin in horses is almost identical. For a host species such as the horse—where widely different experimental protocols are used and where many species of parasites are involved—the compilation of data is cumbersome; and for practical purposes it may be more useful to tabulate the species or "claims" for which approval has been granted by major governmental regulatory agencies. This approach has the advantage not only of simplicity but of subsuming the elements of statistical probability and host safety that are integral parts of the registration process. Table 17.1 lists the "approved claims" for the oral use of ivermectin at 200 μg/kg in horses. The following summary of efficacy against individual species is limited to orally administered drug, except where data obtained using the injectable formulation are needed to introduce or supplement data obtained with the paste.

B. *Parascaris equorum*

When given orally in a paste formulation, ivermectin at 200 μg/kg totally eliminated the passage of *P. equorum* eggs in naturally infected horses

TABLE 17.1. Horse parasites for which ivermectin oral paste has been approved at a dosage of 0.2 mg/kg.[1]

Large strongyles	
	Strongylus vulgaris, adult and arterial larval stage
	S. edentatus, adult and tissue stage
	S. equinus, adult
	Triodontophorus spp., adult
Small strongyles	
	Cyathostomum spp., adult and L_4 stage
	Cylicocyclus spp., adult and L_4 stage
	Cylicostephanus spp., adult and L_4 stage
	Cylicodontophorus spp., adult and L_4 stage
	Gyalocephalus sp., adult and immature[2]
Other nematodes	
	Parascaris equorum, adult, L_3 and L_4 stage
	Oxyuris equi, adult and L_4 stage
	Trichostrongylus axei, adult
	Habronema muscae, adult and cutaneous L_3 stage
	Draschia spp., cutaneous L_3 stage[2]
	Onchocerca sp., microfilaria
	Dictyocaulus arnfieldi, adult and L_4 stage
Bots	
	Gastrophilus spp., oral and gastric stages

[1] Unless otherwise specified, approval refers to the Food and Drug Administration of the United States of America.
[2] Approved in country or countries other than United States.

(Corba *et al.* 1986), illustrating that the oral paste, like the injectable solution, is active against adult *P. equorum*. An effect on the passage of eggs was also observed by Puccini and colleagues (1984). In another study, fecal ascarid egg counts in 14 naturally infected horses were negative following treatment with ivermectin oral paste and remained at zero for 10 to 12 weeks following treatment, while egg counts in the 6 control horses were substantially unchanged (E.T. Lyons, unpublished data). Efficacy against adult ascarids was demonstrated more directly and definitively in controlled studies in which ascarid burdens were determined at necropsy (French *et al.* 1988b; DiPietro *et al.* 1987). In both studies ivermectin paste at 200 μg/kg was 100% effective against the adult worms.

Ivermectin is also active against the immature stages of *P. equorum*. In two studies in naturally infected ponies, larval burdens were determined at necropsy following treatment with the paste at 200 μg/kg. When necropsy was performed 2 weeks after treatment, the reduction in lung larval burden was 100% (French *et al.* 1988b) and the reduction in intestinal larval burden was also 100% (French *et al.* 1988b; DiPietro *et al.* 1987). When necropsy was delayed until 5 weeks after treatment, larvae were recovered from the intestines; and, since treatment is highly active against the early migrating stage, this probably reflected reinfection, despite effort taken in one of the trials to prevent it. In one of the trials, treatment was not associated with clear-cut improvement in clinical condition but was associated with improved weight gain (French *et al.* 1988b).

To define the efficacy of ivermectin against immature *P. equorum* more precisely, 2 trials were conducted on experimentally induced infections. Groups of 6 horses were treated with ivermectin paste or liquid at 200 μg/kg, or were maintained as untreated or vehicle-untreated controls (DiPietro *et al.*, in press; French *et al.*, in press). Treatment was administered on Day 11 of infection, when the majority of the parasites would be in the migratory L_3 larval stage. (Necropsy of indicator horses at that time revealed larvae in the lungs but not in the small intestine). At necropsy, 14 days after treatment, the efficacy of ivermectin against *P. equorum* was determined to be 100% in both trials and with both formulations ($P < 0.001$). It is not possible to conclude from the data whether all of the larvae were killed in the lungs or on early entry into the small intestine.

To determine efficacy against the later (L_4) stage of *P. equorum*, 4 trials were conducted with experimentally induced infections (A. Batty, unpublished data; J.L. Duncan, unpublished data; T.R. Bello 1985; and DiPietro *et al.*, in press). Treatment was given on Day 28 or 29 of infection. At necropsy on Day 42 or 43 of infection (14 days after treatment), the immature ascarids in the small intestine were counted, revealing reductions of 62%, 95%, greater than 99%, and greater than 99% in the paste-treated groups in the 4 trials, respectively. In 2 of the trials, ivermectin liquid was also tested, and reductions of greater than 99% were recorded in both (DiPietro *et al.*, in press; J.L. Duncan, unpublished data). Using an appropriate statistical method (Friedman's test) to allow for heterogeneity of variances among treatments, the overall reduction was calculated as 98.4% ($P > 0.001$). In the trial by DiPietro and colleagues (in press), gross examination of lung and liver revealed similar lesions in the treated and untreated foals, but the ascarids recovered from the treated animals were significantly smaller than those from the controls. Thus treatment evidently affected the parasites adversely, perhaps by interfering with feeding, but did not kill them.

Thus the paste and liquid ivermectin formulations have been shown to be highly active against both the early (L_3) tissue phase and against the later intestinal (L_4) phase. The significance and differences of opinion associated with this efficacy have been discussed by Boraski (1987).

C. *Strongylus vulgaris*, *S. edentatus*, *S. equinus*

The oral paste formulation, used at 200 μg/kg, was 100% active against adult *S. vulgaris*, as was the injectable formulation which was tested in the same experiment (Klei *et al.* 1984).

The migratory fourth stage larvae of *S. vulgaris* are of special importance because (1) they cause lesions of certain arteries (especially the mesenteric), often giving rise to serious clinical signs; and (2) they are particularly hard to eliminate by chemotherapeutic means. Extensive studies by Slocombe and his colleagues (Slocombe *et al.* 1982; Slocombe and McGraw 1984; Slocombe *et al.* 1984) showed that the injectable formulation of ivermectin is highly active against the migratory fourth stage larvae. He further showed that efficacy against late fourth stage larvae may not be demonstrable if necropsy is performed only 2 weeks after treatment; and he cautioned that treatment appeared to cause some larvae to become situated more deeply in the wall of the ileocolic artery, prompting a concern about the eventual fate of such larvae and the impact of their putative slow disintegration within the arterial wall—especially after repeated cycles of infection and treatment. Studies by Klei and his colleagues (Klei *et al.* 1984a; Klei *et al.* 1984b) confirmed that the interval between treatment and necropsy is critical for demonstrating the efficacy of ivermectin against the migratory larvae of *S. vulgaris*. In their experience, the oral paste (and the injectable formulation) at 200 μg/kg was 99% effective against 8-week-old larvae, as revealed by necropsy 5 weeks after treatment. Klei also commented on the potential impact of dead or dying larvae on the arterial walls. He noted,

> Killing *S. vulgaris* larvae with ivermectin not only promoted a remarkable resolution of arterial lesions, but also prevented their progression into the lesions observed in the nontreated controls. Although ivermectin clearly kills intravascular *S. vulgaris* larvae, nematode bodies persist for some time following treatment, as indicated by the numbers of dead larvae recovered. It is interesting to note that the presence of the inactive or paralyzed worms alone does not provoke the arterial lesions associated with *S. vulgaris* migrations. Observations of lesions in livers and lungs in control animals confirm and extend previous observations that *S. vulgaris* migrations are not restricted to the predilection sites in the mesenteric vasculature. The severity and occurrence of lesions in extravascular sites were markedly reduced in the ivermectin-treated foals, indicating that resolution of these lesions also occurs within the 5-week period following treatment.

Repeated cycles of infection and ivermectin therapy have not resulted in clinical disease or unique lesions (T.R. Klei, unpublished data). It is not known whether ivermectin is active against the earliest parasitic (L_3) stage of *S. vulgaris,* but there is evidence that the drug (at least when given intramuscularly) is effective prophylactically. A foal treated 2 weeks before inoculation with larvae and necropsied 4 weeks after inoculation had no evidence of arterial infection, whereas the arteries of control foals showed clear signs of the infection (Slocombe *et al.* 1984). Apparently the ivermectin persisted in sufficient concentration to affect the third or fourth stage larvae at some time during the 4-week period following inoculation with infective larvae.

Ivermectin was tested at 0.2 μg/kg against adult *S. edentatus* in horses. In 5 trials, side-by-side comparison of the paste and injectable formulations gave reductions in worm burden of greater than 99% and 100%, respectively (T.R. Klei, D.H. Wallace, T.A. Yazwinski, and J.L. Duncan, unpublished data). Against the L_4 migratory stage of this species, an efficacy of 100% was recorded for both formulations (J.L. Duncan, unpublished data).

In 4 trials, the paste and injectable formulations were 100% effective in removing adult *S. equinus* at a dosage of 0.2 μg/kg (T.R. Klei, T.A. Yazwinski, and D.H. Wallace, unpublished data).

D. Small Strongyles

The efficacy of ivermectin paste against strongyles in general, as determined by fecal examination, was reported by Asquith, Plue, and Seward (1983). Baker and colleagues (1984) gave ivermectin at 200 μg/kg in the paste formulation (or the injectable formulation) to horses in which benzimidazole treatment had already been shown to have little effect on the output of strongyle eggs. The egg counts were reduced by 100% at 14 days after treatment, and remained reduced by 90% or more for at least 2 months. Similarly, Burrows, Thomson, and Lindsey (1985) used fecal examination to demonstrate the efficacy of the paste formulation against benzimidazole-resistant small strongyles and showed that egg counts remained zero for at least 3 weeks. French and colleagues (1985) reported that treatment with the paste formulation at 200 μg/kg resulted in egg counts "at or near zero for 8 to 10 weeks." These data have been supplemented by data from controlled trials (based on necropsy and recovery of parasites from treated and untreated horses) in which the efficacy of the paste formulation was compared directly with that of the injectable product. Against adult *Cyathostomum* spp., both formulations were more than 99% effective (D.H. Wallace and J.L. Duncan, unpublished data). Against adult *Poteriostomum* the injectable product was 63% effective while the paste was 100% effective (T.A. Yazwinski, unpublished data). Against unidentified species of small strongyle, immature and mature, both formulations were more than 99% effective (D.H. Wallace and J.L. Duncan, unpublished data). Thus the activity of the paste formulation at least equals the activity of the injectable product in these trials and in the trials previously reported (for references, see Campbell and Benz, 1984).

E. *Dictyocaulus arnfieldi* (Lungworm)

Ivermectin paste was administered orally (200 μg/kg) to ponies experimentally infected with *D. arnfieldi* (Britt and Preston 1985). On the basis of fecal examination and necropsy, the treatment was judged 100% effective against the adult and immature stages (including inhibited forms). Lyons, Drudge, and Tolliver (1985) also reported evidence of efficacy against *D. arnfieldi* in donkeys.

F. *Draschia* sp. and *Habronema* sp.

The cutaneous lesions ("summer sores") caused by third stage larvae of *Draschia* sp. and *Habronema* sp. have been notoriously difficult to cure by means of chemotherapy, but Herd and Donham (1984) showed that 1 or 2 intramuscular doses of ivermectin at 200 μg/kg were highly effective. A lindane ointment was used to prevent reinfection, and under these circumstances "the typical summer sore was replaced by healthy pink granulation tissue at 7 days and this healed after 1 to 5 weeks." Biopsy was used to demonstrate the absence of larvae after treatment. One dose was sufficient in 86% of the 31 horses treated, while the remaining horses—which apparently became reinfected despite precautions—required a second dose. In a subsequent trial with the oral paste formulation, the results were difficult to assess quantitatively—because of spontaneous cures in some of the untreated control animals—but did support the finding of efficacy against cutaneous *Habronema* sp. in horses (V.E. Reuter-Dallman, unpublished).

G. *Onchocerca cervicalis*

Ivermectin is not known to be active against the adult stage of any species of *Onchocerca* in any host species, and its lack of efficacy in the case of *Onchocerca* spp. in the horse has been documented (Lyons, Drudge, and Tolliver 1988). However, its activity against the skin-dwelling microfilariae of the genus *Onchocerca* has been known since Egerton and colleagues (1981) demonstrated that a single subcutaneous injection at 200 μg/kg was highly effective against the microfilariae of *O. cervicalis* in horses. Subsequent studies have shown that intramuscular administration of the same dosage is highly effective; and Herd and Donham (1983) have reviewed the parasitological and clinical significance of the finding.

The efficacy of the paste formulation against the microfilariae of *O. cervicalis* has also been reported (French *et al.* 1988a; Foil *et al.*, 1985; and Pollitt *et al.* 1986). In these studies, treatment resulted in both the disappearance of microfilariae from the skin and the resolution of the associated lesions. In the experience of Pollitt and colleagues (1986), "a single oral dose of ivermectin caused all microfilariae of *Onchocerca spp.* to disappear from the skin and all the horses showed marked clinical improvement of their dermatitis 1 to 2 weeks after treatment. By 4 to 6 weeks it was impossible to determine the original sites of the lesions." These authors went on to point out that ivermectin did not reduce lesions attributed to hypersensitivity to midge bites, and therefore it could be used in horses to differentiate between that form of dermatitis and onchocercal dermatitis. The presence of *O. cervicalis* microfilariae in the skin is by no means always associated with dermatitis, but where dermatitis occurs, it can be treated successfully with ivermectin.

H. Other Helminths

Ivermectin at 200 μg/kg, given orally in the paste formulation, was effective against *Strongyloides westeri* in foals (Ryan and Best 1985; Schlichting and Stoye 1985). This observation is in accord with earlier studies using the injectable formulation (see reviews cited previously). Ponies with naturally acquired infections of *Setaria equina* were treated intramuscularly with ivermectin. Dosages of 200 to 500 μg/kg gave moderate efficacy (80%–88%) (Klei, Torbert, and Ochoa 1980). Ivermectin was given to a pony with severe jaw disease attributed to invasion of the tissue by *Micronema deletrix,* but the disease was not alleviated (Keg *et al.* 1984). A pony continued to pass *Anoplocephala* spp. eggs in the feces after treatment with ivermectin paste (Torbert, Kramer, and Klei 1982), as would be expected in view of the lack of efficacy of this drug against tapeworms in general.

I. *Gastrophilus* spp. (Bots)

The efficacy of parenterally administered ivermectin against the parasitic larvae (stomach bots) of *Gastrophilus intestinalis* and *G. nasalis* was reported by Egerton and colleagues (1981), who showed that subcutaneous dosages as low as 20 μg/kg were highly effective. The effectiveness of the broad-spectrum intramuscular dosage of 200 μg/kg has been demonstrated by several groups (see reviews cited previously). The oral paste is as effective as the injectable formulation, as illustrated by a trial in which a single dose of the paste at 200 μg/kg removed 99% of *G. intestinalis* larvae and 100% of *G. nasalis* larvae (Torbert, Kramer, and Klei 1982) and a trial in which the same dosage removed 100% of second and third stage larvae of *G. intestinalis* (Britt and Preston 1985).

J. *Sarcoptes scabiei*

Ivermectin was highly effective against *Sarcoptes scabiei* (of goat origin) in experimentally infected donkeys, *Equus asinus* (Abu-Samra *et al.* 1985). Similarly, systemic ivermectin treatment in conjunction with a topical acaricidal dressing was reported curative against sarcoptic mange (perhaps of fox origin) in horses (Christensson *et al.* 1984).

References

Abu-Samra MT, Ali BH, Musa BE, Ibrahim KEE (1985) Experimental infection of the domestic donkey (*Equus asinus asinus*) with a goat strain of *Sarcoptes scabiei,* and treatment with ivermectin. *Acta Tropica* 42:217–224.

Asquith RL, Plue RE, Seward RL (1983) Field performance of the equine parasiticide, ivermectin, in an oral paste. *Equ. Vet. J.* 3:90–91.

Baker NF, Miller JE, Madigan JE, Fulton R, Seward RL (1984) Anthelmintic action of ivermectin, oxibendazole, and pyrantel pamoate against thiabendazole-resistant small strongyles of horses. *Equ. Pract.* 6:8–19.

Bello TR (1985) Proc. 30th Ann. Mtg., Am. Assoc. Vet. Parasit., University of North Carolina.

Boraski EA (1987) Ivermectin, efficacy against ascarids—new information. *Calif. Vet.* 41:16–17.

Britt DP, Preston JM (1985) Efficacy of ivermectin against *Dictyocaulus arnfieldi* in ponies. *Vet. Rec.* 116:343–345.

Burrows RO, Thomson BM, Lindsey MJ (1985) Efficacy of ivermectin against nematodes of horses including small strongyles resistant to benzimidazole. *Austral. Vet. J.* 61:343–344.

Campbell WC (1985) Ivermectin: An update. *Parasit. Today* 1:10–16.

Campbell WC, Benz GW (1983) Ivermectin: A review of efficacy and safety. *J. Vet. Pharm. & Therap.* 7:1–16.

Christensson D, Lindstedt E, Wierup M, Aropsenius J (1984) Sarcopotic mange in horses in Sweden. *Svensk Vet.* 36:15–17 (in Swedish).

Corba J, Andrasko H, Stoffa P, Holakovsky P (1986) Efficacy of Eqvalan™ and Panacur™ paste against gastrointestinal nematodes of horses. *Veterinarstvi* 36:79–80 (in Slovak).

DiPietro JA, Lock TF, Todd KS, Davis JL (in press) Evaluation of ivermectin for larvacidal effect in experimentally induced *Parascaris equorum* infections in pony foals. *Am. J. Vet. Res.*

DiPietro JA, Lock TF, Todd KS, Reuter VE (1987) Evaluation of ivermectin paste in the treatment of ponies for *Parascaris equorum* infections. *J. Am. Vet. Med. Assoc.* 190:1181–1183.

Egerton JR, Brokken ES, Suhayda D, Eary CH, Wooden JW, Kilgore RL (1981) The antiparasitic activity of ivermectin in horses. *Vet. Parasit.* 8:83–88.

Egerton JR, Seward RL, Robin B (1984) Ivermectin as an antiparasitic agent for horses. Proc. MDS AGVET Symposium: Recent Developments in the Control of Animal Parasites, XXII World Veterinary Congress, Perth, Australia, Aug. 25–26, 1983, pp. 49–55.

Foil LD, Klei TR, Miller RI, Foil CS, French DD (1985) Pathogenesis of equine ventral midline dermatitis and its association with *Onchocerca cervicalis* and *Haematobia irritans*. Abst. 196, 11th Conf. World Assoc. Adv. Vet. Parasitol., Rio de Janeiro, Brazil, Aug. 5–9, 1985.

French DD, Klei TR, Chapman MR, Torbert BJ (1985) Field evaluation of ivermectin against benzimidazole resistant strongyles in Louisiana horses. Abst. 197, 11th Conf. World Assoc. Adv. Vet. Parasitol.

French DD, Klei TR, Foil CS, Miller RI, Foil LD, Chapman MR, McClure JJ (1988a) Efficacy of ivermectin in paste and injectable formulations against microfilariae of *Onchocerca cervicalis* and resolution of associated dermatitis in horses. *Am. J. Vet. Res.* 49:1550–1554.

French DD, Klei TR, Taylor HW, Chapman MR, Wright FR (1988) Efficacy of ivermectin in the oral paste formulation against naturally acquired adult and larval stages of *Parascaris equorum* in pony foals. *Am. J. Vet. Res.* 49:1000–1003.

French DD, Klei TR, Chapman MR and Taylor HW (in press) Efficacy of ivermectin in the oral paste and oral drench formulations against migrating larvae of *Parascaris equorum*. Am. J. Vet. Res.

Herd RP, Donham JC (1983) Efficacy of ivermectin against *Onchocerca cervicalis* microfilarial dermatitis in horses. *Am. J. Vet. Res.* 44:1102–1105.

Herd RP, Donham JC (1984) Control of equine cutaneous nematodiasis by ivermectin. Proc. MSD AGVET Symposium: Recent Developments in the Control of Animal Parasites, XXII World Vet Congr., Perth, Australia, Aug. 25–26, 1983, pp 286–295.

Klei TR, Torbert BJ, Chapman MR and Turk MAM (1984a) Efficacy of ivermectin in injectable and oral paste formulations against eight-week-old *Strongylus vulgaris* larvae in ponies. Am. J. Vet. Res. 45:183–185.

Klei TR, Torbert BJ, Onchoa R (1980) Efficacy of ivermectin (22,23-dihydro-avermectin B_1) against adult *Setaria equina* and microfilariae of *Onchocerca cervicalis* in ponies. *J. Parasit.* 66:859–861.

Klei TR, Turk MAM, Torbert BJ, Chapman MR (1984a) Ivermectin in parenteral and oral paste formulations: efficacy against gastrointestinal parasites, migrating larvae of *Strongylus vulgaris,* and post-treatment responses of infected ponies. Proc. MSD AGVET Symposium: Recent Developments in the Control of Animal Parasites, XXII World Vet., Congr., Perth, Australia, Aug. 25–26, 1983, pp 271–285.

Leaning WHD (1984) The efficacy and safety evaluation of ivermectin as a parenteral and oral antiparasitic agent in horses. In Milne FJ (ed) Proceedings of the Twenty-Ninth Annual Convention of the American Association of Equine Practitioners, Las Vegas, Nevada, Dec. 1983.

Lyons ET, Drudge JH, Tolliver SC (1985) Ivermectin: treating for naturally occurring infections of lungworms and stomach worms in equids. *Vet. Med.* 80:58–64.

Lyons ET, Drudge JH, Tolliver SC (1988) Verification of ineffectual activity of ivermectin against adult *Onchocerca spp.* in the ligamentum nuchae of horses. *Am. J. Vet. Res.* 49:983–985.

Madigan JE (1984) Ivermectin use in the horse, reviewed. *Calif. Vet.* 38:29–32, 35.

Pollitt CC, Holdsworth PA, Kelly WR, Meacham CS, Sheahan B (1986) Treatment of equine onchocerciasis with ivermectin paste. *Austral. Vet. J.* 63:152–156.

Puccini V, Tassi P, Lo Storto E, Troiano P (1984) Field evaluation of the efficacy of ivermectin paste against intestinal helminths in horses. *Obiettivi e Documenti Vet.* 5:53–55 (in Italian).

Ryan WG, Best PJ (1985) Efficacy of ivermectin paste against *Strongyloides westeri* in foals. *Vet. Rec.* 117:169–170.

Schlichting CK, Stoye, M (1985) Effect of ivermectin on *Strongyloides westeri* in foals. Prakt. Tierarzt. 66:128–130 (in German).

Slocombe JOD, McCraw BM, Pennock PW and Vasey J (1982) Effectiveness of ivermectin against later 4th-stage *Strongylus vulgaris* in ponies. Am. J. Vet. Res. 43:1525–1529.

Slocombe JOD, McCraw BM, Pennock PW, Vasey J (1984) Ivermectin in the control of *Strongylus vulgaris* in the equine. Proc. MSD AGVET Symposium: Recent Developments in the Control of Animal Parasites, XXII World Vet. Congr., Perth, Australia, Aug 25–26, 1983, pp 265–270.

Slocombe JOD and McGraw BM (1984) Evaluation of ivermectin against later 4th-stage *Strongylus vulgaris* in ponies at two and five weeks after treatment. Canadian J. Comp. Med. 48:343–348.

Torbert BJ, Kramer BS, Klei TR (1982) Efficacy of injectable and oral paste formulations of ivermectin against gastrointestinal parasites in ponies. *Am. J. Vet. Res.* 43:1451–1453.
Weiss J (1984) Value of ivermectin in treating certain parasitoses of horses. *Rev. Med. Vet.* 135:425–433 (in French).

CHAPTER 18

Use of Ivermectin in Dogs and Cats

W.C. Campbell

I. DOGS
   A. Products
      1. Heartgard 30
      2. Heartgard 30 chewable
   B. Antiparasitic efficacy
      1. Endoparasites
         a. *Dirofilaria immitis* (heartworm)
         b. *Dipetalonema reconditum*
         c. *Toxocara canis*
         d. *Toxascaris leonina*
         e. *Ancylostoma caninum* (hookworm)
         f. *Uncinaria stenocephala* (hookworm)
         g. *Strongyloides stercoralis*
         h. *Filaroides osleri*
         i. *Capillaria spp.*
         j. *Trichuris vulpis* (whipworm)
      2. Ectoparasites
         a. *Sarcoptes scabei*
         b. *Demodex canis*
         c. *Otodectes cynotis*
         d. *Ctenocephalides cati*
II. CATS
   A. Products
   B. Antiparasitic efficacy
      1. Endoparasites
         a. *Aelurostrongylus abstrusus*
         b. *Toxocara cati*
         c. *Ancylostoma* spp.
         d. Other helminths
      2. Ectoparasites
         a. *Nodoedres cati*
         b. *Otodectes cynotis*
         c. *Ctenocephalides cati*

I. Dogs

A. Products

1. Heartgard 30™

This is a product for the prevention of heartworm disease in dogs. It is for use by, or on the order of, a licensed veterinarian, and consists of color-coded packages of white, hard tablets containing ivermectin in the amount of 65 μg (blue code, for dogs weighing up to 25 lb), 136 μg (green code, for dogs weighing 26 to 50 lb), or 272 μg (brown code, for dogs weighing 51 to 100 lb). When administered according to this schedule, the tablets provide a minimum ivermectin dosage of 6 μg/kg.

The product is to be administered at monthly intervals, beginning within one month after the first expected exposure to mosquitoes and ending within a month after the last potential exposure. The indication for use in heartworm prevention is based on efficacy studies summarized below.

The product is not recommended for dogs under 6 weeks of age. Certain dogs, particularly Collies, are exceptionally susceptible to ivermectin toxicity (see Chapter 10). In such dogs, adverse reactions have been reported when ivermectin was given under experimental conditions at 200 μg/kg but not when given at 50 μg/kg.

2. Heartgard 30 Chewable™

The chewable formulation consists of tablets that are designed to be readily accepted by dogs when proffered to them, thus obviating the need to insert the medication into the dog's mouth. In other respects the product's use is similar to that of Heartgard 30™.

B. Antiparasitic Efficacy

1. Endoparasites

a. *Dirofilaria immitis* (heartworm):

Immatures. Ivermectin prevents the maturation of the immature (precardiac) stages of heartworm, thus preventing heartworm disease. The studies that have demonstrated this efficacy are listed in Table 18.1 and have been reviewed in detail elsewhere (Campbell 1987).

When treatment (50 μg/kg) was given 1 day after inoculation of dogs with infective larvae, heartworm subsequently failed to appear in the heart (Blair, Jacob, and Ewanciw 1982). Because the third stage larva is believed to molt about 2 days after inoculation, the success of treatment was probably due to efficacy against the third stage larva. It is possible, however, that the quantity of drug remaining in the dog's tissues after the worms had molted was sufficient to affect the fourth stage directly.

TABLE 18.1. Prophylactic efficacy of ivermectin against *D. immitis* when given to experimentally infected dogs at various intervals after inoculation.

Time of Treatment	Dosage (μg/kg)	Efficacy[1]	Investigators
1–2 days	50 po × 1	100%	Blair *et al.* 1982
1 month	3.0 po × 1[2]	Poor	McCall *et al.* 1986
	3.0 po × 1	None	Paul *et al.* 1986a
	1.0 po × 1	Poor	McCall *et al.* 1986
	1.0 po × 1	Poor	Paul *et al.* 1986a
	2.0 po × 1	100%	McCall *et al.* 1986
	3.0 po × 1[2]	100%	McCall *et al.* 1986
	3.3 po × 1	High	Paul *et al.* 1986a
	3.0 po × 1	100%	McCall *et al.* 1981
	12.5 po × 1	100%	McCall *et al.* 1981
	50 po × 1	100%	Blair and Campbell 1980
	50 po × 1	100%	McCall *et al.* 1981
	200 po × 1	100%	McCall *et al.* 1981
	200 sc × 1	100%	McCall *et al.* 1981
	400 po × 1	100%	McCall *et al.* 1981
1.5 months	2.0 po × 1	Poor	Paul *et al.* 1986a
	2.0 po × 1	Variable	McCall *et al.* 1986
	3.3 po × 1	High[3]	Paul *et al.* 1986b
	6.0 po × 1	100%	Paul *et al.* 1986b
	12 po × 1	High[4]	Paul *et al.* 1986b
	25 po × 1	100%	Paul *et al.* 1986b
	50 po × 1	100%	Paul *et al.* 1986b
2 months	3.3 po × 1	Variable	McCall *et al.* 1986
	6.0 po × 1	100%	McCall *et al.* 1986
	12 po × 1	High	McCall *et al.* 1986
	25 po × 1	100%	McCall *et al.* 1986
	50 po × 1	100%	McCall *et al.* 1986
	50 po × 1	100%	Blair and Campbell. 1980
	200 po × 5	100%	Egerton *et al.* 1980
3 months	50 po × 1	Variable	Blair and Campbell 1980
	50 po × 1	Variable	McCall *et al.* 1981
	100 po × 1	Variable	McCall *et al.* 1981
	200 po × 1	Variable	McCall *et al.* 1981

Abbreviations: po, orally; sc, subcutaneously.

[1] 100%, no worms found in any treated animal; high, 95% to 100% reduction in all treated animals; variable, 100% reduction in some treated animals and <95% reduction in others; poor, <95% reduction in all treated animals.

[2] Dogs held for 1 year after treatment instead of usual 1/2 year.

[3] Two male worms in 1 of 8 dogs.

[4] One male worm in 1 of 8 dogs.

When treatment is given 1 month after inoculation of dogs with infective larvae, the subsequent absence of worms in the heart can be attributed to efficacy against the fourth stage larvae (references in Table 18.1). This stage is extraordinarily susceptible to the action of ivermectin—perhaps more so than any stage of any other helminth. Single oral doses as low as 1 μg/kg have been highly active, but administration of such a dosage has not given uniform results, and in practice of dosage of 6 μg/kg is used to ensure complete prophylaxis in all cases.

A marked falling-off in efficacy is observed when treatment is delayed until 3 months after inoculation (Table 18.1), and this probably reflects the increasing proportion of the worm population that has molted to the fifth stage and become refractory to the drug.

Repeated cycles of infection and ivermectin treatment have been used to demonstrate the immunogenicity of immature *D. immitis* (Blair and Campbell 1981; Blair, Jacob, and Ewanciw 1982).

Adults. In contrast to the exceptional susceptibility of the immature stages in the body tissues of infected dogs is the apparently total refractoriness of the adult worms in the lumen of the heart and associated blood vessels. Even dosages approximating the maximum tolerated dosage for dogs have not resulted in the death of the adult worms. The adult worms are undoubtedly exposed to the drug because the drug is demonstrably present in the blood plasma of treated animals in general. The drug may not reach the inside of the worms, however, and may not affect them adversely even if it does. Ivermectin does not kill or paralyze adult heartworm *in vitro* (Anantaphruti *et al.* 1982); and it has also been shown that, under *in vitro* conditions, radiolabeled ivermectin does in fact get widely distributed in the tissues of the worms but does not affect them adversely in any visible way (R. E. Howells, unpublished data). Despite these indications of the insusceptibility of adult *D. immitis* to ivermectin, certain observations suggest that the drug may have a suppressive effect on the reproduction of the worm following *in vivo* treatment (Anantaphruti *et al.* 1982; Knight *et al.* 1986; Lok *et al.* 1988). The nature of this effect is unclear. While Anantaphruti and colleagues observed a scarcity of advanced microfilariae in the anterior part of the uteri, Lok and colleagues observed an accumulation of fully developed microfilariae and a decrease in the early embryonic stages. The latter authors suggested that treatment of the host dog with ivermectin might block an early stage in the embryogenesis of *Dirofilaria* within that host, without preventing the more advanced embryos from continuing their development into microfilariae. Alternatively, or in addition, the accumulation of fully developed microfilariae within the uteri might be due to blockade of the mechanism by which microfilariae are expelled from the vulva (Lok *et al.* 1988).

Microfilariae. The microfilariae of *D. immitis* are highly susceptible to ivermectin, and the use of ivermectin as a microfilaricide has been discussed in detail elsewhere (Jackson 1987). Many authors have reported the suppression of peripheral microfilaremia after the treatment of dogs with ivermectin at various dosages (Table 18.2). This could reflect paralysis and sequestration of microfilariae, but evidence of killing—at

TABLE 18.2. Dosages of ivermectin found capable of reducing or eliminating microfilariae of *D. immitis* in dogs. Degree and duration of effect depend on various factors; see text.

Dosage (μg/kg)	Investigators
Various	Jackson and Seymour 1981
2.0 po × 3[1]	Schlotthauer *et al.* 1986
3.1 po × 1[2]	Blair *et al.* 1983
10 po × 3[1]	Schlotthauer *et al.* 1986
12.5 po × 1	Blair *et al.* 1983
12.5 po × 1	Swartz 1985
50 po × 1[2]	Blair *et al.* 1983
50 po × 1	Boreham *et al.* 1983
50 po × 1[2]	Jackson 1984
50 po × 1[2]	Jackson *et al.* 1986
200 po × 1[2]	Blair *et al.* 1983
200 po × 1	Anantaphruti *et al.* 1982
200 sc × 1	Plue *et al.* 1983
200 sc × 1	Simpson and Jackson 1985
250 po × 1[2]	Knight *et al.* 1986
400 po × 3[1]	Schlotthauer *et al.* 1986
500 sc × 1	McManus and Pulliam 1984

Abbreviations: po, orally; sc, subcutaneously.
[1] At intervals of approximately 1 month.
[2] Preceded by adulticide treatment in at least some groups.

least at higher dosages—has been found by examination of various visceral tissues at biopsy or necropsy of treated dogs (McManus and Pulliam 1984; Simpson and Jackson 1985).

Following the administration of a single dose of ivermectin at 250 or 500 μg/kg *per os* (p.o.), suppression of microfilaremia was barely detectable at 4 hours, significant at 8 hours, and very marked at 18 hours (Knight *et al.* 1986; McManus and Pulliam 1984). The time required for suppression following lower dosages has not been determined precisely, but 90% of dogs receiving 50 μg/kg p.o. became microfilaria-negative within 3 weeks, and the remainder became negative within 4, or (in a few cases) more weeks (Jackson 1987). Of the 121 dogs so treated, 96% became negative after a single dose, and 100% were negative after receiving multiple doses.

If microfilaricidal treatment is not preceded or followed by adulticidal treatment, the suppression of microfilaremia will be temporary. Treatment may reduce the reproductive capacity of the adults (Anantaphruti *et al.* 1982), but they will again shed microfilariae if given sufficient time.

Although ivermectin at 50 μg/kg is used routinely as a microfilaricide by some veterinarians, this use has not been approved by government regulatory agencies. Such approval has not been sought by the manufacturer of the drug, and no recommendation or claim is made by the manufacturer with respect to microfilaricidal use.

As in the case of adult *D. immitis,* the microfilariae are not killed by ivermectin *in vitro* (Devaney and Howells 1984) although preliminary data suggest that ivermectin can be lethal to microfilariae when host leukocytes are present in the medium (E. C. McManus, unpublished data). Further work is needed to determine why both stages are virtually unaffected *in vitro,* while one is susceptible in the blood-vascular system of the host and the other is not.

b. *Dipetalonema reconditum*

Lindemann and McCall (1983) gave ivermectin orally at 250 μg/kg to three Beagle dogs experimentally infected with *D. reconditum.* Treatment was followed by a reduction of more than 99% in the number of circulating microfilariae. When the dogs were necropsied, no adult *D. reconditum* were found in the abdominal cavity or connective tissues, but the authors cautioned that the absence of adult worms in this experiment is not necessarily a reflection of drug efficacy.

c. *Toxocara canis*

Treatment of patent naturally acquired infections of *T. canis* in dogs reduced the worm burden by 91% when the ivermectin dosage was 200 μg/kg subcutaneously (s.c.) and 97% when the dosage was 400 μg/kg s.c. (Anderson and Roberson 1982).

The immature stages of *T. canis* are important in two quite different contexts—the intestinal and the extraintestinal. Against the intestinal fourth stage larvae (in dogs treated 2 weeks after inoculation with infective eggs) ivermectin was 97% effective at 200 μg/kg s.c. and 98% effective at 400 μg/kg s.c. (Anderson and Roberson 1982). Dosages of 50 and 100 μg/kg s.c. gave no significant reduction in worm burden. Yazwinski, Tilley, and Greenway (1982) also treated dogs 2 weeks after inoculation with infective eggs of *T. canis,* but they reported 100% efficacy at dosages of 100 μg/kg s.c. and even 50 μg/kg s.c. This discrepancy may be due to the difference in intensity of infection, the mean control worm burden being 232 in the former trial and only 5.4 in the latter.

The importance of the extraintestinal (L_2) larvae of *T. canis* lies in their role in transuterine and transmammary transmission from bitch to pup; and it has been notably difficult to block this transmission by chemotherapy. Using experimentally infected mice as a model, Abo-Shenada (1982) found that L_2 larvae were affected by ivermectin at high dosage (2000 μg/kg) given p.o. or s.c. on Days 2 to 7 post inoculation. In mice so treated the larvae failed to migrate from the host liver to the brain and muscles; but when treatment was given after the larvae had completed their migration (Days 8 to 13) even that very high dosage failed to reduce their number. Studies in dogs, however, suggest that it is possible to affect *T. canis* in the tissues in such a way that pups born to treated bitches are essentially free of infection. Bitches inoculated with *T. canis* eggs were treated with ivermectin around the 42nd day of gestation (when the larvae are reactivated from the tissues) and the pups subsequently born to those bitches were necropsied either at birth or at weaning (Shoop *et al.* 1988). Treatment regimens that resulted in greater than 99% reduction in worm burden and in the passage of eggs in the feces were: 1000 μg/kg s.c. on Days 20 and 42 of gestation; 500 μg/kg s.c. on Days 38, 41, 44, and 47 of gestation; or 1000 μg/kg s.c. on Day 20 followed by 500 μ/kg on Days 42, 47, and 53 of gestation.

d. *Toxascaris leonina*

T. leonina appears to be less sensitive to ivermectin than *T. canis,* but very little comparative information is available. Using experimentally infected dogs, Anderson and Roberson (1982) found that dosages up to 400 μg/kg s.c. did not give satisfactory activity against the adult worms. Yazwinski, Tilley, and Greenway (1982) treated dogs 4 weeks after inoculation with *T. leonina* eggs (when the worms would have been in the L_4 stage). They recorded 100% efficacy with a dosage of 200 μg/kg s.c., but the mean number of worms recovered from control dogs was small.

c. *Ancylostoma caninum* (hookworm)

The canine hookworms are among the most susceptible of parasites to the action of the avermectins. In a controlled trial against adult *A. caninum* in dogs, abamectin was 98% effective at 5 μg/kg, and avermectin B_{2a} was 100% effective at 3 μg/kg (Blair and Campbell 1978). Ivermectin, too, was found to be highly active against hookworms (Table 18.3). Yazwinski, Tilley, and Greenway (1982) reported high activity at 50 μg/kg, subcutaneously, but did not test lower dosages. Egerton, Eary, and Suhayda (1985) reported that a single oral or subcutaneous dose at 24 μg/kg was more than 99% effective against both the L_4 and adult stages.

In one study, ivermectin at 10 μg/kg p.o. not only resulted in the expulsion of all of the hookworms but affected the eggs within the female worms (Wang *et al.*, in press). Eggs were teased out of the uterine tissue of female worms passed in the feces of treated dogs (and from female worms recovered from untreated dogs at necropsy) and cultured under conditions suitable for hatching and development of infective larvae. Such larvae were recovered from cultures of eggs obtained from untreated dogs but not from dogs treated with ivermectin at dosages varying from 10 to 100 μg/kg. Similarly, when ivermectin was added directly to

TABLE 18.3. Dosages of ivermectin reported to be at least 95% effective in reducing the numbers of various nematode parasites in dogs. All treatments refer to single dose; p.o. = oral, s.c. = subcutaneous.

Parasite	Dosage (μg/kg)	Reference
Toxocara canis		
L_4 stage	50 s.c.	Yazwinski *et al.* 1982
L_4 stage	200 s.c.	Anderson and Roberson 1982
adult	400 s.c.	Anderson and Roberson 1982
Toxascaris leonina		
immature	200 s.c.	Yazwinski *et al.* 1982
adult	400 s.c.	Anderson and Roberson 1982
Ancylostoma caninum		
L_4 stage	24 p.o.	Egerton *et al.* 1985
L_4 stage	50 s.c.	Anderson and Roberson 1982
L_4 stage	12 s.c.	Egerton *et al.* 1985
L_4 stage	50 s.c.	Yazwinski *et al.* 1982
adult	50 s.c.	Anderson and Roberson 1982
adult	12 p.o.	Egerton *et al.* 1985
adult	12 s.c.	Egerton *et al.* 1985
adult	10 p.o.	Wang *et al.* in press
Ancylostoma braziliense		
adult	50 s.c.	Anderson and Roberson 1982
Uncinaria stenocephala		
L_4 stage	24 p.o.	Egerton *et al.* 1985
L_4 stage	12 s.c.	Egerton *et al.* 1985
adult	24 p.o.	Egerton *et al.* 1985
adult	24 s.c.	Egerton *et al.* 1985
Trichuris vulpis		
immature	10 s.c.	Yazwinski *et al.* 1982
adult	10 s.c.	Anderson and Roberson 1982
Capillaria aerophila		
See text.		
Strongyloides stercoralis		
See text.		

cultures of *A. caninum* eggs, development was suppressed by 95% at 10 μg/ml and by 100% at 100 μg/ml (Wang *et al.*, in press). These same authors showed that ivermectin was lethal to infective (L_3) larvae of *A. caninum in vitro* at 0.025 μg/ml, and immobilized or killed adult *A. caninum in vitro* at concentrations ranging from 0.7 to 7.0 μg/ml—the severity of the effect being proportional to the concentration of drug in the medium.

f. *Uncinaria stenocephala* (hookworm)

Egerton, Eary, and Suhayda (1985), using similar techniques for each species, found *U. stenocephala* to be only slightly less susceptible than *A. caninum* to the therapeutic effect of ivermectin. Dosages that gave at least 95% reduction in the number of *U. stenocephala* are listed in Table 18.3. Against the adult stage, treatment at 12 μg/kg was 80% effective when given orally but 90% effective when given subcutaneously (Egerton, Eary, and Suhayda 1985). When given by either route, a dosage of 24 μg/kg was more than 96% effective against the adults and against L_4 larvae (Egerton, Eary, and Suhayda 1985).

g. *Strongyloides stercoralis* spp.

In a preliminary probe, ivermectin was given as a single oral dose at 800 μg/kg to 1 of 2 dogs that had severe (corticosteroid-enhanced) strongyloidiasis. The untreated dog, when necropsied 6 days after treatment, yielded 56,556 adult intestinal worms and 976,185 intestinal larvae. The treated dog yielded no intestinal adults and only 2 larvae (L.M. Aikens and G.A. Schad, personal communication 1988). Negligible numbers of worms or larvae were recovered from extraintestinal sites in either dog.

h. *Filaroides osleri*

There seems to be no published evidence of the efficacy of ivermectin against *F. osleri,* but Clayton (1983) mentioned *en passant* that a single injection at 400 μg/kg had shown "promising results in a limited number of experimental *F. osleri* infections."

i. *Capillaria* spp.

A single dog with nasal capillariasis (*C. aerophilia*) was given ivermectin orally at 200 μg/kg. The nasal discharge stopped within 7 days and the feces became free of eggs within 14 days. There was no relapse for at least 8 months (Evinger, Kazacos, and Cantwell 1985). A single dog with urinary capillariasis (*C. plica*) was injected subcutaneously with ivermectin at 200 μg/kg (after temporary alleviation of clinical signs had been achieved by fenbendazole therapy). The ivermectin treatment was followed by apparent clinical and parasitological cure (passage of eggs in urine ceased within 7 days) (Kirkpatrick and Nelson 1987).

j. *Trichuris vulpis* (whipworm)

When tested against immature (4-week-old) *T. vulpis* in experimentally infected dogs, ivermectin was 100% effective at 100 μg/kg s.c. (Yazwinski, Tilley, and Greenway 1982), but the control dogs had a mean of only 6.0 worms. Against mature *T. vulpis,* treatment was more than 99% effective at 100 μg/kg s.c., and more than 95% effective at 200 μg/kg p.o. (J. R. Egerton, unpublished data).

2. Ectoparasites

a. *Sarcoptes scabiei*

Dogs with natural infestations of *Sarcoptes scabiei* were treated subcutaneously with ivermectin at various dosages. At 200 μg/kg or higher, treatment resulted in complete cure by Day 7 after treatment. Dosages as low as 50 μg/kg were also effective but took 2 to 3 weeks to achieve their full effect (Yazwinski *et al.* 1981). The efficacy of ivermectin was confirmed in a clinical trial involving almost 300 dogs. Despite confinement of the dogs "in a heavily contaminated environment which was conducive to repeated reinfestation during treatment," 2 doses of the drug at 200 μg/kg s.c., given 14 days apart, provided marked clinical improvement and complete parasitological cure 2 weeks after the second injection (Scheidt *et al.* 1984). Additional evidence of efficacy was provided by Gravino, de Caprariis, and Agresti (1985), who used 400 μg/kg s.c., and gave 3 treatments at 8-day intervals.

b. *Demodex canis*

Despite anecdotal reports of ivermectin's efficacy in demodectic mange, there is little or no scientific evidence to support it. In one clinical study, ivermectin was administered subcutaneously to 4 dogs with generalized amitraz-resistant demodecosis. The dosage was 400 μg/kg and was repeated weekly for a total of 8 treatments. Despite this rather intensive treatment, and despite the apparent clinical and parasitological cure of 1 dog, no reduction in mite number could be demonstrated in the remaining 3 dogs (Scott and Walton 1985). All 4 dogs, however, showed some clinical improvement, and the authors suggested that this might be a reflection of decreased mite activity in the skin. Perhaps the dosage used in that study was not high enough, because Gravino, de Caprariis, and Giglio (1985) reported a favorable response in an (uncontrolled?) study in which 20 dogs were given 600 μg/kg s.c. at weekly intervals for a total of 5 treatments. On the other hand, Belot, Parent, and Pangui (1984) reported that demodectic mange responded to 2 doses of ivermection at 400 μg/kg s.c. given 15 days apart. These 3 trials were conducted in the United States, Italy, and France, respectively, so there may be geographical strains with different degrees of susceptibility. Additional controlled studies are needed to clarify the matter.

c. *Otodectes cynotis*

The efficacy of ivermectin versus *O. cynotis* was demonstrated by Yazwinski and colleagues (1981) in a controlled clinical trial using natural infections. A single subcutaneous injection at 200 μg/kg gave complete cure in 14 days, while a single treatment at 400 μg/kg resulted in cure in 7 days. Similarly, Molina (1986) found that a single injection at 200 μg/kg gave complete cure in 14 days, and Chauve (1984) also found that dosage to be fully effective.

d. *Ctenocephalides cati*

Despite anecdotal reports of efficacy, neither abamectin nor ivermectin has been shown to have significant activity against fleas on dogs. In a controlled study, ivermectin was given orally, at 50 μg/kg/day or

500 μg/kg/week, to dogs exposed repeatedly to *C. cati*. The treatment neither reduced the number of fleas to a detectable degree, nor prevented reinfestation (Blair, Egerton, and Ewanciw 1984).

II. Cats

A. Products

Ivermectin has not been approved by regulatory agencies for use in cats in any form, nor has any application for such use been submitted by the manufacturer.

B. Antiparasitic Efficacy

1. Endoparasites

a. *Aelurostrongylus abstrusus*

Blagburn and colleagues (1987) gave ivermectin orally at various dosages to cats with natural infection of *A. abstrusus,* but there was little if any evidence of efficacy. Kirkpatrick and Megella (1987) tested ivermectin against the same parasite in a single naturally infected cat. After an injection of ivermectin at 200 μg/kg, larvae continued to be detectable in the feces. After a second injection at 400 μg/kg larvae could no longer be found in the feces, but no improvement in the pulmonary disease could be demonstrated radiographically, and the findings in this single animal are of doubtful significance.

b. *Toxocara cati*

In a single treated cat, the passage of *T. cati* eggs in the feces ceased after treatment of the cat with ivermectin at 200 μg/kg s.c. (Kirkpatrick and Megella 1987). The limited evidence of efficacy provided by this single instance is supported by observations made by Blagburn and colleagues (1987) in several cats with very light natural *T. cati* infection. In those cats, oral treatment at 100 or 300 μg/kg appeared to be highly effective, but additional studies would clearly be needed to determine the efficacy of ivermectin against this common ascarid.

c. *Ancylostoma* spp.

Hookworms in cats, like those in dogs, appear to be very sensitive to ivermectin. Using cats with very light natural infections, Blagburn and colleagues (1987) obtained evidence that dosages ranging from 10 to 300 μg/kg p.o. and s.c. were active against *A. braziliense*; and in one cat infected with *A. tubaeforme,* a dosage of 10 μg/kg p.o. appeared to be effective.

d. Other Helminths

It is not known whether ivermectin is effective against *Capillaria* sp. in cats. Ivermectin is not known to be active against any species of flukes or tapeworms, and the incidental observations of Blagburn and colleagues (1987) on several tapeworm species in cats are in accord with this general finding.

2. Ectoparasites

a. *Nodoedres cati*

According to Bigler, Waber, and Pfister (1984), a single s.c. injection of ivermectin at 1000 μg/kg was effective in controlling an outbreak of notoedric mange. This was a clinical report, not the record of a laboratory trial, but all 17 treated cats were judged completely cured. Suarez and Bertero (1986) used the same high dosage successfully against *N. cati* and reported that all skin scrapings were negative for mites 7 and 30 days after treatment.

b. *Otodectes cynotis*

Chauve (1984) reported that ivermectin at 200 μg/kg s.c. was effective against naturally acquired *O. cynotis* infection in cats. Chauve and Reynaud (1984) extended this observation to experimentally induced infestations, and showed that mites disappeared 14 days after the cats had received a single injection at 666 μg/kg. Further clinical reports of the effectiveness of the 200 μg/kg s.c. dosage, and of a dosage of 400 μg/kg s.c., were provided by Church (1985) and Franc, Dorchies, and Soubeyroux (1985), respectively.

c. *Ctenocephalides cati*

In a clinical note, Bigler, Waber, and Pfister (1984) reported that adult populations of fleas (presumably *C. cati*) were "decimated" by an injection of ivermectin at the very high dosage of 1000 μg/kg. However, there appears to be no evidence, obtained under controlled conditions, of the efficacy of ivermectin against fleas on cats.

References

Abo-Shenada MN (1982) The effect of some anthelmintics on the second stage larvae of *Toxocara canis*. *Parasitol.* 85:xiii (in Soc. Proc.).

Anantaphruti M, Kino H, Terada M, Ishii AI, Sano M (1982) Studies on chemotherapy of parasitic helminths (XIII): Efficacy of ivermectin on the circulating microfilariae and embryonic development in the female worm of *Dirfilaria immitis*. *Jap. J. Parasitol.* 31:517–530.

Anderson DL, Roberson EL (1982) Activity of ivermectin against canine intestinal helminths. *Am. J. Vet. Res.* 43:1681–1683.

Belot J, Parent R, Pangui JL (1984) Canine demodectic mange: Clinical observations in a treatment trial with ivermectin. *Point Vet.* 16:618–620.

Bigler B, Waber S, Pfister K (1984) Successful treatment of *Notoedres cati* infestation with ivermectin. *Schweiz. Arch. Tierheilkd.* 126:365–367 (in German).

Blagburn BL, Hendrix CM, Lindsay DS, Vaughan JL (1987) Anthelmintic efficacy of ivermectin in naturally parasitized cats. *Am. J. Vet. Res.* 48:670–672.

Blair LS, Campbell WC (1978) Efficacy of avermectins against *Ancylostoma caninum* in dogs. *J. Helminthol.* 52:305–307.

Blair LS, Campbell WC (1979) Efficacy of avermectin B_1a against microfilariae of *Dirofilaria immitis*. *Am. J. Vet. Res.* 40:1031–1032.

Blair LS, Campbell WC (1981) Immunization of ferrets against *Dirofilaria immitis* by means of chemically abbreviated infections. *Para. Immunol.* 3:143–147.

Blair LS, Egerton JR, Ewanciw EV (1984) *Ctenocephalides felis*: failure of ivermectin given *per os* in miglyol vehicle to control experimental flea infestations of dogs in a double blind controlled trial. *Proc. Amer. Assoc. Vet. Parasitol.* July 15–17, New Orleans, LA.

Blair LS, Jacob L, Ewanciw DV (1982) Immunization of dogs against *Dirofilaria immitis* by means of chemically abbreviated infections. *Mole. Biochem. Parasit.*, Supplement, p. 678.

Blair LS, Malatesta PF, Ewanciw DV (1983) Dose-response study of ivermectin against *Dirofilaria immitis* microfilariae in dogs with naturally acquired infections. *Am. J. Vet. Res.* 44:475–477.

Blair LS, Williams E, Ewanciw DV (1982) Efficacy of ivermectin against third-stage *Dirofilaria immitis* larvae in ferrets and dogs. *Res. Vet. Sci.* 33:386–387.

Boreham PFL, Atwell RB (1983) Absence of shock-like reactions to ivermection in dogs infected with *Dirofilaria immitis*. J Helminthol 57:279–281.

Campbell WC (1987) Ivermectin and heartworm. *Sem. Vet. Med. & Surg.* (*Sm. Anim.*) 2:48–55.

Chauve C (1984) Prospects for a parenteral treatment for otodectic mange in dogs and cats. *Sci. Vet. Med. Comp.* 86:41–43.

Chauve C, Reynaud M-C (1984) Parenteral treatment of otodectic mange in cats: efficacy of ivermectin. *Sci. Vet. Med. Comp.* 86:189–192 (in French).

Church D (1985) Treat and control infestations of ear mites. *Vet. Med.* 54:4.

Clayton HM (1983) The management and treatment of respiratory nematode infections in small animals. *Vet. Ann.*, 23rd issue, pp 254–259.

Devaney E, Howells RE (1984) The microfilaricidal activity of ivermectin *in vitro* and *in vivo*. *Trop. Med. Parasit.* 35:47–49.

Egerton JR, Eary CH, Suhayda D (1985) Dose-titration studies of ivermectin against experimental *Ancylostoma caninum* and *Uncinaria stenocephala* infections. *Am. J. Vet. Res.* 46:1057–1059.

Evinger JV, Kazacos KR, Cantwell HD (1985) Ivermectin for treatment of nasal capillariasis in a dog. *J. Am. Vet. Med. Assoc.* 186:174–175.

Franc M, Dorchies PH, Soubeyroux H (1985) Studies on the treatment of otoacariasis in cats with ivermectin. *Rev. Med. Vet.* (France) 136:685–686 (in French).

Gravino AE, deCaprariis D, Agresti A (1985) Impiego della 22,23-diidroavermectina nel trattamento dello rogna sarcoptica del cane. *Acta Med. Vet.* 31:43–47.

Gravino AE, deCaprariis D, Giglio M (1985) Impiego della 22,23-diidroavermectina nel trattamento della Demodicosi del cane. *Acta Med. Vet.* 31:185–189.

Jackson RF (1987) Microfilaricides. *Sem. in Vet. Med. & Surg.* (*Sm. Anim.*) 2:44–47.

Jackson RF (1984) Ivermectin again. Am Heartworm Soc Bull 10:9.

Jackson RF, Seymour GW (1981) Efficacy of avermectins against microfilariae of *Dirofilaria immitis*. In Otto GF (ed) *Proceedings of the Heartworm Symposium 1980*. Vet. Med. Pub. Co., Edwardsville, KS, pp 131–136.

Jackson RF, Seymour WG, Beckett R (1986) Routine use of 0.05 mg/kg ivermectin as a microfilaricide, in Otto GF (ed): Proceedings of the Heartworm Symposium, 1986. Washington, DC, American Heartworm Society, pp 37–39.

Kirkpatrick CE, Megella C (1987) Use of ivermectin in treatment of *Aelurostrongylus abstrusus* and *Toxocara cati* infections in a cat. *J. Am. Vet. Med. Assoc.* 190:1309–1310.

Kirkpatrick CE, Nelson GR (1987) Ivermectin treatment of urinary capillariasis in a dog. *J. Am. Vet. Med. Assoc.* 191:701–702.

Knight DH, Campbell WC, Weiner DJ, Washabau RJ (1986) Microfilaricidal efficacy of ivermectin in adulticide treated and untreated heartworm infected dogs. In Otto GF (ed) *Proceedings of the Heartworm Symposium 1986*. American Heartworm Society, Washington, D.C., pp 19–27.

Lindemann BA, McCall JW (1983) Microfilaricidal activity of ivermection against *Dipetalonema reconditum*. *J. Vet. Pharm. & Therap.* 6:75–76.

Lok JB, Harpaz T, Knight DH (1988) Abnormal patterns of embryogenesis in *Dirofilaria immitis* treated with ivermectin. *J. Helminthol.* 62:175–180.

McCall JW, Lindemann BE, Porter CA (1981) Prophylactic activity of avermectins against *Dirofilaria immitis*, in Otto GF (ed): Proceedings of the Heartworm Symposium, 1980. Edwardsville, KS, Veterinary Medicine, pp 126–130.

McCall JW, Dziminanski MT, Plue RE (1986) Ivermectin in heartworm prophylaxis: Studies with experimentally induced and naturally acquired infections. In Otto GF (ed) *Proceedings of the Heartworm Symposium 1986*. American Heartworm Society, Washington, D.C., pp 9–13.

McManus EC, Pulliam JD (1984) Histopathologic features of canine heartworm microfilarial infection after treatment with ivermectin. *Am. J. Vet. Res.* 45:91–97.

Molina CG (1986) The activity of ivermectin against *Octodectes cynotis* in naturally infested dogs. *Vet. Mex.* 17:39–40.

Paul AJ, Todd KS, Sundberg JP (1986a) Efficacy of ivermectin against *Dirofilaria immitis* larvae in dogs 30 and 45 days after induced infection. *Am. J. Vet. Res.* 47:883–884.

Paul AJ, McCall JW, Todd KS (1986b) Efficacy of ivermectin against *Dirofilaria immitis* larvae in dogs forty-five days after induced infection. In Otto GF (ed) *Proceedings of the Heartworm Symposium 1986*. American Heartworm Society, Washington, D.C., pp 33–35.

Plue RE, Seward RL, Acre KE, Cave JS, Schlotthauer JC, Stromberg BE (1983) Clearance of *Dirofilaria immitis*, microfilariae in dogs using 200 mcg/kg ivermectin subcutaneously, in Otto GF (ed): Proceedings of the Heartworm Symposium, 1983, Edwardsville, KS, Veterinary Medicine, pp 153–160.

Scheidt VJ, Medleau L, Seward RL, Schwartzman RM (1984) An evaluation of ivermectin in the treatment of sarcoptic mange in dogs. *Am. J. Vet. Res.* 45:1201–1202.

Schlotthauer JC, Stromberg BE, Paul AJ (1986) Safety and acceptability of ivermectin in dogs with naturally acquired patent infection of *Dirofilaria immitis*. In Otto GF (ed) *Proceedings of the Heartworm Symposium 1986*. American Heartworm Society, Washington, D.C., pp 29–32.

Scott DW, Walton DK (1985) Experiences with the use of amitraz and ivermectin for the treatment of generalized demodicosis in dogs. *Am. Anim. Hosp. Assoc.* 21:535–541.

Shoop WL, Egerton JR, Eary CH, Suhayda D (1988) Control of *Toxocara canis* transmission from bitch to offspring with ivermectin. Program and Abstracts, *Am. Soc. Parasitol.*, Winston-Salem, NC, pp 59–60.

Simpson CF, Jackson RF (1985) Lesions in the liver and kidney of *Dirofilaria immitis*-infected dogs following treatment with ivermectin. Zeitschrift fur Parasitenkunde 71:97–105.

Swartz EO (1985) Treating for microfilaremia caused by heartworms. Vet Med 80:59.

Suarez CJM, Bertero SI (1986) Tratamiento de la sarna notoedrica del gato con ivermectina. *Vet. Argent.* 3:340–344.

Wang C, Huang XX, Zhang YQ, Yen QY, Wen Y (in press) Efficacy of ivermectin in hookworms as examined in *Ancylostoma caninum* infections. *J. Parasit.*

Yazwinski TA, Pote L, Tilley W, Rodriguez C, Greenway T (1981) Efficacy of ivermectin against *Sarcoptes scabiei* and *Otodectes cynotis* infestations of dogs. *Vet. Med. Small Anim. Clinic.* 76:1751.

Yazwinski TA, Tilley W, Greenway T (1982) Efficacy of ivermectin in the treatment of artificially induced canine, mixed, gastrointestinal helminthiasis. *Vet. Med. Small ANim. Clinic.* 77:225–226.

CHAPTER 19

Use of Ivermectin in Laboratory and Exotic Mammals and in Birds, Fish, and Reptiles

M.D. Soll

III. Wild, Zoo and Exotic Pet Animals
- A. Rodents
- B. Hedgehogs
- C. Carnivores
  - 1. Foxes
    - a. Endoparasites
    - b. Ectoparasites
  - 2. Wolves
  - 3. Cape Hunting Dog
- D. Ungulates
  - 1. Camels
    - a. Endoparasites
    - b. Ectoparasites
  - 2. Alpacas and Llamas
  - 3. Reindeer
  - 4. Deer
    - a. Endoparasites
    - b. Ectoparasites
  - 5. Bighorn sheep
  - 6. Impala
  - 7. Other Antelope
  - 8. Bison
  - 9. Buffalo
  - 10. Wild boar
  - 11. Other species
- E. Elephants
- F. Nonhuman primates
  - 1. Mite infections
  - 2. Nematode infections

IV. Birds
- A. Nematodes
  - a. *Ascaridia*
  - b. *Capillaria*
  - c. *Pelecitus*
  - d. *Oxyspirura*
  - e. *Syngamus*
- B. Mites
  - a. *Dermanyssus* and *Ornithonyssus*
  - b. *Cnemidocoptes* spp.
  - c. *Sternostoma tracheolum*
  - d. *Cytodites nudus*
  - e. *Pterolichidae*

V. Fish
- A. Copepods
- B. Nematodes

I. Introduction

The first observations on the antiparasitic properties of the avermectins were made in laboratory animal screens. Ivermectin is potent (allowing for administration of very small doses); it can be administered either orally or parenterally; and it is effective against both arthropod and nemathelmintic endo- and ectoparasites. These attributes have led to the extensive use of the compound for treating parasitic infections in a variety of laboratory, wild, zoo, and exotic mammals, as well as in reptiles, birds, and fish. Apart from domestic animals, ivermection has been approved by various regulatory authorities for use in camels and reindeer only. The treatment of any other species with the product is considered to be "extralabel" usage.

II. Laboratory Animals

A. Mice

Ivermectin's efficacy has been tested in mice against naturally acquired parasite infections as well as in a number of mouse-parasite model systems.

1. Endoparasites

a. *Aspiculuris tetraptera*

Ivermectin added to the drinking water for 24 hours to provide a dose of 1.0 to 1.6 mg/kg body weight was fully effective in removing naturally acquired infections of this parasite from laboratory mice (Hasslinger and Wiethe 1987).

b. *Nematospiroides dubius*

Oral treatment at 5 mg/kg on Days 3 or 6 post infection was reported to remove all worms present (Sayles and Jacobson 1983); Rajasekariah and colleagues (1986) reported that a much lower dose of 0.3 mg/kg completely eliminated adult worms from mice.

c. *Strongyloides* spp.

Grove (1983) reported that, following ivermectin treatment of mice with .01 mg on Days 0 and 1 (migration phase) and 3 and 4 (intestinal phase) after infection with *S. ratti,* the treated animals subsequently passed no larvae in the feces. Moreover, he found that a single dose of .05 mg 6 days after infection eradicated intestinal adult worms. Rajasekariah and colleagues (1986) reported that 2 treatments at 0.3 mg/kg are required to eliminate adult parasites from mice.

Grove (1983) reported that *S. stercoralis* responds similarly to ivermectin: daily doses of .01 mg of ivermectin on Days 0, 1, 2, and 3 after infection greatly reduced parasite numbers in the muscles, while a single dose of 0.1 mg given 1 hour or 6 days after infection completely eradicated larvae from the muscles.

d. *Syphacia obvelata*

Ostlind, Nartowicz, and Mickle (1985) reported that feeding a diet containing 0.0005% ivermectin for 6 days to mice naturally infested with pinworms was more than 99% effective against both adult and immature worms; moreover, a single oral treatment at a dose rate of 2 mg/kg was 94% to 100% effective against adult and 86% to 97% effective against immature *S. obvelata*.

e. *Toxocara canis*

Treating mice harboring immature *T. canis* with ivermectin at 2 mg/kg for 2 to 7 days after infection (Abo-Shenada and Herbert 1984), or 0.4 mg/kg on Days 15 to 28 after infection (Carillo and Barriga 1987) alters the distribution of the larvae: Larvae are retained in the liver and lungs, and fewer migrate to the brain. None of these dose rates completely eradicated the parasite from the tissues, however.

f. *Trichinella* spp.

Treating mice with avermectin at a dose rate of 3 mg/kg reduced the number of intestinal *T. spiralis* 80% to 90% (Campbell, Blair, and Lotti 1979). The number of parasites was not reduced significantly, however, following ivermectin treatment (5–10 mg/kg) of mice harboring the migrating and muscle stages of a number of *Trichinella* spp. (Sanmartin-Duran *et al.* 1986). Ivermectin was effective against intestinal forms of *T. nelsoni* and *T. nativa* in this study, reducing their number by 91% to 96% (relative to controls), following treatment at 2 and 5 mg/kg on Days 1 and 6 post infection.

g. *Trichuris muris*

Although some degree of efficacy was apparent after a repeated dose of ivermectin at 10 mg/kg, mice treated for *T. muris* infestation were not completely cured (Rajasekariah *et al.* 1986).

2. Microfilariae

Ivermectin's microfilaricidal activity has been demonstrated against immature stages of a number of filarial parasites in mice.

Single doses of ivermectin as low as 0.2 mg/kg destroyed 100% of *Onchocerca lienalis* microfilariae within 5 days after treatment. The same dose, administered at various times prior to microfilariae infection, reduced parasite recoveries by 92% for infection 4 days after treatment (Bianco *et al.* 1986).

Devaney an Howells (1984) reported that *Brugia pahangi* microfilaremia was reduced by 87% 24 hours after treatment of mice orally at 5 mg/kg; the peritoneal microfilariae of this species were unaffected. *O. lienalis* larvae in the cutaneous and subcutaneous tissues, and *Dirofilaria immitis* microfilariae in the blood of mice were also killed at this dose.

Zahner and colleagues (1987) reported that subcutaneous treatment of *Dipetalonema viteae*-infected *Mastomys natalensis* with ivermectin at 0.1 mg/kg once or 0.05 mg/kg on 5 consecutive days reduced microfilaremia 100% over a 42-day trial period. Higher doses (0.2 mg/kg once or 5×1.5 mg/kg) were required to remove microfilariae of *Litomosoides carinii*. Lower doses removed circulating microfilariae of both species for shorter periods of time. Activity against adult *D. viteae* was demonstrated following 5 consecutive daily treatments at 0.2 mg/kg and higher; ivermectin did not affect the numbers of adult *L. carinni* at these dose rates.

3. Ectoparasites

The efficacy of ivermectin has been evaluated against some parasitic arthropod species in the mouse.

a. Mites

Silverman, Blatt, and Lerro (1983) reported that feeding mice a commercial diet containing 2 mg of ivermectin/kg of feed for two 6-day periods, 1 week apart, effectively eliminated *Myobia musculi* mites. Efficacy of the product against murine mites was confirmed by Wing, Courtney, and Young (1985), who demonstrated that 2 subcutaneous injections at 0.2 mg/kg, given 1 week apart, effectively eliminated *Mycoptes musculinus* and *Myobia musculi* from laboratory mice. Single treatments reduced infections only temporarily.

Baumans *et al.* (1988) reported that spraying mice with a .01% solution of ivermectin was effective in eliminating symptoms of mite infection for 12 weeks after treatment.

b. Triatomid bugs

Treating mice with ivermectin at 0.2 mg/kg was reported to have caused high mortality and a reduction in egg-laying potential of *Rhodnius prolixus* and *Hemiptera triatominae* feeding on these animals (Azambuja *et al.* 1985).

c. *Cuterebra fontinella*

The *C. fontinella*/mouse model was used to demonstrate the systemic insecticidal efficacy of the avermectins. Ostlind, Cifelli, and Lang (1979) reported an avermectin mixture to be effective at dose levels of 0.15 mg/kg and higher. Drummond (1980) subsequently confirmed this activity using ivermectin in mice with induced *C. fontinella* infections.

B. Rats

Rats have been used as a model system to assess ivermectin's basic toxicology, as well as for extensive studies on the drug's mode of action, pharmacology, and pharmacokinetics (Calcott and Fatig 1984; Chiu *et al.* 1986; Olsen and Snowman 1985; Pong and Wang 1980; Pong, Wang, and Fritz 1980; Williams and Yarbrough 1979).

Antiparasitic evaluation has been limited to a few endoparasite–rat models, although efficacy has been demonstrated against natural pinworm infestations.

a. *Angiostrongylus cantonensis*

Although treatment of 6-week-old infections of *A. cantonensis* at a dose of 0.1 mg/kg resulted in a lower fecal egg and larval count in rats (indicating an effect on the fecundity of the parasite), ivermectin did not have a demonstrable vermicidal effect at this level. Oral treatment at the higher dose of 1 mg/kg, 3 days after induced infection, did result in a significant reduction in the number of worms recovered (Ishii *et al.* 1983).

b. *Trichinella spiralis*

Although treatment at 0.3 mg/kg was only 84% effective against migrating larvae and 83% effective against encysted forms, increasing the dose rate to 3 mg/kg was reported to increase efficacy to 94% and 99% respectively, against these 2 stages of *T. spiralis* (Rapic, Dzakula, and Matic-Piantanida 1982). Daily treatment at 0.6 mg/kg for 3 days was found to be only 54% effective against intestinal *T. spiralis* (Alcaino, Gorman, and Imbert 1984).

c. *Syphacia muris*

Treatment of rats with ivermectin at 0.2 mg/kg/day for 5 consecutive days was 99% effective against natural infections of this parasite (Battles *et al.* 1987). There was no difference in body weight between treated and control animals, and no toxic signs were observed after treatment.

C. Guinea Pigs

1. Ticks

In screening tests, ivermectin has been shown to be completely effective against the lone star tick (*Amblyomma americanum*) when adult ticks are fed on treated guinea pigs (Hunt 1982). Efficacy has also been demonstrated against larval, nymphal, and adult *Rhipicephalus sanguineus*—as well as *A. americanum*—when these ticks were fed on guinea pigs treated at dose rates of up to 2.0 mg/kg (Wilkins *et al.* 1981).

2. Tsetse Flies

Mortality of tsetse flies (*Glossina palpalis*) occurred among flies fed exclusively on guinea pigs treated with ivermectin at dose rates greater than 2.0 mg/kg (Distelmans, D'Haeseleer, and Mortelmans 1983).

3. Mange Mites

Ivermectin has been used successfully to treat mange caused by the mite *Trixacarus caviae* in a guinea pig colony. The compound was administered at 0.2 mg/kg subcutaneously on 3 occasions with 7-day intervals (Harvey 1987).

D. Hamsters

Ivermectin's efficacy against the human hookworm *Necator americanus* was evaluated against a strain of the parasite adapted to laboratory hamsters. Doses of 30 mg/kg once, or 10 mg/kg twice, were required for complete clearance of immature *N. americanus*; lower doses of 15 mg/kg once, or 7.5 mg/kg twice, completely eliminated infestation in hamsters carrying adult parasites (Rajasekariah *et al.* 1986).

E. Gerbils

The avermectin's efficacy against *Trichostrongylus colubriformis* was assessed in gerbils early in the development phase of these compounds. A mixture of avermectin B_{1a} and B_{2a} was found to be 100% effective against 6-day-old *T. colubriformis* when administered at 0.03 mg/kg (Ostlind and Cifelli 1981).

F. Rabbits

The resolution of lesions on the ears of rabbits caused by psoroptic mite infestation gave the first indication of the potential activity of this class of compounds against arthropods (Wilkins *et al.* 1980). Numerous studies have subsequently been conducted to demonstrate ivermectin's efficacy against natural and induced mange mite infections in rabbits. The rabbit has also been used as a model to assess the systemic effect of ivermectin on tsetse flies and ticks feeding on treated animals.

1. Mange Mites

Although subcutaneous injection of ivermectin at 0.2 mg/kg is reported to be effective for treating rabbits naturally infected with psoroptic and sarcoptic mange mites (Ashmawy and Fahmy 1987; Macchioni, Marconcini, and Sbrana 1983); Mousa *et al.* 1986a), some investigators have found that a single treatment at 0.2 or 0.4 mg/kg does not always eliminate psoroptic mites (Wright and Riner 1985; Prosl and Kanout 1985). Wright and Riner (1985) suggest that the susceptibility of 2 psoroptic mite species, *Psoroptes ovis* and *P. cuniculi,* to ivermectin treatment in rabbits may be different. Romero and Valentini (1984) report that 2 treatments at 0.25 mg/kg, 7 days apart, were effective in eradicating psoroptic and sarcoptic mite infection; Prosl and Kanout (1985) recommend 2 treatments at 0.4 mg/kg, 4 to 6 days apart, for eradication of *P. cuniculi* infection. Curtis, Housley, and Brooks (1988) report that 2 ivermectin treatments at 0.4 mg/kg with an 18-day interval are safe and effective for treating rabbits with ear mite infections but suggest that subsequent injections may be necessary in rabbitries with poor sanitation. Two subcutaneous ivermectin treatments 3 weeks apart are also reported to be effective against *Notoedres cati* infection in rabbits (Manurang, Partoutomo, and Stevenson 1985).

2. Tsetse Flies

The reproductive capacity of *Glossina palpalis* fed on rabbits treated with ivermectin at 2.0 mg/kg has been shown to be significantly reduced (Abbeele, D'Haeseleer, and Goossens 1986).

3. Ticks

In an assessment of the suitability of the rabbit as a model for testing systemic ascaricides, ivermectin has been shown to be effective against induced infestations of *Ornithodoros moubata* for up to 7 days after treatment at dose rates of 0.1 to 0.4 mg/kg (Frossard 1981).

G. Ferrets and Jirds

Because the ferret (*Mustela putorius*) is susceptible to infection with the canine heartworm *Dirofilaria immitis,* this species was initially used to assess the effect of ivermectin on the precardiac stages of heartworm. Ferrets, artificially infected with *D. immitis* 2 to 42 days prior to treatment, were given ivermectin at dose rates between 0.0125 and 2.0 mg/kg (Blair and Campbell 1980; Blair, Williams, and Ewanciw 1982). The results of these studies suggest that the minimum effective dose for suppression of maturation of *D. immitis* larvae in ferrets lies between .0125 and 0.05 mg/kg, which is higher than the dose required for this purpose in dogs.

In contrast to the exquisite sensitivity of the precardiac stages of *D. immitis* to ivermectin, this compound has not been shown to be effective in preventing the development of adult *Brugia pahangi* in the jird (Campbell 1982; Denham 1982).

III. Wild, Zoo, and Exotic Pet Animals

Although ivermectin is a useful antiparasitic agent for the treatment of a variety of parasitic diseases encountered in wild, zoo, and exotic pet animals, its overall usage in these species is relatively small and does not warrant full-scale development projects to assess all aspects of safety and efficacy for the numerous species represented here.

The injectable formulation is registered for use in camels in Algeria, Jordan, Morocco, and Sudan; it has also been approved under an IR4 (minor species) development program for use in reindeer in the United States. Apart from these applications, none of the commercially available formulations is registered for use in other nondomesticated species; considerable extra-label usage of these products does occur, however. This section reviews the reported use of ivermectin in these species.

A. Rodents

In addition to the treatment of natural and induced parasitic infections of a number of rodent species under laboratory conditions, squirrels have been successfully treated with ivermectin for mite infestation (*Notoedres douglassi*). Subcutaneous treatment at a dose rate of 0.5 mg/kg resulted in almost complete resolution of skin lesions within 5 days; no mites were recovered from subsequent multiple skin scrapings (Evans 1984).

B. Hedgehogs

Ivermectin is reported to be effective against *Crenosoma striatum* (95.9%) and *Capillaria* spp. (100%) when administered at dose rate of 3 mg/kg to hedgehogs (Barutzki, Laubmeier, and Forstner 1987).

C. Carnivores

1. Foxes

a. Endoparasites

Blagburn and colleagues (1986) report a study in which wild foxes were trapped and an assessment of helminth infection made by fecal flotation. Animals were then divided into groups and treated with a number of anthelmintics, including ivermectin at 0.4 mg/kg. Of the 9 foxes positive for *Ancylostoma* spp. eggs prior to ivermectin treatment, none was positive by 3 weeks after treatment.

In a study involving more than 500 female arctic and silver foxes, those treated with ivermectin subcutaneously at 0.2 mg/kg had better conception and parturition rates than untreated animals (Kopczewski *et al.* 1987). The numbers of cubs with *Toxocara canis* eggs in the feces at 30, 60, and 75 days of age was approximately 50% lower for those cubs born to ivermectin-treated vixens than for those born to controls.

b. Ectoparasites

The efficacy of ivermectin has been assessed against 2 mite species—*Sarcoptes scabiei* var *canis* and *Cheyletiella blakei*—in foxes.

Sarcoptic mange mites were eradicated from foxes treated with ivermectin at dose rates of 0.2 or 0.4 mg/kg once or 0.2 mg twice with a 5-week interval (Berge and Smeds 1984). These authors recommend a treatment regimen involving an initial dose of 0.4 mg/kg, followed by a second dose of 0.2 mg/kg, 2 to 3 weeks later, to control this parasite in foxes.

In a study involving polar foxes, Malczewski and colleagues (1984) reported that 6 months after 2 subcutaneous ivermectin treatments at dose rates up to 0.5 mg/kg, 6 weeks apart, no *C. blakei* mites were recovered from treated animals; these foxes were also free from clinical signs of infestation after treatment.

2. Wolves

Treatment of captive wolves with ivermectin by intramuscular injection, the direct oral route, or in treated meat was found to kill the adult and nymphal stages of the biting louse, *Trichodectes canis* (Taylor and Spraker 1983). Free-ranging packs were subsequently successfully treated with injections and treated meat. Offspring of previously infested, treated adults were also reported to be free of lice.

3. Cape Hunting Dog

Following treatment of adult heartworm (*Dirofilaria immitis*) with thiacetarsamide sodium, a single oral dose of ivermectin at 0.2 mg/kg was used as a microfilaricide in 2 Cape hunting dogs (Loomis and Lee 1984). These authors warn that heartworm should be considered when importing canines to or from an enzootic heartworm area; they suggest that ivermectin at 0.005 mg/kg once a month be considered for prophylactic treatment.

D. Ungulates

Because wild ungulates are physiologically similar to the domestic species for which the ivermectin products are registered and because they harbor parasites similar to those found in cattle, sheep, pigs, and horses, many ungulate species are treated with ivermectin.

1. Camels

Ivermectin given at 0.2 mg/kg subcutaneously effectively treats and controls gastrointestinal nematodes and sarcoptic mange mites in camels (*Camelus dromedarius*) (Ibrahim *et al.* 1981; Tager-Kagan and Robin 1986; Jones 1987). Studies have demonstrated a wide safety margin, but specific trials have not been done to demonstrate safety in breeding camels. Camels should not be treated within 28 days of slaughter for human consumption.

a. Endoparasites

Efficacy against endoparasites was established in 3 controlled studies involving 32 camels (Robin, Koenig, and Anstey, in press). Treatment at the recommended dose rate of 0.2 mg/kg provided effective control of the following gastrointestinal nematodes:*

Haemonchus spp. (adults)	*H. contortus* *H. lonistipes*
Ostertagia spp. (adults)	
Trichostrongylus spp. (adults)	*T. axei* *T. colubriformis* *T. probolurus* *T. vitrinus*
Camelostrongylus mentulatus (adults and L4)	
Impalaia tuberculata (adults)	
Nematodirus spathiger (adults)	
Chabertia ovina (adults)	
Oesophagostomum spp. (adults)	*O. columbianum* *O. venulosum*

In these studies, efficacy was also demonstrated against *Cooperia* spp., although the control animals had only small numbers of these parasites.

Boyce and colleagues (1984) report that for 4 trials in which ivermectin was administered to camels at 0.2 mg/kg the number of trichostrongylid eggs (*Haemonchus, Trichostrongylus,* and *Cooperia*) was effectively reduced in the feces. Although subcutaneous treatment had no effect on the number of *Trichuris* spp. eggs in the feces up to 10 weeks after treatment, oral treatment reduced *Trichuris* egg counts by more than 85%. Robin, Koenig, and Anstey (in press) reported variable efficacy against *Trichuris globulosa* following subcutaneous treatment at 0.2 mg/kg.

b. Ectoparasites

A single injection of ivermectin at 0.2 mg/kg subcutaneously markedly reduces the numbers of *Sarcoptes scabiei* var *cameli* and frequently leads to resolution of clinical signs of scab. Two injections may be necessary to provide complete control. The efficacy of 2 treatments with a 14- to 16-day interval was confirmed by Hashim and Wasfi (1986), and Opferman (1985), who report the absence of live mites on animals 3 weeks to 12 months after treatment.

---

* Data on file, MSDRL

Variable efficacy has been demonstrated against the oestrid larvae of *Cephalopina titillator* in the nasal passages of camels treated at 0.2 mg/kg (Tager-Kagan and Robin 1986; Robin, Koenig, and Anstey 1988).

2. Alpacas and Llamas

Ivermectin, injected subcutaneously at 0.2 mg/kg, has been used to successfully treat sarcoptic mange in alpacas (Alva and Guerrero 1986). In llamas, this dose was effective against lice infestation (*Microthoracius* spp.) (Fowler 1986) and nasal myaisis caused by the oestrid larvae of *Cephenemya* sp. (Fowler and Murphy 1985).

Administration of ivermectin at 0.2 mg/kg once a month for 6 months was used to treat a herd of llamas prophylactically for *Parelaphostrongylus tenuis* infection (Krogdahl, Thilsted, and Olsen 1987). These authors recommended that prophylactic treatment at 2 two-monthly intervals should be considered if llamas are grazed on pastures inhabited by deer (*Odocoileus virginianus*).

3. Reindeer

Ivermectin, administered subcutaneously at 0.2 mg/kg, is approved for treating and controlling warbles (*Oedemagena tarandi*) in reindeer (*Rangifer tarandus*) in the United States. Under an IR4 (minor species) development project conducted in Alaska, a high degree of efficacy was established in extensive studies (Dieterich 1985). Safety was demonstrated and no adverse reactions were elicited following treatment of animals at 5 and 10 times the recommended dose. The withdrawal period is 56 days.

Ivermectin's efficacy in reindeer is supported by a field study conducted in Sweden (Nordkvist *et al.* 1984). Grazing reindeer treated with ivermectin at 0.2 mg/kg were returned to pasture for 150 days during the winter. Efficacy, determined by slaughtering and processing 5 treated and 5 control animals at the end of this time, was reported to be at or near 100% against *Oedemagena tarandi, Cephenemyia trompe, Dictyocaulus viviparus,* and *Elaphostrongylus rangiferi.* The high level of efficacy, despite the long treatment/slaughter interval, is due to the reindeers' decreased exposure to infective larvae in the winter months. The average weight loss of the treated group over the winter was significantly less than that of the controls.

4. Deer

Ivermectin's efficacy has been evaluated against various endo- and ectoparasites in red deer (*Cervus elaphus*), white-tailed deer (*Odocoileus virginianus*), and mule deer (*O. hemionus*).

a. Endoparasites

Dictyocaulus viviparus. The high level of efficacy of ivermectin against lungworm in domestic animals has also been demonstrated in red deer. Treatment at 0.1 mg/kg subcutaneously 1 to 4 weeks after induced infections was 100% effective against this parasite (Mackintosh and Mason 1985). Oral treatment (0.2 mg/kg) of red deer on pasture reduced fecal larval counts to low levels by 20 days after each of 4 treatments (Bowie, Mackintosh, and Mason 1987). Mean larval output and proportion of deer shedding *D. viviparus* larvae at 27 and 33 days after treatment were significantly lower for ivermectin-treated animals than for those treated with oxfendazole.

Parelaphostrongylus. In white-tailed deer, ivermectin has been shown to be effective against certain immature stages of *Parelaphostrongylus tenuis* (the meningeal nematode), but not against the adults. Kocan (1985) reports that treatment at 0.1 or 0.2 mg/kg subcutaneously is effective against larvae penetrating the abomasum. Treatment on Days 10 and 30 after infection was ineffective. This could be due to the apparent inability of the avermectins to cross the blood-brain barrier, and the fact that the larvae of this parasite are generally located in the spinal cord by Day 10 after infection. Fecal larval output was reduced completely by 10 days after treatment of deer with patent infections, but larvae reappeared in the feces by Day 28. These findings, together with the absence of eggs and larvae in the lungs of animals slaughtered 12 days after treatment, indicate activity against first stage larvae in the lungs and possibly an effect on egg production (Kocan 1985).

Samuel and Gray (1988) report that ivermectin treatment (0.2 or 0.4 mg/kg) of white-tailed deer artificially infected with the muscle nematode *Parelaphostrongylus andersoni,* eliminated first stage larvae from the feces for up to six weeks. This was attributed to suppressed larval production by adult females and/or destruction of larvae in the lungs.

Oral ivermectin treatment had little effect on the adults of another metastrongyloid nematode *Elaphostrongylus cervi* in red deer (Watson 1986).

b. Ectoparasites

Lice. Treatment of mule and white-tailed deer with ivermectin at 0.2 mg/kg intramuscularly was reported to reduce the number of *Linognathus africanus* by 90% within 7 days of treatment. A second treatment 21 days later further reduced louse numbers but did not eradicate them (Foreyt, Rice, and Kim 1986). The interval between treatments in this case was probably too long relative to the life cycle of the parasite to completely eliminate the infection.

Fly Strike. Treatment of a single red deer stag suffering from fly strike with 40 mg of ivermectin subcutaneously (total dose) reportedly aborted the strike within 3 days (Fletcher 1984).

Warbles. Ivermectin treatment has been reported to be effective for treatment of warbles in farmed deer (Rafferty 1982). Petrov and colleagues (1986) report the use of a "briquette containing salt and a larvacide such as ivermectin" for treatment and prophylaxis of warbles in wild deer in the hunting areas of Bulgaria.

5. Bighorn Sheep

Desert bighorn sheep (*Ovis canadensis*), naturally infested with *Psoroptes ovis,* were successfully treated for scabies with ivermectin administered intramuscularly at 0.5 or 1.0 mg/kg—either as a single or repeated dose with a 14-day interval (Meleney, Wright, and Guillot 1980; Kinzer *et al.* 1983). Ivermectin was also effective against this parasite in free-roaming sheep treated by administering 35 mg of the drug loaded in frozen gelatin "bullets" and fired from a modified rifle (Meleney, Wright, and Guillot 1980).

Activity against lungworm has also been demonstrated. Under laboratory conditions, Miller and colleagues (1987) report that a single subcutaneous injection (0.2 mg/kg) eliminated first stage *Protostrongylus* larvae from the feces of bighorn sheep examined 4 weeks after treatment. Good efficacy was confirmed by monitoring fecal larval counts of bighorns treated subcutaneously (0.5 mg/kg) at the time of translocation, over an extended period of time (Miller and Hobbs 1988).

6. Impala

Horak and colleagues (1984) evaluated the efficacy of ivermectin against the endo- and ectoparasites of free-living impala treated subcutaneously at 0.2 mg/kg. Based on parasite recoveries, a high level of efficacy was demonstrated against the nematode parasites *Longistrongylus sabie, Haemonchus krugeri, Trichostrongylus thomasi, T. colubriformis, Impalia tuberculata, Gaigeria pachyscelis,* and *Oesophagostomum columbianum*. Activity was variable against *Cooperia hungi, Cooperoides hamiltoni,* and *Strongyloides* spp.

Of the 4 tick species present on these animals, only *Boophilus decoloratus* was markedly affected by treatment. The efficacy of ivermectin at this dose was high against the sucking lice *Linognathus aepycerus* and *L. nevilli* but poor against the biting lice *Damalinia aepycerus* and *D. elongata*.

This spectrum of activity is similar to that observed against gastrointestinal nematodes and lice on goats treated at 0.2 mg/kg subcutaneously (unpublished).

7. Other Antelope

Based on fecal egg counts, ivermectin at 0.2 mg/kg is reported to be effective against gastrointestinal nematodes of the genera *Nematodirus, Trichuris, Trichostrongylus, Ostertagia, Cooperia, Haemonchus,* and

Chabertia, as well as sarcoptic mange mites. Studies were conducted on 8 unspecified antelope species, under zoo conditions, (Frolka and Rotinska 1985).

8. Bison

Studies have been conducted to provide data on the use of ivermectin at 0.2 mg/kg subcutaneously for controlling and treating hypodermosis (*Hypoderma bovis*) in the American buffalo (*Bison bison*), under the auspices of the IR4 (minor species) system (Schillhorn, Sikarskie, and Braselton 1987). These studies demonstrated safety at doses at 0.2 mg/kg and 1.0 mg/kg. Efficacy against *Hypoderma bovis* was evaluated under field conditions, by treating animals at 0.2 mg/kg in the fall. The mean number of grub lesions in treated animals the following spring was zero compared to 11.3 for the control animals (Schillhorn, Sikarskie, and Braselton 1987). The efficacy of ivermectin against *Hypoderma* in the bison is therefore comparable to that established in cattle for this parasite.

9. Buffalo

The efficacy of ivermectin against louse infection (*Haematopinus tuberculatus*) has been assessed in buffaloes (Lau and Singh 1985). Subcutaneous treatment at 0.2 mg/kg was less effective (85%) than treatment at 0.4 mg/kg (100%) on evaluation 7 to 14 days later. Efficacy waned to 45% to 50% by 33 days after treatment in this study. It was suggested that a second treatment 7 to 14 days after the first may result in better efficacy over a longer period of time.

10. Wild Boar

Kutzer (1986) reports that ivermectin (0.5 mg/kg administered as a single oral dose) was effective against *Sarcoptes suis, Ascaris suum, Metastrongylus* spp, and *Oesophagostomum* spp in wild boar. Efficacy against *Trichuris* and *Capillaria* was poorer. The drug was also administered by mixing in feed. In the case of severe mange infestation, and where animals are treated in game reserves and hunting grounds, retreatment is recommended after 7 days (Kutzer 1986).

11. Other Species

Numerous anecdotal accounts exist for the use of ivermectin for treating parasitic infections in a wide variety of other ungulate species. The low dose volume required to obtain a high level of endo- and ectoparasitic efficacy, even following intramuscular or oral administration, has resulted in ivermectin's widespread use in projectile darts, or mixed with feed or lick formulations, for treating parasitic conditions in a number of other ungulates both in the wild and in zoos.

E. Elephants

Five Asian and 4 African elephants infested with lice (*Haematomyzus elephantis*) were treated with 2 doses of ivermectin orally at levels between .059 and .087 mg/kg, 5 to 6 weeks apart (Karesh and Robinson 1985). The authors selected the oral route because, previously, injection had produced local inflammation at the site of administration. Although no lice were found 7 days after the first treatment, some were present prior to the second. No reinfestation occurred following the second treatment.

Ivermectin treatment (0.2 mg/kg intramuscularly) was effective in reducing fecal egg counts and improving the physical condition of approximately 70 orphaned African elephant calves (P. R. Trembath, personal communication 1988).

F. Nonhuman Primates

The efficacy of ivermectin for treating primates naturally infected with arthropod and nematode parasites has been evaluated. Primates have also been used in a study to evaluate the efficacy of the compound against induced filarial infections.

1. Mite Infections

Joseph and colleagues (1984) reported that rhesus macaques with pulmonary acariasis (*Pneumonyssus*) treated with ivermectin at 0.2 mg/kg subcutaneously had only dead, fragmented mites in their lungs at necropsy, while control monkeys had numerous live mites. Histopathologically, inflammatory lesions were most severe in control animals and decreased progressively with time in treated monkeys. Efficacy against lung mites in this species has also been reported by Brack and Rietschel (1986).

Efficacy has been demonstrated against *Psorergates* mites in stump-tailed macaques (Bowman and Griffith 1987).

2. Nematode Infections

Feeding thiabendazole-medicated pellets for 1 week to rhesus monkeys infected with *Strongyloides fuelleborni* did not eliminate the infection. Brack and Rietschel (1986) subsequently treated the animals with ivermectin at 0.2 mg/kg subcutaneously for lung mite infections and found this treatment to be effective against both the mites and the persisting *Strongyloides* infection. No eggs were present in the feces 1 month after treatment. Efficacy has been reported against natural *Strongyloides* spp. infection in squirrel-monkeys (Battles, Greiner and Collins 1988).

An apparently healthy cymologous monkey (*Macaca fusicularis*) which died after routine inhalation anesthesia was found to be infected with the filarioid nematode *Edesonfilaria malayensis* (Kornegay *et al.* 1986). The animal had been treated with ivermectin 17 days prior to surgery: the authors postulated that treatment had killed many of the nematodes, resulting in parasitic emboli which led to pulmonary infarction. The authors advised that this potential complication should be considered when monkeys with filariasis are treated prior to anesthesia. The apparent effect on the adult parasite is surprising given the fact that other adult filarid parasites are relatively refractory to ivermectin treatment (except at high doses).

In an induced infection study, ivermectin given orally at 0.2 and 0.3 mg/kg was ineffective in preventing development of *Brugia malayi* infective larvae innoculated into leaf monkeys (*Presbytis cristata*) at the time of treatment (Mak *et al.* 1987). This is in line with the finding of Denham (1982) and Campbell (1982), who reported ivermectin to be ineffective against the developing stages of *Brugia pahangi* in jirds.

IV. Birds

Ivermectin, administered orally, topically, and by injection, has been used for the treatment of mite and nematode infestations in wild and domesticated birds. Coles (1987) considers the drug to work equally well in these species when given orally or by injection and recommends oral dosing.

In chickens, somnolence has been observed at doses of 5.4 mg/kg (Zeman 1987). Listlessness and ataxia occurred at 16.2 mg/kg, but a dose of 48.6 mg/kg was required to cause mortality. Mousa and colleagues (1986b) reported that doses of 0.1 to 15.0 mg/kg of ivermectin were nontoxic to chickens.

A. Nematodes

a. *Ascaridia*

A single oral ivermectin treatment at 0.1, 0.2, or 0.4 mg/kg was found to be ineffective against the tissue phase of *Ascaridia galli* in chickens infested 12 days before treatment. These dosages were, however, 96% to 100% effective against adult worms present 40 days after infection (Mousa *et al.* 1986b). These authors therefore recommended a repeated treatment with a 30-day interval for controlling this parasite. The inclusion of ivermectin in poultry feed at a level of 4 ppm was 84% effective against a challenge infection of *A. galli* (R. L. Kilgore, unpublished data). Successful treatment of *Ascaridia columbae* infection in pigeons required 2 oral doses (1.5 mg) 3 weeks apart (Schepkens, Duchatel, and Vindevogel 1985).

Okaema (1988) reports that subcutaneous injection of guinea fowl

(*Numidia meleagris*) at 0.14 mg/kg was effective in controlling natural infections of *Ascaridia galli, Heterakis gallinarum,* and *Sublura suctoria.*

b. *Capillaria*

A single ivermectin treatment, administered orally (1.5 mg, total dose) or by intramuscular injection (0.3 mg, total dose) was effective in removing *Capillaria* spp. from naturally infected pigeons (Schepkens, Duchatel, and Vindevogel 1985).

Intramuscular treatment (0.4 mg/kg) of 28 raptors (7 genera) reduced the numbers of *Capillaria* spp. eggs in the feces by 96%, 8 weeks after treatment (Kollias, Griener, and Heard 1987). These authors recommended a repeat treatment 3 to 4 weeks after the first for controlling this parasite.

c. *Pelecitus*

Oral treatment with ivermectin at 0.2 mg/kg did not result in complete resolution of lesions attributable to subcutaneous filariasis (*Pelecitus* sp.) in a yellow-collared macaw (Allen *et al.* 1985). Although a needle aspirate revealed dead microfilariae 14 days after treatment, surgery was required to remove adult worms.

d. *Oxyspirura*

Artificial infections of *Oxyspirura* sp. in the eyes of chickens were treated successfully with a single dose (.05 mg) of ivermectin instilled into the eye (Thomas-Baker 1986). A dose of .01 mg/bird was not effective against this parasite when administered orally or intramuscularly. Natural infections in the eyes of wood partridges were also removed by intraocular administration of .05 mg.

e. *Syngamus trachea*

Seagulls infected with *S. trachea* have been successfully treated with oral ivermectin (Rowley 1987).

B. Mites

a. *Dermanyssus* and *Ornithonyssus*

Although a noticeable effect was seen on mites (*Dermanyssus gallinae*) on fowls treated intraabdominally with ivermectin at 0.6 mg/kg, dose rates of 1.8 to 5.4 mg/kg were required to obtain adequate efficacy (Zeman 1987).

Neither ivermectin treatment at 0.5 mg/kg subcutaneously nor the inclusion of the compound in the feed at levels of 0.4, 2.0, or 4.0 ppm for 28 days was effective against northern fowl mites (*Ornithonyssus sylviarum*) on hens (R. L. Kilgore, unpublished data). These findings are supported by those of DeVaney (1985), who reported that low levels of ivermectin were not effective against this mite.

b. *Cnemidocoptes* spp.

Ivermectin has been used by intramuscular injection (0.2 mg/kg) and topical application to treat "scaly-leg" in cage birds ranging in size from budgies to macaws (Kelso 1984; Tassi 1984; Hogan *et al.* 1984; Ryan 1986). Heavily infested birds may require a second injection (Kelso 1984; Hogan *et al.* 1984) or 2 oral treatments at 0.2 mg/kg 10 to 16 days apart (Ryan 1987). Topical application of a 1% solution to crusts on the beak, eyelids, legs, and pericloacal areas of affected birds was reportedly effective in all but the most severe cases (Tassi 1984). Kummerfeld and Nolte (1987) reported effective spot treatment of budgerigars for *Cnemidocoptes pilae* infestation at levels of 0.4 to 20.0 mg of ivermectin/kg.

c. *Sternostoma tracheolum*

Dead mites were recovered from the lungs and air sacs of canaries injected intramuscularly with .02 to .06 mg of ivermectin per bird (Brownell 1984). In this study, clinical recovery occurred 10 days after treatment, and the birds began singing 4 days later. Although no mortality occurred in birds treated at these high levels, immobility was reported.

d. *Cytodites nudus*

Subcutaneous injection of golden pheasants infested with this air-sac mite was effective only at high doses (50 mg/kg) (Grimm and Centurier 1986).

e. *Pterolichidae*

Three doses of ivermectin (0.2 mg/kg orally) at 4-week intervals were effective for the treatment of quill mite infestation in an adult ostrich (Hoover, Lochner, and Mullins 1988).

V. Fish

Ivermectin has been used to control parasitic copepods on fish; the drug has shown some efficacy against nematodes. Dosage levels in fish are critical: the toxic level is close to the therapeutic level in some species. Although no mortalities or toxic effects were reported following oral ivermectin treatment of Atlantic salmon or rainbow trout at 0.2 mg/kg, the margin of safety is narrow, with mortalities occurring at twice this dose (Palmer *et al.* 1987). Mortality of mottled sculpin, 5.5 cm in length, was reported to have occurred after injection of more than .05 ml of a .05% ivermectin solution (Heckman 1985).

A. Copepods

Compared to untreated controls, numbers of parasitic copepods (*Lepeopthirus salmonis* and *Caligus elongatus*) on Atlantic salmon and the numbers of fish with skin lesions were reduced by Day 60 following administration of ivermectin in feed pellets at intervals of 14 to 21 days (Palmer *et al.* 1987). These copepods were also reduced in number following a single oral dose of ivermectin at 0.2 mg/kg. In this study, ivermectin was mainly active against adult copepods and, although reinfestation with juveniles occurred, they did not survive to the adult stage.

Lernea spp. on goldfish given an intramuscular injection of a .00008% solution of ivermectin, administered at a dose rate of 0.1 ml/50 g, began to disintegrate 4 days after treatment. After 6 days, the fish were clear of parasites. Ulcers at the point of attachment were healed by Day 10 (Hyland and Adams 1987).

B. Nematodes

Ivermectin administered intramuscularly or in the water was moderately effective against *Rhabdochona* sp. in mottled sculpin (Heckman 1985). Although subcutaneous treatment at dose rates of 0.1 to 10.0 mg/kg was effective against *Anguillicola crassus*—a nematode found in the air bladder of eels—all ivermectin-treated eels died within 2 weeks (Tarachewski, Renner, and Mehlhorn 1988).

IV. Reptiles

Although adverse reactions were not recorded in snakes given ivermectin at 0.2 mg/kg (Lawrence 1984; Stanchi and Grisolia 1986), and the corn snake (*Elapha guttata*) tolerated doses of up to 1.0 mg/kg without apparent adverse clinical signs, chelonians were found to be sensitive to the effects of the compound at much lower levels (Teare and Bush 1983). Red-footed tortoises were killed by treatment at 0.4 mg/kg; paralysis occurred with doses as low as 0.05 mg/kg when it was repeated within 72 hours. Doses which induced minimal signs of toxicosis ranged from 0.025 mg/kg in leopard tortoises to 0.1 mg/kg in box tortoises. A dose of 0.05 mg/kg was considered safe in red-footed tortoises if treatment intervals were not less than 7 days (Teare and Bush 1983).

A. Snakes

Ivermectin treatment at 0.2 mg/kg subcutaneously was effective in the treatment of snakes for mite infestation and pythons for tick infestation (Lawrence 1984). This dose was reported to be 83% effective against

Ophinyssus sp. mites by Stanchi and Grisolia (1986). These authors recommended that treated snakes should be placed in parasite-free housing after treatment.

B. Chelonians

Repeated treatment at .05 mg/kg weekly for 2 to 6 weeks reduced shedding of eggs and larvae (*Proatracti* sp. and *Kolicephalus* sp.) in the feces of red-footed tortoises (Teare and Bush 1983).

Conclusion

Ivermectin is efficacious against a wide-range of endo- and ectoparasites, in a wide variety of hosts, and is formulated in a variety of dosage forms.

Although mammals tolerate ivermectin very well, it must be emphasized that the safety of the drug for nondomestic species—with the exception of camels and reindeer—has not been proven in controlled studies. Use in nonmammalian species is not without risk, especially for reptiles and fish, where the therapeutic dose may be close to the toxic level.

Similarly, because the compound's efficacy against the wide array of parasites infecting laboratory, zoo, wild, and exotic animals has not been proven in controlled studies, clinical response to "extra-label" usage of the product should be monitored closely.

References

Abbeele J van den, D'Haeseleer F, Goossens M (1986) Efficacy of ivermectin on the reproductive biology of *Glossina palpalis*. *Annales de la Societe Belge de Medicine Tropicale 66:167–172.*

Abo-Shenada MN, Herbert IV (1984) Anthelmintic effect of levamisole, ivermectin, albendazole and fenbendazole in larval *Toxocara canis* infection in mice. *Res. Vet. Sci. 36:87–91.*

Alcaino H, Gorman T, Imbert R (1984) Treatment of experimental trichinelliasis in the rat with febantel and ivermectin. *Parasitologie al Dia* 8:79–83.

Allen JL, Kollias GV, Griener EC, Boyce W (1985) Subcutaneous filariasis (*Pelecitus* sp.) in a yellow collared macaw. *Avian Dis.* 29:891–894.

Alva J., Guerrero C (1986) Use of ivermectin against sarcoptic mange in alpacas. IVITA, *Boletin de Divulgacion* No. 21:23–27.

Ashmawy K, Fahmy MM (1987) Acaricidal efficiency of Ivomec against psoroptic and sarcoptic mites infesting rabbits. *J. Egypt. Vet. Med. Assoc.* 47:315–319.

Azambuja PD, Lima Gomes JEP, Lopes F, Garcia ES (1985) Efficacy of ivermectin against the bloodsucking insects *Rhodnius prolixus* and *Hemiptera triatominae*. *Memoirs of the Institute Oswaldo Cruz* 80:439–442.

Barutzki D, Laubmeier E, Forstner MJ (1987) Endoparasite infestation of hedgehogs with a contribution to therapy. *Tierarztl. Prax.* 15:325–331.

Battles AH, Adams SW, Courtney CH, Mladinich CRT (1987) Efficacy of ivermectin against natural infection of *Syphacia muris* in rats. *Lab. Ani. Sci.* 37:791–792.

Battles AH, Greiner EC, Collins BR (1988) Efficacy of ivermectin against natural infection of *Strongyloides* spp. in squirrel-monkeys. *Lab. Ani. Sci.* 38:474–485.

Baumans V, Havenaar R, Van Herck H, Rooymans TP (1988) The effectiveness of Ivomec and Neguvon in the control of murine mites. *Lab. Anim.* 22:243–245.

Berge GN, Smeds E (1984) Efficacy of ivermectin against *S. scabiei* infestations of foxes. *Nord. Vet. Med.* 36:156–161.

Bianco AE, Nwachukwa MA, Townson S, Doenhoff MJ, Muller RL (1986) Evaluation of drugs against *Onchocerca microfilariae* in an inbred mouse model. *Trop. Med. Parasit.* 37:39–45.

Blagburn BL, Swango LJ, Hendrix CM, Lindsay DS (1986) Comparative efficacies of ivermectin, febantel, fenbendazole and mebendazole against helminth parasites of gray foxes. *J. Am. Vet. Med. Assoc.* 189:1084–1085.

Blair LS, Campbell WC (1980) Suppression of maturation of *Dirofilaria immitis* in *Mustela putorius* by a single dose of ivermectin. *J. Parasit.* 66:691–692.

Blair LS, Williams E, Ewanciw DV (1982) Efficacy of ivermectin against third stage *Dirofilaria immitis* larvae in ferrets and dogs. *Res. Vet. Sci. 33:386–387.*

Bowie, JY, Mackintosh CG, Mason PC (1987) Effect of ivermectin and oxfendazole on shedding of larvae of the lungworm *Dictyocaulus viviparus* by Deer. *New Zeal. Vet. J.* 35:8–10.

Bowman TA, Griffith JW (1987) Comparison of treatments for *Psorergates* mites in stumptailed macaques. *Lab. Ani. Sci.* 37;100–102.

Boyce W, Kollias G, Courtney CH, Allen J, Chalmers E (1984) Efficacy of ivermectin against gastrointestinal nematodes in dromedary camels. *J. Am. Vet. Med. Assoc.* 185:1307–1308.

Brack M, Rietschel W (1986) Ivermectin for the control of *Strongyloides fuelleborni* in rhesus monkeys. *Kleintierpraxis* 31:29.

Brownell JR (1984) *Sternostoma tracheolum*—continuing studies. *Proc. 33rd Western Poultry Disease Conf.*, Davis, CA, pp 91–93.

Calcott PH, Fatig RO (1984) Avermectin modulation of gamma-aminobutyric acid binding to membranes of rat brain, brine shrimp and a fungus. *J. Antibiot.* 37:797–801.

Campbell WC (1982) Efficacy of the avermectins against filarial parasites. *Vet. Res. Commun.* 5:251–262.

Campbell WC, Blair LS, Lotti VJ (1979) Efficacy of avermectins against *Trichinella spiralis* in mice. *J. Helminthol.* 53:254–256.

Carrillo M, Barriga O (1987) Anthelmintic effect of levamisole hydrochloride and ivermectin on tissue toxocariasis of mice. *Am. J. Vet. Res.* 48:281–283.

Chiu SHL, Sestokas E, Taub R, Buhs RP, Green M, Sestokas R, VandenHeuval WJA, Arison BH, Jacobs TA (1986) Metabolic disposition of ivermectin in tissues of cattle, sheep and rats. *Drug Metab. & Dispos.* 14:590–600.

Coles BH (1987) Ivermectin for birds. *Vet. Rec.* 120:604.

Curtis SK, Housley R, Brooks DL (1988) The use of ivermectin in rabbits for the treatment of ear mites. *Proc. 125th Mtg. AVMA,* Portland, Oregon, Abstr. 113.

Denham DA (1982) The effects of some avermectins on the growth of *Brugia pahangi. Meth. & Find. Exper. Clin. Pharmacol.* 4:347–350.

Devaney E, Howells RE (1984) The Microfilaricidal activity of ivermectin in vitro and in vivo. *Trop. Med. Parasit.* 35:47–49.

DeVaney JA (1985) Progress on control of northern fowl mites on caged laying hens. *Vet. Parasit.* 18:289–295.
Dieterich RA (1985) An overview of Alaskan reindeer diseases and current control methods. In Fennessy PF, Drew KR (eds) *Biology of Deer Production,* Proc. of Intern. Conf., Dunedin, NZ, pp 97–100.
Distelmans W, D'Haeseleer D, Mortelmans J (1983) Efficacy of systemic administration of ivermectin against tsetse flies. *Annales de la Societe Belge de Medecine Tropicale* 63:119–120.
Drummond RO (1980) Mouse–*Cuterebra* animal systemic insecticide tests. *Proc. Entomol. Soc. Am.* 5:230–231.
Evans RH (1984) Ivermectin treatment of notoedric mange in two fox squirrels. *J. Am. Vet. Med. Assoc.* 185:1437–1438.
Fletcher J (1984) Ivermectin in fly strike. *Vet. Rec.* 115:475.
Foreyt WJ, Rice DH, Kim KC (1986) Pediculosis of mule deer and white-tailed deer fawns in captivity. *J. Am. Vet. Med. Assoc.* 189:1172–1173.
Fowler ME (1986) Lice in llamas. *Avia/Exotic Prac.* 3:22–25.
Fowler ME, Murphy J (1985) *Cephenemya* sp. infestation in the llama. *Calif. Vet.* 39:10–12.
Frolka J, Rotinska J (1985) Possible use of Ivomec and Eqvalan in the treatment of parasitic diseases of animals in zoological gardens. *Veterinarstvi* 35: 415–416.
Frossard TL (1981) Studies on the suitability of rabbits as a model for testing systemic acaricides under laboratory conditions. Thesis, Munich University, 39 pp.
Grimm F, Centurier C (1986) *Cytodites nudus*—an air sac mite in golden pheasants. *Praktische Tierarzt* 67:198–199.
Grove DI (1983) The effects of 22,23 dihydroavermectin B_1 on *Strongyloides ratti* and *S. stercoralis* infections in mice. *Ann. Trop. Med. Parasit.* 77:405–410.
Harvey RG (1987) Use of ivermectin for guinea pig mange. *Vet. Rec.* 120:351.
Hashim DH, Wasfi IA (1986) Ivermectin treatment of camels naturally infected with sarcoptic mange. *World Ani. Rev.* 57:26–29.
Hasslinger MA, Wiethe T (1987) Oxyurids of small laboratory animals and their control with ivermectin. Tierarzt. Prax. 15:93–97.
Heckmann RA (1985) The efficacy of ivermectin against nematodes of fish. Proceed. of the 60th Annual Mtg. of the Am. Soc. for Parasit. Abstract 24.
Hogan HL, Joseph B, Henrickson R, Lowenstine L (1984) Efficacy and safety of ivermectin for scaly leg mite infestation in parakeets. *Proc. of Annual Mtg. of the Am. Assoc. of Zoo Veter.* Abstract 156.
Hoover JP, Lochner FK, Mullins SB (1988) Quill mites in an osrich with rhinitis, sinusitis and air saculitis. *Compan. Anim. Pract.* 2:23–26.
Horak IG, Boomker J, Kingsley SA, De Vos V (1984) The efficacy of ivermectin against helminth and arthropod parasites of impalla. *J. S. Afr. Vet. Assoc.* 54:251–253.
Hunt LM (1982) Guinea pig-*Amblyomma americanum* animal systemic insecticide test. *Proc. Entomol. Soc. Am.* 7:253.
Hyland KPC, Adams SJR (1987) Ivermectin for use in fish. *Vet. Rec.* 120:539.
Ibraham MS, Mohamed AR, El-Balkemy FA, Omran H, El-Mekkauri MF (1981) Studies on the relation between the effect of IvomecT as a parasitic control and the general health condition of camels. *Res. Bull.* No. 375, Oct. 1981, Zagazig Univ., Egypt.

Ishii AI, Terada M, Kwo H, Hayashi M, Sano M (1983) Studies on chemotherapy of parasitic helminths; effects of avermectin B_1a on *Angiostrongylus cantonensis* in rats. *Intl. J. Parasit.* 13:491–498.

Jones PGH (1987) Recent advances in parasite control as an aid to increasing livestock health and productivity. J. Egypt. Vet. Med. Assoc. 47:347–364.

Joseph BE, Wilson DW, Hendrickson RV, Robinson PT, Benirschke K (1984) Treatment of pulmonary acariasis in rhesus macaques with ivermectin. *Lab. Ani. Aci.* 34:360–364.

Karesh WB, Robinson PT (1985) Ivermectin treatment of lice infestations in two elephant species. *J. Am. Vet. Med. Assoc.* 187:1235–1236.

Kelso PC (1984) Ivermectin cures scaly mite infestation. *Vet. Med.* 79:446.

Kinzer HG, Meleney WP, Lange RE, Houghton WE (1983) Preliminary evaluation of ivermectin for control of *Psoroptes ovis* in desert bighorn sheep. *J. Wildlife Dis.* 19:52–54.

Kocan AA (1985) The use of ivermectin in the treatment and prevention of *Paralephostrongylus tenuis* in white-tailed deer. *J. Wildlife Dis.* 21:454–455.

Kollias GV, Griener EC, Heard D (1987) The efficacy of ivermectin and praziquantel against gastrointestinal nematodes and trematodes in raptors. Proc. of 1st Conf. in Zool. and Avian Med., Florida, pp 408–409.

Kopczewski A, Malczewski A, Wroblewska M, Zdunkiewicz T (1987) Effect of ivermectin on the fertility and health of foxes. *Med. Weterynaryjna* 43:102–104.

Kornegay RW, Giddens WE, Morton WR, Knitter GH (1986) Verminous vasculitis pneumonia and infarction in a cymologous monkey after treatment with ivermectin. *Lab. Ani. Aci.* 36:45–47.

Krogdahl DW, Thilsted JP, Olsen SK (1987) Ataxia and hypermetria caused by *Parelaphostrongylus tenuis* infection in llamas. *J. Am. Vet. Med. Assoc.* 190:191–193.

Kummerfeld N, Nolte CS (1987) Treatment of mite infestation in budgerigars and finches using ivermectin spot-on methods. *Kleintierpraxis* 32:293–296.

Kutzer E (1986) Zur behandlung der Sarcoptesraude bei wild- und hausschweinen mit ivermectin. *Dtsch. tiearztl. Wschr.* 93:426–429.

Lau HD, Singh NP (1985) Efficacy of ivermectin in the control of the louse *Haematopinus turberculatus* in buffaloes. *Proc. of 11th Conf. of the WAAVP,* Abstract 47.

Lawrence LJ (1984) Ivermectin as an ectoparasiticide in snakes. *Vet. Rec.* 115:441–442.

Loomis MR, Lee CD (1984) Canine heartworm infection in African Cape Hunting Dogs. *Annual Mtg. of the Am. Assoc. of Zoo Veter.* p. 137.

Macchioni G, Marconcini A, Sbrana L (1983) Sarcoptic mange in the domestic rabbit and guinea pig. Annali della Facolta di Medicina Veterinaria de Pisa 36:287–294.

Mackintosh CG, Mason PC (1985) Anthelmintics and lungworm in deer. In Fennesy PF, Drew KR (eds) *Biology of Deer Production,* Proc. of Conf., Dunedin, N.Z. pp 131–133.

Mak JW, Lam PL, Rain An, Suresh K (1987) Chemoprophylactic studies with ivermectin against subperiodic *Brugia malayi* infection in the leaf monkey. *J. Helminthol.* 61:311–314.

Malczewski A, Kopczewski A, Malczewski M, Zielinski J (1984) Mange due to *Cheyletiella blakei* in polar foxes in Poland. *Zentralblatt fur Bakteriologie Mikrobiologie und Hygiene* 258:412–413.

Manurang J, Partoutomo S, Stevenson P (1985) Treatment of rabbit ear mange caused by *Notoedres cati* with ivermectin and neguvon. Panyakit Hewan 17:308–311.

Meleney WP, Wright FC, Guillot FS (1980) Identification and control of psoroptic scabies in bighorn sheep. *Proc. 84th Annual Mtg. of the U.S. Ani. Health Assoc.*, Louisville, Kentucky, pp 403–407.

Miller MW, Hobbs NT (1988) Ivermectin for treating lungworms in mountain sheep: an appropriate technology with a specific utility. *Wildl. Soc. Bull.* 16:236–238.

Miller MW, Hobbs NT, Rutherford WH, Miller LLW (1987) Efficacy of injectable ivermectin for treating lungworm infections in mountain sheep. *Wildl. Soc. Bull.* 15:260–263.

Mousa S, Gad N, Sokkar I, Raheem MA (1986a) Efficacy of a single injectable dose of ivermectin for psoroptic and sarcoptic mange in rabbits. *Assiut Vet. Med. J.* 17:237–239.

Mousa S, Gad N, Sokkar I, Raheem MA (1986b) Investigations on the efficacy of ivermectin for ectoparasites and nematodes in chickens. *Assiut Vet. Med. J.* 17:225–233.

Nordkvist M, Christensson D, Rehbinder C (1984) A deworming field trial with ivermectin in reindeer. *Rangifer* 4:10–15.

Okaeme AN (1988) Ivermectin in the control of helminthiasis in guinea fowl. *Vet. Q.* 10:70–71.

Olsen RW, Snowman AM (1985) Avermectin B_1a modulation of gamma aminobutyric acid benzodiazapine receptor binding in mammalian brain. *J. Neurochem.* 44:1074–1082.

Opferman RR (1985) Treatment of sarcoptic mange in a dromedary camel. *J. Am. Vet. Med. Assoc.* 187:1240–1241.

Ostlind DA, Cifelli S (1981) Efficacy of thiabendazole, levamisole and the major natural avermectins against *Trichostrongylus colubriformis* in the gerbil. *Res. Vet. Sci.* 31:255–256.

Ostlind DA, Cifelli S, Lang R (1979) Insecticidal activity of the antiparasitic avermectins. *Vet. Rec.* 105;168.

Ostlind DA, Nartowicz MA, Mickle WG (1985) Efficacy of ivermectin against *Syphacia obvelata* in mice. *J. Helminthol.* 59:257–261.

Palmer R, Rodger H, Drinan E, Dwyer C, Smith PR (1987) Preliminary trials on the efficacy of ivermectin against parasitic copepods of Atlantic salmon. *Bull. Europ. Assoc. Fish Pathol.* 7:47–54.

Petrov D, Nedelchev N, Meshkov S, Rusev I, Yuzer P, Paliiski E (1986) A study of hypodermatosis in wild ruminants. *Vet. Sbirka* 84:26–28.

Pong SS, Wang CC (1980) The specificity of high affinity binding of avermectin B_1a to mammalian brain. *Neuropharm.* 19:311–317.

Pong SS, Wang CC, Fritz LC (1980) Studies on the mechanism of action of avermectin B_1a. *J. Neurochem.* 34:351–358.

Prosl H, Kanout AG (1985) Treatment of ear mange in rabbits with ivermectin. *Berliner und Munchener Tierarztliche Wochenschrift* 98:45–47.

Rafferty GC (1982) Red deer endoparasites. *Vet. Rec.* 111:565.

Rajasekariah GR, Deb BN, Dhage KR, Bose S (1986) Response of laboratory-adapted human hookworm and other nematodes to ivermectin. *Ann. Trop. Med. Parasit.* 80:615–621.

Rapic D, Dzakula N, Matic-Piantanida D (1982) Anthelmintic activity of ivermectin against *Trichinella spiralis* larvae in rats. *Vet. Arh.* 52:131–139.

Robin B, Koenig K, Anstey MD (in press) Efficacy of ivermectin against internal parasites in dromedaries (*Camelus dromedarius*). *Revue Scientifique et Technique*.

Romero JR, Valentini HG (1984) Efficacy of avermectin in the treatment of mange in rabbits. *Vet. Argent.* 1:871–874.

Rowley J (1987) *Syngamus trachea* in three seagulls. *Compan. Anim. Pract.* 1:46.

Ryan T (1986) Cnemidocoptic mite infestation in cage birds. *Mod. Vet. Prac.* 67:525–526.

Ryan T (1987) Cnemidocoptic mite infestation in cage birds. *Clinc. Ins.* 2:305–306.

Samuel WM, Gray JB (1988) Efficacy of ivermectin against *Parelaphostrongylus andersoni* in white-tailed deer. J. Wildl. Dis. 24:491–495.

Sanmartin-Duran ML, Sernandez L, Yebra MJ, Santamarina MT, Ubeira FM (1986) Anthelmintic effect of ivermectin on the endogenous cycle of *Trichinella*. *Revista Iberica de Parasitologia* 46:189–193.

Sayles PC, Jacobson RH (1983) Effects of various anthelmintics on larval stages of *Nematospiroides dubius*. *J. Parasit.* 69:1079–1083.

Schepkens E, Duchatel JP, Vindevogel H (1985) Treatment of *Ascarida columbae* and *Capillaria spp. infestations in pigeons with ivermectin. Ann. Med. Vet.* 129:475–485.

Schillhorn van Veen TW, Sikarskie JG, Braselton WE (1987). Safety, efficacy and tissue residues of ivermectin used to control hypodermosis in Bison. *Proc. Conf. of Res. Workers in Ani. Dis.*, Chicago, IL, Abstraact 205.

Silverman J, Blatt H, Lerro A (1983) Effect of ivermectin against *Myobia musculi*. *Lab. Ani. Sci.* 33:487.

Stanchi NO, Grisolia CX (1986) Use of ivermectin in the treatment of snake mite infection. *Vet. Argent.* 3:26.

Tager-Kagan P, Robin B (1986) Results of a trial of ivermectin against parasites of dromedaries in Niger. *Rev. Elev. Med. Vet. Pays Tropic.* 39:333–340.

Taraschewski H, Renner C, Mehlhorn H (1988) Effects of levamisole hydrochloride, metrifonate, fenbendazole, mebendazole and ivermectin on *Anguillicola crassus* pathogenic in the air bladder of eels. *Parasit. Res.* 74:281–289.

Tassi P (1984) Topical treatment for scaly mites. *Vet. Med. Small Ani. Clinic.* 79:1447.

Taylor WP, Spraker TH (1983) Management of a biting louse infestation in a free ranging wolf population. Proc. Annual Mtg. Am. Assoc. of Zoo Veterin. pp 40–41.

Teare JA, Bush M (1983) Toxicity and efficacy of ivermectin in chelonians. *J. Am. Vet. Med. Assoc.* 183:1195–1197.

Thomas-Baker B (1986) Ivermectin as a treatment for ocular nematodiasis in birds. Proc. Annual Mtg. of Am. Assoc. Zoo Veterin. pp 99–100.

Watson TG (1986) Efficacy of drenching deer and wapiti with particular reference to *Elaphostrongylus cervi* and *Dictyocaulus viviparus*. Proc. N.Z. Vet. Assoc. Deer Branch Course No. 3, Rotorua: 170–182.

Wilkins CA, Conroy J, Ho P, O'Shanny WJ, Capizzi T (1981) The effect of ivermectin on the live mass, period of attachment and percent control of ticks. In Whitehead GB, Gibson JD (eds) *Tick Biology and Control*, Rhodes University, Grahamstown, SA, pp 137–142.

Wilkins CA, Conroy JA, Ho P, O'Shanny WJ, Malatesta PF, Egerton JR (1980) Treatment of psoroptic mange with avermectins. *Am. J. Vet. Res.* 41:2112–2113.

Williams M, Yarbrough GG (1979) Enhancement of in vivo binding of diazepam by a novel anthelmintic agent, avermectin B_1a. *Eur. J. Pharmacol.* 56:273–276.

Wing SR, Courtney CH, Young MD (1985) Effect of ivermectin on murine mites. J. Am. Vet. Med. Assoc. 187:1191–1192.

Wright FC, Riner JC (1985) Comparative efficacy of injection routes and doses of ivermectin against *Psoroptes* in rabbits. *Am. J. Vet. Res.* 46:752–754.

Zahner H, Sanger I, Lammler G, Muller HA (1987) Effect of ivermectin on *Dipetalonema viteae* and *Litomosoides carinii* infections of *Mastomys natalensis. Trop. Med. Parasit.* 38:117–122.

Zeman P (1987) Systemic efficacy of ivermectin against *Dermanyssus gallinae* in fowls. *Vet. Pathol.* 23:141–146.

Chapter 20

Abamectin Use in Crop Protection

Richard A. Dybas

I. Introduction

Initial indications that the avermectins possessed activity against arthropods were obtained in studies with avermectin B_{1a} against the confused flour beetle (*Tribolium confusum*) and the sheep blowfly larva (*Lucilia cuprina*). Evaluation of the 8 major natural avermectins and several hundred semisynthetic avermectin analogs and derivatives showed that avermectin B_1, the major component of the fermentation of *Streptomyces avermitilis,* was extremely toxic to acarines and to a wide range of insects, including members of the orders Diptera, Homoptera, Coleoptera, and Lepidoptera (Putter *et al.* 1981). Avermectin B_1 (MK-936), with the common name abamectin, was selected for use against arthropod pests of economic importance in horticulture and agriculture.

II. Products

A. AVID®, AGRI-MEK®, VERTIMEC®

Abamectin for use in foliar spray applications is formulated as a 1.8% w/v emulsifiable concentrate containing 0.15 lb abamectin per U.S. gallon. The oral LD_{50} of this product in rats is 650 mg/kg body weight, while the dermal LD_{50} in rabbits is greater than 2000 mg/kg body weight. Rabbits exhibit slight-to-moderate eye irritation and very slight–to-slight skin irritation. Skin sensitization was not observed in guinea pigs with the emulsifiable concentrate formulation.

The product is being developed for use on a number of horticultural and agronomic crops to control phytophagous mites and insects. It is recommended at rates in the range of 0.005 to 0.025 lb abamectin/acre (5.4 to 27 grams ai/hectare), in volumes of water ranging from 5 to 1000 gallons per acre, depending on the crop to be treated and application equipment. For certain crop applications, e.g., for control of mites and insects on citrus, pear, and deciduous tree nuts, the product is recommended in combination with a 0.25% narrow-range paraffinic oil in dilute sprays or a minimum of 1 gallon oil per acre (9.5 liters/ha) in concentrate sprays.

The maximum recommended application rate for citrus, pears, and deciduous tree nuts is 0.025 lb active ingredient (ai)/acre (20 fl oz AGRI-MEK®/acre). The maximum recommended rate for ornamental plants, cotton, vegetables, and strawberries is 0.02 lb ai/acre (16 fl oz AGRIMEK®/acre).

A maximum of 0.075 lb ai/acre per growing season will be allowed on citrus, pears, and tree nuts, and 0.20 lb ai/acre on vegetable crops.

With the exception of mild symptoms of phytotoxicity to certain ferns, and slight spotting of carnation foliage, crops tolerate the product well when the recommended application directions are followed. This applies to abamectin sprayed in water or, where recommended, in combination with paraffinic spray oils (Green *et al.* 1985a).

B. AFFIRM®

Abamectin for use in controlling the red imported fire ant (*Solenopsis invicta*) is formulated as a bait containing 0.011% w/w abamectin in soybean oil on pregelled defatted corn grits. The oral LD_{50} in rats and dermal LD_{50} in rabbits is greater than 2000 mg/kg, and the product is nonirritating to rabbit skin.

AFFIRM® is intended for use at a rate of 1.0 lb of bait per acre for broadcast application through ground or aerial equipment, or 5 to 7 tablespoons of bait for treatment of individual fire ant mounds. The product is recommended for nonagricultural lands such as lawns, turf, golf courses, and parks. The U.S. EPA-approved label restricts bait application to land other than pastures, range lands and crop land.

III. Applications

A. Red Imported Fire Ant (*Solenopsis invicta*)

The red imported fire ant is an important pest in the southern United States. The worker ants inflict painful stings to humans, they feed directly on crops, and the ant mounds cause damage to farm machinery. Any successful control strategy requires eliminating the worker ants and/or the physogastric queen, who is responsible for the reproductive capacity of the colony.

Studies conducted in the USDA's Gainesville, FL, laboratory demonstrated that abamectin exhibits a rate-related delayed toxicity to red imported fire ant (RIFA) workers. This delayed effect is an important criterion for efficacy of a bait toxicant against RIFA, since the worker ants must gather the bait toxicant and distribute it throughout the colony before the effects of treatment are observed.

In laboratory studies, abamectin at a concentration of 0.1% killed more than 75% of RIFA workers after 10 days exposure. Delayed toxicity to worker ants was observed; less than 10% kill occurred 1 day after treatment at that concentration (Lofgren and Williams 1982; Williams 1983). When entire colonies were treated in the laboratory, 0.0025% abamectin in soybean oil caused loss of all brood production and sterility of the RIFA queen. Abamectin effects at this concentration appeared irreversible. Lower abamectin concentrations—for example, 0.00025% in soybean oil—caused a reduction in brood production; however, the effects were transient, with a return to normal egg production in 16 weeks.

Histological examination of the ovaries of sterile queens showed several tissue and cell abnormalities. The damage was characterized by hypertrophy of the squamous epithelium that sheaths the ovarioles, and pycnosis of the nurse-cell nuclei. According to the authors, the lack of eggs containing yolk, the very small number of eggs produced, and the small size of the eggs all point to an effect on the neurosecretory cells (Glancey, Lofgren, and Williams 1982).

Abamectin applied at 1 lb of bait per acre (50 mg ai/acre) resulted in virtually complete elimination in worker brood (> 95%) and a significant reduction in colony ant populations (> 85%) at 6 to 12 weeks post treatment. Consistent with the irreversible effects on RIFA queens noted in the laboratory, the USDA researchers found no worker brood in treated colonies 18 weeks after application (Lofgren and Williams 1982; Williams 1985).

Treating individual fire ant mounds with abamectin bait provided high colony mortality, in the range of 55% to 82%, 12 to 21 weeks after treatment with 1, 4, and 7 tablespoons bait per mound. The 7-tablespoon rate provided the fastest kill, although by 21 weeks there was no difference in colony mortality between the 4- and 7-tablespoon rates. The 7-tablespoon rate of AFFIRM® is recommended for use by homeowners, since more rapid kill of worker ants and elimination of fire ant colonies is expected in this market (Greenblatt *et al.* 1986). Apperson, Powell, and Browne (1985) and Lemke and Kissam (1987) also reported that AFFIRM® provided greater than 80% reduction in colonies with brood and colony mortality following treatment of individual mounds.

Preliminary evidence from field trials suggests that fire ants do not rapidly recolonize abamectin-treated areas. The gradule elimination of worker populations and the presence of live sterile queens in treated colonies may prevent adoption and establishment of newly mated physogastric queens in abamectin plots (Greenblatt *et al.* 1986). Therefore, the slow action of abamectin appears to offer the advantage of providing high mortality to treated colonies while delaying or preventing reinfestation of treated areas.

B. Citrus

1. Citrus Rust Mite (*Phyllocoptruta oleivora*)

The eriophyid citrus rust mite is an important pest in the United States, Brazil, and other humid citrus-growing areas, causing extensive fruit russeting, reduced fruit size and juice quality, and decreased internal solids. When tested under laboratory conditions, abamectin was highly toxic by contact to *P. oleivora* on leaf discs, with an LC_{90} of 0.02 ppm (McCoy, Bullock, and Dybas 1982). Mortality was slow, especially at low doses, requiring 48 to 72 hours to achieve maximum kill. No toxicity to *P. oleivora* eggs was observed up to 25 ppm, the highest concentration tested.

Preliminary field trials conducted on citrus indicated that abamectin was effective in reducing initial *P. oleivora* populations to below economic threshold levels, at application rates of 0.0125 to 0.05 lb ai/acre (13.5–54.0 g ai/ha). Residual control of citrus rust mites was very short, however, with reinfestation of treated fruit occurring 4 weeks post treatment under some conditions.

Laboratory and field studies with tetranychid and eriophyid mites showed that low, nonacaricidal concentrations of emulsified paraffinic oil were effective in enhancing abamectin's contact and residual toxicity against mite species (Dybas 1985). Subsequently, several authors reported that applications of abamectin at 0.0125 to 0.025 lb ai/acre (13.5–27.0 g ai/ha), in combination with a minimum of 1 gallon oil per acre, resulted in enhanced activity and provided greater than 90% reduction of initial rust mite populations. Furthermore, rust mite populations and fruit damage were controlled at these rates for up to 16 weeks under the demanding conditions of Florida and Texas (McCoy, Bullock, and Dybas 1982; Childers and Sorrell 1983; French 1984; Childers 1985). These results clearly show that abamectin, when applied in combination with a paraffinic oil on citrus, can control rust mite populations below economic thresholds at one half to one quarter the rates effective without oil.

Thus, abamectin combined with oil is recommended to control *P. oleivora* infestations on all varieties of citrus, including lemons, orange, grapefruit, and tangerines. Using this practice, essentially russet-free fruit is obtained with abamectin treatments under virtually all application conditions. There has been no evidence of phytotoxicity or fruit injury from use of abamectin 0.15 EC formulation at recommended rates in combination with paraffinic crop oil.

2. Broad Mite (*Polyphagotarsonemus latus*)

Abamectin is highly toxic to *Polyphagotarsonemus latus* adults on fruit under laboratory conditions, with an LC_{90} of 0.05 ppm (Dybas and Green 1984). Brown reported that abamectin was not toxic to *P. latus* eggs (unpublished); however, abamectin residues on citrus fruit treated at 0.1 ppm provided 100% mortality to emerging larvae. Lower concentrations were less effective against the immatures, with 50% mortality observed at 0.025 ppm.

Abamectin was effective against *P. latus* infestations in field trials at rates of 0.0125 to 0.025 lb ai/acre in combination with 0.25% emulsified paraffinic oil. Initial mite populations were reduced by greater than 90%, with residual protection of fruit for 4 weeks or longer. Abamectin was more effective against *P. latus* when applied in combination with oil, consistent with the results obtained with *P. oleivora* (Brown, unpublished).

3. Citrus Red Mite (*Panonychus citri*)

Citrus red mite feeding causes serious injury to citrus foliage, including impaired photosynthesis and respiration and increased leaf drop. In laboratory bioassays, abamectin had an LC_{90} of 0.24 ppm against adult *Panonychus citri* (Dybas and Green 1984; Table 20.1).

Several researchers have reported that abamectin applied at rates of 0.0125 to 0.05 lb ai/acre reduced initial *P. citri* populations by 70% or more within 7 to 14 days post treatment. In these trials, low doses of paraffinic oil extended abamectin's residual mite control. However, field trial results are inconsistent and have shown that residual control of *P. citri* on foliage is highly variable, ranging from 2 to 6 weeks under typical growing conditions (Elmer and Morse 1985; French 1986; Elmer and Morse 1984; Brown and Jesser 1982; Brown and Jesser 1981; Childers and Sorrell 1984; Hare 1986). Results of laboratory bioassays of field-treated foliage have confirmed abamectin's short residual activity on citrus. The LT_{50} for abamectin residues, applied to orange trees at 0.025 lb ai/acre plus oil, for citrus red mite was 3 days or less (Dybas, unpublished). Because abamectin's effect on *P. citri* is inconsistent, the manufacturer has decided not to seek a label claim for control of this spider mite at this time.

Abamectin is unstable in the presence of sunlight. Several studies have shown that when abamectin is exposed to light as a thin film on glass or on foliage, it degrades rapidly, with a half-life ($t_{1/2}$) of 4 to 6 hours (MacConnell *et al.*, in press; Dybas *et al.*, in press). The limited nature of abamectin's residual activity against *P. citri* in field trials is due to the rapid decomposition and weak translaminar movement of the drug in

TABLE 20.1 Activity of abamectin against insect larvae and adult mites and aphids.

Mite Species (Contact effect against adult mites)	LC_{90} (ppm)[A]
Phyllocoptruta oleivora (Ashmead) (citrus rust mite)	0.02
Tetranychus urticae Koch (twospotted spider mite)	0.03
Panonychus ulmi (Koch) (European red mite)	0.04
Polyphagotarsonemus latus (Banks) (broad mite)	0.05
Tetranychus turkestani (Ugarov & Nikolski) (strawberry spider mite)	0.08
Tetranychus pacificus (McGregor) (Pacific spider mite)	0.16
Panonychus citri (McGregor) (citrus red mite)	0.24
Insect Species (Foliar residue bioassay)	**LC_{90} (ppm)[A]**
Manduca sexta (L.) (tobacco hornworm)	0.02
Leptinotarsa decemlineata (Say) (Colorado potato beetle)	0.03
Heliothis virescens (F.) (tobacco budworm)	0.10
Epilachna varivestis Mulsant (Mexican bean beetle)	0.40
Trichoplusia ni (Huebner) (cabbage looper)	1.0
Heliothis zea (Boddie) (cotton bollworm)	1.5
Spodoptera eridania (Cramer) (southern armyworm)	6.0
Spodoptera frugiperda (J.E. Smith) (fall armyworm)	25.0

[A] Mortality assessed 72–96 hours after exposure. Dybas, R.A., Green, A. St. J. (1984) Avermectins: Their Chemistry and Pesticidal Activity. Proceedings, 1984 British Crop Protection Conference—Pests and Diseases, Brighton, England 31:947–954.

citrus foliage (Wright *et al.* 1985a). In metabolism studies with tritium-labeled product, Iwata and colleagues (1985) noted the short half-life of abamectin on citrus fruit and foliage, while Bull and colleagues (1984) demonstrated that abamectin applied to cotton foliage decomposed with a half-life less than 1 day. Bull found 82% loss of abamectin by 2 days and 98% degradation by 8 days post application, indicating that the rate of abamectin decomposition is rapid and unaffected by foliage type.

4. Citrus thrips (*Scirtothrips citri*)

In laboratory studies the LC_{95} of abamectin to first instar *Scirtothrips citri* exposed to 1-day-old foliar residues was 10.9 ppm (Grout and Morse 1986). Abamectin was less toxic to adult female *S. citri* than to immatures. The LC_{90} of 2-hour foliar residues to 3 field colonies of adult female thrips ranged from 40 to 192 ppm (Morse and Brawner 1986).

Experience to date indicates that abamectin is only moderately toxic to *S. citri*. Several field trials conducted in California demonstrated that single applications of abamectin at 0.01 to 0.02 lb ai/acre provided only fair control of *S. citri* populations and fruit scarring on sensitive navel oranges in the San Joaquin Valley (Morse and Brawner 1983; Morse, Elmer, and Brawner 1984; Morse, Grout, and Brawner 1986; Morse and Brawner 1987). More recent studies, however, have shown that sequential applications of abamectin at these rates, at petal fall and 7 days later, may provide effective control of *S. citri* populations and maintain fruit scarring and injury below economic levels for several weeks. Because of the critical timing for abamectin citrus thrips sprays, additional experience is required under a variety of conditions to better define its utility against this citrus pest.

5. Beneficial Organisms

Abamectin exhibits a relatively low order of intrinsic toxicity to the predatory mite *Euseius tularensis* (LC_{90} 9.5 ppm) compared to its activity on citrus red mite (LC_{90} 0.30 ppm) in slide-dip bioassays. These data (Brown, unpublished) provide a safety factor of 31.7 based on the LC_{90} ratio for predator to prey and a safety factor of 54.6 at the LC_{50} level. In a field trial by Brown (unpublished), populations of the predatory mite *E. tularensis* rebounded rapidly following an application of abamectin at 0.025 lb ai/acre plus 1% crop oil. The numbers of predatory mites had declined at 3 days following application but were reestablished to control-plot levels by 6 days.

Morse and colleagues (1987) reported that field-aged foliar residues of abamectin were relatively innocuous to selected beneficial arthropods of citrus. One-day-old residues of abamectin, applied to lemon foliage at 0.025 lb ai/acre (the highest rate recommended on the product's label) in combination with 0.5% narrow-range oil, showed less than 10% mortality to the hymenopterous scale parasite, *Aphytis melinus,* the mealybug destroyer, *Cryptolaemus montrouzieri,* and the predator mite, *Eusieus stipulatus.* These results are consistent with many earlier observations that applying abamectin to citrus foliage at recommended rates is not likely to disrupt natural beneficial populations and is compatible with grower Integrated Pest Management (IPM) practices (Morse and Elliot 1985; Grafton-Cardwell and Hoy 1983; Hoy and Cave 1985; Lienk, unpublished).

Under laboratory conditions on agar medium, abamectin at 1.5 ppm reduced growth of *Hirsutella thompsonii* by 28% but had no effect on *Aschersonia aleyroidis* conidial growth and germination at that concentration. In field applications, however, abamectin has not had a negative impact on growth nor disrupted the ability of these parasitic fungi to control *P. oleivora* or the citrus whitefly, *Dialeuroides citri,* (McCoy, Bullock, and Dybas 1982).

The cumulative results of studies on abamectin's effects on beneficials, including predators, parasites, and entomophagous fungi, strongly support the utility of the product in established Integrated Pest Management programs.

C. Ornamentals

1. Twospotted Spider Mite (*Tetranychus urticae*)

Abamectin showed high intrinsic toxicity to *Tetranychus urticae* adults under laboratory conditions in contact bioassays. The contact LC_{90} to adults on bean plants was 0.03 ppm (Table 20.1). Abamectin is toxic to all stages of *T. urticae* except the egg stage.

Abamectin did not kill eggs at concentrations up to 4.5 ppm in the laboratory; however, slight reduction in hatch of 3-day-old eggs laid on bean leaves was observed. This effect was likely due to abamectin's ability to penetrate the egg chorion at that age, resulting in paralysis of the developing larvae and inhibition of eclosion (Green and Dybas 1984).

Abamectin (AVID®) has displayed long residual activity in controlling *T. urticae* populations on foliage in laboratory and greenhouse studies. Because abamectin is nonovicidal at standard application rates, foliar persistence is important in controlling larvae hatching from eggs present at the time of application. In a laboratory bioassay on roses, abamectin applied at 4.5 ppm provided 84% mortality to *T. urticae* adults 10 days after treatment and 44% kill after 21 days (Green and Dybas 1984). Long residual control of *T. urticae* was observed under commercial greenhouse application conditions. Abamectin applied at 4.5 ppm in a full-cover spray on roses maintained *T. urticae* populations below a threshold of 1 mite per leaf for at least 28 days. Similarly, on chrysanthemum the same concentration of abamectin held populations below 2 adults per leaf for over 42 days (Green and Dybas 1984; Green *et al.* 1985b). Several authors have reported on abamectin's long residual control of mites on chrysanthemum, carnation, and roses (Robb, Virzi, and Parrella 1985; Mollet *et al.* 1986).

The penetration of abamectin's residues into the cuticle of plants has been demonstrated in our laboratories (Presier, unpublished). This translaminar movement provides a reservoir of abamectin within the mesophyll, accounting for the long residual activity to mites and insects feeding on plant tissue. Green and colleagues (1985b) reported that abamectin applied at 4.5 ppm showed translaminar activity in the control of *T. urticae* on rose foliage in laboratory and greenhouse studies. Greater than 80% mortality was observed at 7 days to *T. urticae* adults and immatures feeding on the ventral side of leaves, following application of abamectin to the dorsal surface. Similarly, Wright and colleagues (1985a) reported control of *T. urticae,* but not aphids (*Aphis fabae* or *Aphis gossypii*), due to translaminar action by abamectin on chrysanthemum. The LC_{50} for abamectin residues applied to either the dorsal or ventral leaf surface was 30.1 to 33.4 ppm for *T. urticae;* however, higher concentrations, 450 ppm or greater, were required to achieve 50% mortality of aphids. While aphids feed selectively on the phloem, phytophagous mites such as *T. urticae* feed within the leaf parenchyma and are likely to ingest a higher concentration of abamectin than the aphids.

2. Leafminer (*Liriomyza trifolii*)

Abamectin is highly toxic to adult *Liriomyza trifolii* and early instar larvae mining within leaf tissue. When applied to newly eclosed larvae on chrysanthemum, abamectin provided 100% control at a 12 ppm concentration. Greater than 90% control of third stage *L. trifolii* larvae was obtained at that concentration; however, 48 ppm was required to provide 100% kill of third stage larvae and complete inhibition of pupation and adult emergence (Parrella 1983).

Abamectin is not toxic to *L. trifolii* eggs. However, residues of abamectin within leaf tissue, following application at 4.5 ppm, provided 100% control of newly hatched larvae (Green and Dybas 1984). Abamectin applied on a weekly spray schedule, at concentrations in the range of 4.5 to 24 ppm to chrysanthemum, gerbera daisy, gypsophila, and other flower varieties susceptible to attack by *L. trifolii,* provided over 85% reduction in large mine formation and completed mines. Abamectin is not repellent to *Liriomyza* flies, and in these trials it did not effectively reduce feeding punctures and stippling by adult females (Parrella *et al.* 1988; Green and Dybas 1984; Parrella 1983; Green *et al.* 1985a).

AVID® (abamectin) is recommended at a rate of 0.01 to 0.02 lb ai/acre in full-cover foliar sprays for the control of *Liriomyza trifolii* on flowers and foliage plants. Weekly applications of the product are recommended during periods of continuous fly infestation to obtain high-quality, leafminer-free crops.

3. Thrips Species

Several species of thrips attack ornamental foliage and floral crops worldwide. Because of their secretive feeding habits and protected life stages, these pests are normally difficult to control with nonsystemic, nonfumigant pesticides.

Abamectin was only moderately toxic to adult western flower thrips (*Frankliniella occidentalis*), the most important species affecting ornamentals. Broadbent and Kelly (1987a) reported that in a combined contact and residual toxicity bioassay, abamectin at 40 ppm (the highest concentration tested) produced only 51.9% mortality to adult *F. occidentalis* confined on abamectin residues on petri dishes for 72 hours. Similarly, only 45.6% mortality of adult thrips was observed following 72 hours exposure to abamectin residues on chrysanthemum (Broadbent and Kelly 1987b). The activity against *F. occidentalis* at normal use rates is slow, even when adult thrips are confined and forced to feed on treated foliage.

Oetting (1987) evaluated the toxicity of abamectin at 6 and 12 ppm as a foliar residue on impatiens leaves to *Ecinothrips americanus* under greenhouse conditions. When thrips were introduced onto foliar residues within 24 hours after application, greater than 90% mortality was observed in adult and second instar immatures exposed to 12 ppm abamectin residues for 72 hours. However, the toxicity of abamectin foliar residues decreased rapidly with time. Abamectin provided 60% or less mortality to adult and immature stages of *E. americanus* introduced onto foliar residues aged for 3 days or longer. No significant differences were observed in the sensitivity of adult or immature thrips exposed to abamectin foliar residues at any time period.

Oetting observed that egg hatch was slightly reduced when leaves were sprayed at selected intervals before or after oviposition. The greatest reduction in percent hatch (68%) was observed in eggs that hatched within 3 days following application of abamectin at 12 ppm. Although a few thrips died during eclosion, most first instars emerged completely from the egg and died after crawling on the leaf surface for a short time. The reduction in the number of hatching thrips exposed to 12 ppm abamectin residues was not sufficient for adequate control. In combination with the short residual control of adults, these data suggest the need for multiple applications of the product in commercial greenhouses to break the life cycle of *E. americanus* or other thrips species.

Robb and Parrella (1986) evaluated abamectin for controlling *F. occidentalis* in roses and carnations. The authors observed only moderate activity, an average of 66% control of thrips populations, following 2 applications of abamectin at 0.003 lb ai/100 gallons water, 5 days apart.

In a trial on dahlia against *F. occidentalis,* 3 applications of abamectin at 0.02 lb ai/acre, 7 days apart, completely eliminated a low thrips population. Following the same treatment regime against *F. occidentalis* on carnations, however, abamectin provided only 50.4% control of a heavy thrips population at 7 days after the third application (Taylor, unpublished).

Although abamectin appears to provide useful activity against difficult-to-control thrips species, it has performed erratically in greenhouse trials and has failed to provide consistent control following multiple applications. For these reasons, the manufacturer has decided not to label the product for use against thrips species on ornamental crops until greater experience is obtained.

D. Cotton

1. Spider Mites (*Tetranychus urticae, T. turkestani, T. pacificus, T. cinnabarinus*)

Several studies have shown that abamectin is highly toxic to tetranychid spider mites under laboratory conditions, with LC_{90} values against adult mites in the range of 0.02 to 0.16 ppm (Putter *et al.* 1981; Dybas and Green 1984; Preiser, unpublished).

In another study, Hilton (unpublished) compared the toxicity of abamectin to a field isolate of the carmine spider mite (*T. cinnabarinus*) from Uvalde, TX, and a laboratory colony of the twospotted spider mite (*T. urticae*). Both populations were highly susceptible to abamectin, with an LC_{50} value of 0.0029 ppm for *T. cinnabarinus* compared to an LC_{50} of 0.0087 for the laboratory colony of *T. urticae*. The *T. cinnabarinus* isolate was highly resistant to monocroptophos, which is used extensively in the Uvalde region. For monocroptophos, the LC_{50} for the carmine mite was 11,036 ppm, compared to an LC_{50} of 94.84 ppm for the twospotted spider mite.

In other laboratory bioassays, abamectin was evaluated against 4 field isolates of *T. urticae* from the San Joaquin Valley, CA. Abamectin was equitoxic to all 4 strains, which had varying degrees of resistance to dicofol and propargite, standard miticides used on cotton in the San Joaquin Valley (Hilton and Dybas, in press). Therefore, results of laboratory bioassays indicate that abamectin is effective against spider mites, which are susceptible and resistant to standard cotton miticides. Cross-resistance to abamectin has not been observed in spider mites in limited studies. (Hoy and Cave 1985).

A number of authors have noted abamectin's ability to provide long residual control of spider mites on cotton, despite its rapid photodecomposition following application. This persistence is due to abamectin's translaminar action, which has been observed in both laboratory and field bioassays with spider mites (Wright *et al.* 1985a; Dybas and Green 1984). Bull and colleagues (1984) reported 82% and 98% decomposition of abamectin on cotton after 2 and 8 days, with a half-life of less than 1 day. Rapid penetration of abamectin into cotton foliage was observed within a few hours of application, with 1.3% of the applied dose of tritiated avermectin B1a absorbed into foliage by 8 days.

Results of laboratory bioassays of field-treated foliage have confirmed abamectin's long residual activity on cotton. The LT_{50} for abamectin residues, applied at 0.01 to 0.02 lb ai/acre, to the twospotted spider mite was 21 to 28 days (Dunbar, Dybas, and Norton, in press). Wright and colleagues (1985a) also reported that abamectin applied to cotton leaves at 30 ppm gave 100% kill of adult female *T. urticae* under glasshouse conditions and outdoors for at least 28 days. At 3 ppm abamectin, greater than 95% mortality was maintained for 14 days under glass and greater than 85% control outdoors for 7 days.

The use of emulsified oil in combination with abamectin has been shown to extend the toxicity of abamectin's foliar residues on various crops under greenhouse and field conditions (Dybas 1985). Wright and colleagues (1985b) reported that abamectin applied on cotton at 3 ppm in combination with 0.25% paraffinic oil provided 77% or greater mortality to spider mites for 21 days outdoors and 28 days under glasshouse conditions.

Additionally, Mizell, Schiffhauer, and Taylor (1986), reporting on the complex interaction of host plant, light regime, and additives on the stability of abamectin residues following spray application to a number of crops, noted that the nonionic surfactant, Leaf Act 80A, and paraffinic oil increased the length of abamectin's mite control on bean compared to abamectin alone.

Abamectin has provided excellent control of mites in field trials on cotton. Wynholds and Leigh (1986) reported 90% to 96% knockdown of spider mite populations 13 to 18 days following abamectin applications at 0.008 to 0.009 lb ai/acre, and residual control of 85% to 95% at 41 to 49 days after treatment. These researchers had previously reported 92% to 96% control of mite populations for 46 days following abamectin treatment at 0.02 lb ai/acre (Wynholds and Leigh 1982). Royer and Edelson (1987) showed that abamectin at 0.015 lb ai/acre reduced initial mite populations by 98% at 7 days post treatment and provided 100% control of populations after 21 days. The lower abamectin rate, 0.0075 lb ai/acre, provided 89% to 93% control for the duration of the trial. No control of the cotton aphid, *Aphis gossypii,* was observed with abamectin at these application rates throughout the study. These results confirm laboratory observations on abamectin's weak activity against aphid species on cotton (Wright *et al.* 1985a).

Tuttle and Mullis (1984) evaluated the activity of abamectin against carmine spider mites on cotton applied with and without paraffinic oil. At 0.01 and 0.02 lb ai/acre, abamectin without paraffinic oil gave 92% to 98% control from 3 to 14 days post treatment. In combination with oil, abamectin at 0.01 lb ai/acre provided 98% reduction in mite populations 3 days after application; however, by 14 days, mite populations began to rebound, and only 69% control was observed. The lower rate of abamectin (0.005 lb ai/acre) in this trial was the least effective, providing 84% and 55% control at 3 days and 14 days post application, respectively.

Results obtained from several studies have shown that abamectin at recommended rates of 0.01 to 0.02 lb ai/acre provides 80% or greater reduction of initial spider mite populations by 7 to 10 days post application and greater than 90% reduction by 14 days. Rates below 0.01 lb ai/acre have been slower and less effective in reducing initial mite populations and provide shorter residual control of spider mites (Tuttle and Mullis 1984; Dybas, unpublished).

Field trials have shown that initial reduction of mite populations with abamectin at 0.01 lb ai/acre at 7 days post treatment appears slow. This occurs as a result of abamectin's lack of ovicidal action. Motile spider mites are killed shortly after application; however, eggs present at the time of treatment develop and hatch normally. An additional 3 to 4 days are then required for the newly hatched larvae to accumulate a lethal dose of abamectin.

Abamectin has demonstrated long residual spider mite control on cotton and reduction in crop damage in season-long trials. Statistically significant increases in seed cotton yield per acre over standard acaricide treatments were observed with abamectin treatments of 0.01 lb ai/acre in large-scale field trials conducted in California under a U.S. Environmental Protection Agency (EPA)-approved experimental use permit on cotton (Dunbar, Dybas, and Norton, in press).

2. Lepidoptera

Abamectin is highly selective in its toxicity to lepidopteran larvae, with armyworm species being the least susceptible. Dybas and Green (1984; Table 20.1) reported laboratory foliage bioassays LC_{90} values of 0.02, 1.5, and 6.0 ppm for abamectin against tobacco hornworm (*Manduca sexta*), corn earworm (*Heliothis zea*), and southern armyworm (*Spodoptera eridania*) first instar larvae, respectively, indicating a 300-fold difference in the sensitivity of southern armyworm compared to tobacco hornworm. Similarly, Anderson and colleagues (1986) reported a 400-fold difference in the toxicity of abamectin to *Heliothis virescens* larvae compared to *S. eridania* at the LC_{50} level in a foliage bioassay test. Substantial differences in the susceptibility to abamectin among the noctuid species *H. virescens, H. zea,* and *S. frugiperda* were also noted by Bull (1986). In bioassays against lepidopterans, the first visible symptom of exposure of the first instar larvae to abamectin is paralysis of the hind legs within 24 hours, followed by larval mortality over a 48- to 72-hour period (Wright, Jenkins, and Villavaso, 1985).

Several authors have reported that abamectin is more toxic to lepidopteran larvae via ingestion than by contact with product residues (Anderson *et al.* 1986; Bull 1986; Corbitt, Green, and Wright, in press; Wright, Jenkins, and Villavaso. 1985). In a comparative evaluation, Anderson and colleagues (1986) showed that abamectin was one fourth as toxic as the pyrethroid fenvalerate to *S. eridania* larvae in the foliage ingestion bioassay, whereas by topical application, abamectin was nearly 1000-fold less toxic to *S. eridania* than fenvalerate.

Abamectin was highly toxic to male and female pink bollworm (*Pectinophora gossypiella*) moths under laboratory conditions. Applied topically on either the dorsal thorax or the ventral surface of the last abdominal segment of the moths, abamectin had an LC_{50} of 0.032 to 0.041 ug/insect (Bariola and Lingren 1984). Abamectin prevented mating for up to 72 hours when males or females were treated with an LD_{10} or LD_{50} dose. Additionally, oviposition was completely prevented in female moths treated with an LD_{10} dose. Egg hatch was also significantly reduced by abamectin (Bariola 1984).

In limited field trials conducted to date, abamectin has not provided effective control of noctuid species on cotton (Merck data, unpublished; Mink and Luttrell 1987). Abamectin's rapid photolytic breakdown following application, its weak topical/contact activity against lepidopteran larvae, the limited feeding habits of *Heliothis* species on cotton, and the differential sensitivity among noctuide species are factors that have severely limited the utility of abamectin in the control of Lepidoptera on cotton.

3. Cotton Aphid (*Aphis gossypii*)

Abamectin was shown to be toxic to several aphid species under laboratory conditions in contact bioassays, with LC_{90}'s in the range of 0.4 to 1.5 ppm (Putter *et al.* 1981; Dybas and Green 1984). Abamectin demonstrated poor control of *A. fabae* and *A. gossypii* in foliar translaminar bioassays, with concentrations as high as 450 ppm required to produce 50% mortality in these species.

Aphids feed selectively on the phloem of leaf tissue, and this feeding preference may account for the poor activity of abamectin in the control of aphids compared to spider mites. Royer and Edelson (1987) confirmed the weak activity of abamectin on aphids in a cotton field trial. This study showed initial suppression of *A. gossypii* 7 days after treatment with abamectin applied at 0.01 and 0.02 lb ai/acre; however, essentially no control of cotton aphid populations was observed at 14 and 21 days post treatment. Leigh and colleagues (1988) also showed poor control of a mixed population of *A. gossypii* and *A. craccivora* following a single application of abamectin in the San Joaquin Valley. The limited activity observed against aphids was attributed to biological control, confirming abamectin's safety to beneficial insects.

E. Vegetables (Celery, Tomato, Pepper)

1. *Leafminers* (*Liriomyza trifolii* and *L. sativae*)

Under laboratory conditions abamectin was highly toxic to early instar *L. trifolii* larvae in foliage bioassays. Field-collected adult female *L. trifolii* were allowed to oviposit on California blackeye peas for 4 hours in the laboratory. To evaluate toxicity to the leafminer larvae within the foliage, leaves were dipped in abamectin solutions after eggs had hatched and the larvae developed to the second-third instar. The LC_{95} for *L. trifolii* was found to be 0.746 ppm. The toxicity of abamectin to *L. trifolii* was independent of foliage type, with similar results observed on celery, tomato, and chrysanthemum (Dybas, unpublished).

Schuster and Everett (1983) reported complete control of 1- and 3-day-old larvae in tomato foliage with abamectin applications at 6 and 12 ppm. At these concentrations, abamectin was nonovicidal to *L. trifolii* eggs laid in leaf tissue; however, the treatment resulted in 90% or greater kill of larvae during eclosion due to contact with residues in or on the chorion or in the leaf mesophyll. In addition, abamectin residues of 12 ppm were moderately toxic to the adult flies. Mortality of adult *L. trifolii* exposed in the laboratory to dried abamectin residues on filter paper or tomato foliage was 24% to 38% after 48 hours exposure. Although adult mortality was low, abamectin reduced egg laying and stippling of foliage. Because these functions are initiated by the ovipositor, paralysis of the ovipositor may have occurred as a result of exposure to abamectin residues.

Bioassay of tomato foliage treated with abamectin at 0.01 lb ai/acre showed 40% to 60% mortality of *L. trifolii* males and females exposed to fresh residues for 48 hours. However, little mortality was seen in adult flies exposed to 24-hour field-aged residues, which is consistent with the known rapid breakdown and dissipation of abamectin surface deposits following application (Schuster and Taylor 1987). The field-treated foliar residues were effective in reducing larval growth and survival in tomato leaflets bioassayed 7 days after treatment. The length of residual toxicity to *L. trifolii* larvae noted in this study supports earlier observations regarding the translaminar movement of abamectin in tomato foliage and persistence of internal leaf residues following spray applications (Schuster and Taylor 1987; Wright *et al.* 1985a).

Several authors have reported on the control of *L. trifolii* on tomato, celery, and pepper in field trials with abamectin treatments at the recommended field rates of 0.01 to 0.02 lb ai/acre (Trumble 1983a,b; Carson, Trumble, and Nakakihara 1986; Carson, Nakakihara, and Trumble 1986; Schuster and Everett 1987; Zehnder and Trumble 1984; Schuster 1987; Royer, Edelson, and Cartwright, 1985; Chandler 1985). Greater than 80% reduction in leaf mines and/or pupal emergence has been observed in all trials. Results of limited studies have also shown that, under certain conditions, the addition of the nonionic surfactant, Leaf Act 80A, may improve leafminer control, presumably by enhancing penetration of abamectin into the foliage and thereby extending the period of residual protection (Merck data, unpublished).

2. Twospotted Spider Mite and Tomato Russet Mite (*T. urticae* and *Aculops lycopersici*)

Laboratory studies have shown that abamectin is highly toxic to eriophyid and tetranychid mites (Dybas and Green 1984; McCoy, Bullock, and Dybas 1982). The LC_{90} of abamectin against *T. urticae* adults was 0.03 ppm. Royalty and Perring (1987) found that abamectin was very toxic to *A. lycopersici,* with an LC_{90} of 0.00959 ppm against adults. These authors also noted that abamectin was much less toxic to the predatory mite *Homeopronematus anconai;* thus, abamectin sprays should sufficiently control tomato russet mite without reducing *H. anconai* populations.

Limited field studies have been conducted to date with abamectin for control of mites on tomato with excellent results. Greater than 80% control of mite populations was observed following abamectin applications at 0.01 to 0.02 lb ai/acre (Schuster 1984; Merck data, unpublished).

3. Armyworms (*Spodoptera exigua* and *S. eridania*)

Armyworm species are relatively insensitive to abamectin compared to other insects (Table 20.1). The LC_{90} for abamectin against southern armyworm (*Spodoptera eridania*) was 6.0 ppm in a foliar bioassay (Dybas and Green 1984), 1.96 ppm for beet armyworm (*S. exigua*) by diet incorporation (Trumble *et al.* 1987; Moar and Trumble 1987), and greater than 25 ppm for fall armyworm (*S. frugiperda*) in a foliar bioassay.

In field trials on celery and tomato, abamectin, at rates recommended for leafminer control (0.01 to 0.02 lb ai/acre), was only marginally effective in reducing *Spodoptera* infestations, providing 50% or less control of larval populations and prevention of crop damage in season-long programs (Carson, Trumble, and Nakakihara 1986; Schuster 1987; Trumble 1983a; Trumble 1983b; Waddill 1982; Trumble 1985a; Carson, Nakakihara, and Trumble 1986).

4. Tomato Pinworm (*Keiferia lycopersicella*)

Under laboratory conditions, *K. lycopersicella* larvae were found to be highly susceptible to abamectin. The LC_{95} for first instar larvae exposed to fresh abamectin foliar residues was 0.031 ppm. However, abamectin was shown to be considerably less toxic to pinworm larvae feeding internally within the foliage. In this case, abamectin's LC_{95} was 15.1 ppm or approximately 500-fold higher than obtained for control of *K. lycoper-*

sicella larvae by contact with surface residues (Schuster and Taylor, unpublished).

Limited field studies conducted to date with abamectin on tomato at rates of 0.01 to 0.02 lb ai/acre have provided good results against *K. lycopersicella*. A 93% to 96% reduction of seasonal fruit damage from *K. lycopersicella* was reported following weekly applications of abamectin at 0.01 to 0.02 lb ai/acre (Trumble 1983b). In another trial, 70% to 75% reduction in seasonal damage was observed following 5 weekly applications of abamectin at 0.01 to 0.02 lb ai/acre (Trumble 1985a), while in yet another field trial, 62.5% to 69% reduction in fruit damage was reported following 7 weekly applications (Carson, Trumble, and Nakakihara 1986). Based on the experience obtained to date, abamectin is recommended at a rate of 0.01 to 0.02 lb ai/acre for control of *K. lycopersicella* on tomato.

5. Beneficial Arthropods

Trumble (1985a) reported that weekly treatments of celery with abamectin at 0.01 lb ai/acre (its recommended rate of application for leafminer control) had a minimal effect on both adult and larval stages of the leafminer parasite complex. Abamectin applications did not adversely impact seasonal percent parasitism, adult parasite mortality and survival, or emergence of immature parasites of *Diglyphus intermedius, D. begini, Chrysonotomyia punctiventris, Chrysocharis parksi, C. ainsliei,* and *Halticoptera circulus* from treated foliage.

Abamectin at application rates of 0.01 to 0.02 lb ai/acre also did not adversely affect the beneficial leafminer parasite complex on celery, tomato, and pepper under field use conditions (Zehnder and Trumble 1984; Carson, Nakakihara, and Trumble 1986; Trumble 1985b; Chandler 1985). Parasite mortality from abamectin treatments were not statistically different from the controls.

Results of several field trials support the fact that abamectin has a good safety margin for beneficials and is useful for Integrated Pest Management programs on celery, tomato, and peppers.

F. Pears

1. Pear psylla (*Psylla pyricola*)

Abamectin, at rates of 0.0125 to 0.025 lb ai/acre, has provided significant reduction in *Psylla pyricola* nymphal populations in postbloom sprays on pears. The addition of 0.25% paraffinic oil in dilute sprays, or a minimum of 1 gallon oil per acre, extends abamectin's residual control of psylla nymphs for 4 weeks or longer, and provides effective control of fruit damage.

Burts (1983, 1984) reported that abamectin provided good control of psylla populations throughout the season, and essentially no fruit russeting at harvest due to pear psylla honeydew. Abamectin applied at 0.0125 and 0.025 lb ai/acre plus oil also provided good control of heavy psylla populations, with minimal fruit damage (Burts 1985a,b). In this latter trial, 6% and 2% cull fruit were observed in the low- and high-rate abamectin treatments, compared to 59% in the control plot. Riedl and Shearer (1987) found excellent seasonal control of heavy pear psylla populations following 3 applications of abamectin at 0.0125 and 0.025 lb ai/acre in combination with a paraffinic oil. At harvest, no fruit were downgraded in the high-rate treatment, while only 2.9% fruit damage was observed at the low abamectin rate compared to 21.8% in the control plot. Howitt and Hays (1986) reported that, in a seasonal program, abamectin applied at 0.023 lb ai/acre in combination with superior oil and with superior oil plus the nonionic surfactant, Leaf Act 80A, provided effective control of pyrethroid-resistant psylla populations. At harvest, the sooty fungus rating on leaves was reduced by 96% and 99% in the abamectin oil and oil/surfactant treatments.

Burts (1985a) reported that dormant-season sprays of abamectin at 0.01 lb ai/acre failed to reduce *Psylla pyricola* adult populations below retreatment thresholds even after 2 applications. As a consequence, abamectin is not recommended for prebloom control of overwintered adult *Psylla pyricola*. Abamectin is most effective for control of psylla nymphal populations after petal fall at the recommended rates of 0.0125 to 0.25 lb ai/acre in thorough coverage sprays.

2. Twospotted Spider Mite, European Red Mite, Pear Rust Mite (*Tetranychus urticae, Panonychus ulmi, Epitrimerus pyri*)

The high susceptibility of tetranychid and eriophyid mites to abamectin was discussed in earlier sections of this chapter. The results of several field trials have shown that abamectin, applied at 0.0125 to 0.025 lb ai/acre in combination with 0.025% crop oil in dilute sprays, provides excellent control of *T. urticae, P. ulmi,* and *E. pyri* populations.

Burts (1983, 1984, 1987) reported that abamectin at 0.025 lb ai/acre, in combination with 0.25% oil, provided 89.5% to 97.9%, 95.8% to 100%, and 83.5% to 93.9% control of European red mite, twospotted spider mite, and pear rust mite populations in seasonal programs on pears. Only slightly less control of mite populations was observed in these trials at the 0.0125 lb ai/acre rate: 84% to 90% for European red mite, 90.6% to 100% for twospotted spider mite, and 73.3% to 88.9% for pear rust mite.

Cumulative results from field trials conducted to date indicate that single applications of abamectin at recommended rates of 0.0125 to 0.025 lb ai/acre, in combination with paraffinic oil, reduces initial mite populations by 85% or greater within 7 days after application, and provides control of populations below retreatment levels for 4 weeks or longer.

G. Miscellaneous Crops

1. Strawberry

Limited studies have shown that abamectin is effective against spider mite infestations on strawberry and tree nuts. Carson and colleagues (1987) reported that 7 biweekly applications of abamectin on strawberry at 0.02 lb ai/acre in 50 to 100 gallons of water per acre were effective in reducing *T. urticae* populations throughout the trial. Abamectin's activity was not improved by the addition of 0.1% oil in the spray tank. The authors also reported that abamectin controlled a moderate density of aphids under this spray regime.

Earlier, Trumble and Nakakihara (1984) had reported that abamectin applied to strawberries at 0.04 lb ai/acre, alone and in combination with 0.1% oil, reduced motile spider mite populations by an average of 92.7% and 95.8%, respectively, over an 8-week period following a single application. A second application of abamectin at the same rates, alone and in combination with paraffinic oil, reduced mite levels but was less effective, providing only 30.9% and 72.8% control over a 3-week period.

More recent studies have shown that abamectin controls spider mites very effectively on strawberry following 2 applications, timed on a 7-day spray schedule to kill hatching larvae (Dunbar, unpublished). In 3 replicated field trials, abamectin provided an average of 79% and 68% control of *T. urticae* over a 35-day period when applied twice at 0.02 and 0.01 lb ai/acre, compared to only 52% control of mite populations over the same period from a single application at 0.01 lb ai/acre.

2. Deciduous Tree Nuts

Abamectin applied at 0.00625 lb ai/100 gallons water in a high volume dilute spray to almonds was shown to reduce initial populations of *Tetranychus pacificus* by 85% at 6 days post treatment. Residual control of spider mite populations was obtained for 48 days and was enhanced by the combination of abamectin with a narrow-range spray oil (Sanderson and Barnes 1983). The authors also reported that abamectin treatment did not have a negative impact on beneficial species, including the predatory mite, *Metaseiulus occidentalis,* and six-spotted thrips, *Scolothrips sexmaculatus*. Payne, Dutcher, and Ellis (1985) reported that abamectin applied at a rate of 0.02 lb ai/acre to pecans provided excellent control (95%–100%) of the hickory shuckworm, pecan leaf scorch mite, and pecan weevil. Abamectin, however, provided poor control of yellow aphids and the black aphid in this field trial.

References

Anderson TE, Babu JR, Dybas RA, Mehta H (1986) Avermectin B1: ingestion and contact toxicity against *Spodoptera eridania* and *Heliothis virescens* (Lepidoptera: Noctuidae) and potentiation by oil and piperonyl butoxide. *J. Econ. Entomol.* 79:197–201.

Apperson CS, Powell EE, Browne M (1985) Efficacy of individual mound treatments of MK-936 and amdro against the red imported fire ant (Hymenoptera: Formicidae). *J. Georgia Entomol. Soc.* 19:508–516.

Bariola LA (1984) Pink Bollworms (Lepidoptera: Gelechiidae): Effects of low concentrations of selected insecticides on mating and fecundity in the laboratory. *J. Econ. Entomol.* 77:1278–1282.

Bariola LA, Lingren PD (1984) Comparative toxicities of selected insecticides against pink bollworm (Lepidoptera: Gelechiidae) moths. *J. Econ. Entomol.* 77:207–210.

Broadbent AB, Kelly RF (1987a) Residual toxicity of selected insecticides to western flower thrips. *Pestic. Res. Rep.* E.C.P.U.A., 167.

Broadbent AB, Kelly RF (1987b) Combined contact and residual toxicity of selected insecticides to western flower thrips. Pesticide Research Report E.C.P.U.A., 168.

Brown RD, Jesser MJ (1981) Citrus red mite control in Riverside. *Insectic. & Acaric. Tests* 6:41.

Brown RD, Jesser MJ (1982) Control of citrus red mite with carbamate, pyrethroids, and avermectin B_1. *Insectic. Acaric. Tests* 7:48–49.

Bull DL (1986) Toxicity and pharmacodynamics of avermectin in the tobacco budworm, corn earworm and fall armyworm (Noctuidae: Lepidoptera). *J. Agric. Food Chem.* 34:74–78.

Bull DL, Ivie GW, MacConnell JG, Gruber VF, Ku CC, Arison BH, Stevenson JM, VandenHeuvel WJA (1984) Fate of avermectin B1a in soil and plants. *J. Agric. Food Chem.* 32:94–102.

Burts E (1983) Pear, pest control. *Insectic. & Acaric. Tests* 8:30.

Burts E (1984) Pear, pest control. *Insectic. & Acaric. Tests* 9:45–47.

Burts E (1985a) Pear, pest control. *Insectic. & Acaric. Tests* 10:36–37.

Burts EC (1985b) SN72129 and avermectin B1, two new pesticides for control of pear psylla, *Psylla pyricola* (Homoptera: Psyllidae). *J. Econ. Entomol.* 78:1327–1330.

Burts EC (1987) Pear, pest control. *Insectic. & Acaric. Tests* 12:60–61.

Carson WG, Nakakihara H, Trumble JT (1986) Impact of insecticides on lepidopterous larvae and leafminers on tomatoes. *Insectic. & Acaric. Tests* 11:189–191.

Carson WG, Nakakihara H, Trumble JT, Vath V (1987) Spider mite and aphid control in chemical trials on strawberries. *Insectic. & Acaric. Tests* 12:82.

Carson WG, Trumble JT, Nakakihara H (1986) Effect of insecticides on lepidopterous larvae and leafminers on celery. *Insectic. & Acaric. Tests* 11:109–110.

Chandler LD (1985) Response of *Liriomyza trifolii* (Burgess) to selected insecticides with notes on hymenopterous parasites. *Southwest. Entomol.* 10:228–235.

Childers CC (1985) Citrus rust mite control (CRM). *Insectic. & Acaric. Tests* 10:57–58.

Childers CC, Sorrell RW (1983) Citrus rust mite control (CRM). *Insectic. & Acaric. Tests* 8:34–35.

Childers CC, Sorrell RW (1984) Citrus red mite control (CRM). *Insectic. & Acaric. Tests* 9:69–70.

Corbitt TS, Green A St J, Wright DJ (in press) Relative potency of avermectin B1 against larval stages of *Spodoptera littoralis* Boisd., *Heliothis armigera* Hubu. and *Heliothis virescens* F. (Lepidoptera: Noctuidae). *Crop Protect.*

Dunbar DM, Dybas RA, Norton JA (in press) Abamectin 0.15 EC (ZEPHYR®): Miticide/insecticide for spider mite control on San Joaquin Valley cotton. Beltwide Cotton Insect Research and Control Conference Proceedings.

Dybas RA (1985) Synergistic avermectin combination for treating plant pests. U.S. Patent 4,560,677.

Dybas RA, Green A St J (1984) Avermectins: their chemistry and pesticidal activity. 1984 British Corp Protection Conference, Pests and Diseases 9B-3:947–954.

Dybas RA, Hilton NJ, Babu JR, Preiser FA, Dolce GJ (1989) Novel second generation avermectin miticides and insecticides for crop protection. Topics in industrial microbiology (Demain, Somkuti Hunter-Cevera, and Rossmoore, eds.), chapter 23, 201–210 Elsevier, Amsterdam.

Elmer HS, Morse JG (1984) Citrus red mite pesticide efficacy tests in the San Joaquin Valley. *Insectic. & Acaric. Tests* 9:87–88.

Elmer HS, Morse JG (1985) Citrus red mite pesticide efficacy tests in the San Joaquin Valley. *Insectic. & Acaric. Tests* 10:59–60.

French JV (1984) Rust mite control on Texas citrus. *Insectic. & Acaric. Tests* 9:71.

French JV (1986) Spider mite control on Texas citrus. *Insectic. & Acaric. Tests* 11:98–99.

Glancey BM, Lofgren CS, Williams DF (1982) Avermectin B_{1a}: effects on the ovaries of red imported fire ant queens (Hymenoptera: Formicidae). *J. Med. Entomol.* 19:743–747.

Grafton-Cardwell EE, Hoy MA (1983) Comparative toxicity of avermectin B_1 to the predator *Metaseiulus occidentalis* (Nesbitt) (Acari: Phytoseiidae) and the spider mites *Tetranychus urticae* (Koch) and *Panonychus ulmi* (Koch) (Acari: Tetranychidae) per. J. *Econ. Entomol.* 76:1216–1220.

Green A St J, Dybas RA (1984) Avermectin B_1: Control of mites on ornamentals. 1984 British Crop Protection Conference, Pests and Diseases 11A-7:1129–1133.

Green A St J, Heijne B, Schreurs J, Dybas RA (1985a) Serpentine leafminer (*Liriomyza trifolii*) (Burgess) control with abamectin (MK-936) in Dutch ornamentals, a review of the processes involved in the evolution of the use directions, and a summary of the results of phytotoxicity evaluations. *Med. Fac. Landbouww.* Rijksuniv. Gent 50/2 b:603–622.

Green A St J, Heijne B, Schreurs J, Dybas RA (1985b) Twospotted spider mite (*Tetranychus urticae* Koch) control with abamectin (MK-936) on roses. *Med. Fac. Landbouww.* Rijksuniv. Gent 50/2 b:623–632.

Greenblatt JA, Norton JA, Dybas RA, Harlan DP (1986) Control of the red imported fire ant with abamectin (AFFIRM®), a novel insecticide, in individual mound trials. *J. Agric. Entomol.* 3:233–241.

Grout TG, Morse JG (1986) Insect growth regulators: promising effects on citrus thrips (Thysanoptera: Thripidae). *Can. Ent.* 118:389–392.

Hare J (1986) Citrus red mite pesticide efficacy tests in Riverside. *Insectic. & Acaric. Tests* 11:99–100.

Hilton NJ, Dybas RA (in press) Abamectin (ZEPHYR®): A novel avermectin miticide/insecticide for spider mite control on cotton. Beltwide Cotton Insect Research and Control Conference Proceedings.

Howitt AJ, Hays AR (1986) Pear, full season psylla block test. *Insectic. & Acaric. Tests* 11:71–72.

Hoy MA, Cave FE (1985) Laboratory evaluation of avermectin as a selective acaricide for use with *Metaseiulus occidentalis* (Nesbitt) Acarina: Phytoseiidae). *Exper. & Appl. Acarol.* 1:139–152.

Iwata I, MacConnell JG, Flor JE, Putter I, Dinoff TM (1985) Residues of avermectin B1a on and in citrus fruits and foliage. *J. Agric. Food Chem.* 33:467–471.

Leigh T, Wynholds P, Bentley W, Arrendondo C (1988) Insect pest status in the San Joaquin Valley in 1987. *Cal. Cot. Prog. Rep.* March: 8–9.

Lemke LA, Kissam JB (1987) Evaluation of various insecticides and home remedies for control of individual red imported fire ant colonies. *J. Entomol. Sci.* 22:275–281.

Lofgren CS, Williams CF (1982) Avermectin B_1a: highly potent inhibitor of reproduction by queens of the red imported fire ant (Hymenoptera: Formicidae). *J. Econ. Entomol.* 75:798–803.

MacConnell JG, Demchak RJ, Preiser FA, Dybas RA (in press) A study of the relative stability, toxicity, and penetrability of abamectin and its 8,9-oxide. *J. Agric. Food Chem.*

McCoy, CW, Bullock RC, Dybas RA (1982) Avermectin B_1: a novel miticide active against citrus mites. *Proc. Fla. State Hort. Soc.* 95:51–56.

Mink JS, Luttrell RG (1987) Chemical control of the fall armyworm on cotton. *Insectic. & Acaric. Tests* 12:236–237.

Mizell RF, Schiffhauer DE, Taylor JL (1986) Mortality of *Tetranychus urticae* Koch (Acari: Tetranychidae) from abamectin residues: effects of host plant, light, and surfactants. *J. Entomol. Sci.* 21:329–337.

Moar WJ, Trumble JT (1987) Toxicity, joint action, and mean time of mortality of dipel 2X, avermectin B_1, neem and thuringiensin against beet armyworms (Lepidptera: Noctuidae). *J. Econ. Entomol.* 80:588–592.

Mollet JA, Nelson RD, Norton JA, Dybas RA (1986) Abamectin for control of spider mites on greenhouse carnations and roses Entomological Society of America National Conference, Reno, *NV* Dec. 7–11.

Morse JG, Bellows TS, Gaston LK, Iwata Y (1987) Residual toxicity of acaricides to three beneficial species on California citrus. *J. Econ. Entomol.* 80:953–960.

Morse JG, Brawner OL (1983) Citrus thrips pesticide efficacy tests in California. *Insectic. & Acaric Tests* 8:37–39.

Morse JG, Brawner OL (1986) Toxicity of pesticides to *Scirtothrips citri* (Thysanoptera: Thripidae) and implications to resistance management. *J. Econ. Entomol.* 79:565–570.

Morse JG and Brawner OL (1987) Citrus thrips control trial in California. *Insectic. & Acaric Tests* 12:91–92.

Morse JG, Elliott WG (1985) Citrus red mite pesticide efficacy tests in Riverside. *Insectic. & Acaric. Tests* 10:55–56.

Morse JG, Elmer HS, Brawner OL (1984) Evaluation of unregistered materials for control of citrus thrips in California. *Insectic. & Acaric Tests* 9:91–92.

Morse JG, Grout TG, Brawner OL (1986) Citrus thrips control trials in California. *Insectic. & Acaric Tests* 11:101–102.

Oetting RD (1987) Laboratory evaluation of the toxicity and residual activity of abamectin to *Ecinothrips americanus*. *J. Agric. Entomol.* 4:321–326.

Parrella MP (1983) Evaluations of selected insecticides for control of permethrin-resistant *Liriomyza trifolii* (Diptera: Agromyzidae) on chrysanthemum. *J. Econ. Entomol.* 76:1460–1464.

Parrella, MP, Robb KL, Virzi JK, Dybas RA (1988) Analysis of the impact of abamectin on *Liriomyza trifolii* (Burgess) (Diptera: Agromyzidae). *Can. Ent.* 120:831–837.

Payne JA, Dutcher J, Ellis HC (1985) Performance of pecan insecticides: past, present and future. *Insectic. & Acaric Tests* 10:63–65.

Putter I, MacConnell JG, Preiser FA, Haidri AA, Ristich SS, Dybas RA (1981) Avermectins: novel insecticides, acaricides and nematicides from a soil micro-organism. *Experientia* 37:963–964.

Riedl H, Shearer PW (1987) Pear, insect control with abamectin. *Insectic. & Acaric Tests* 12:66–67.

Robb KL, Parrella MP (1986) Western flower thrips control. *Greenhouse Grower,* September, 94–98.

Robb KL, Virzi JK, Parrella MP (1985) Control of twospotted spider mites on chrysanthemum, California. *Insectic. & Acaric Tests* 10:284.

Royalty RN, Perring TM (1987) Comparative toxicity of acaricides to *Aculops lycopersici* and *Homeopronematus anconai* (Acari: Eriophydae, Tydeidae). *J. Econ. Entomol.* 80:348–351.

Royer TA, Edelson JV (1987) Spider mite and cotton aphid control. *Insectic. & Acaric Tests* 12:251–252.

Royer TA, Edelson JV, Cartwright B (1985) Effect of various soil and foliar applied insecticides on leafminers in bell peppers. *Insectic. & Acaric Tests* 10:127.

Sanderson JP, Barnes MM (1983) Control of spider mites on almonds. *Insectic. & Acaric Tests* 8:91–92.

Schuster DJ (1984) Insect control on fresh market tomatoes in West-Central Florida. *Insectic & Acaric Tests* 9:201–202.

Schuster DJ (1987) Insect control on fresh market tomatoes in West-Central Florida. *Insectic & Acaric Tests* 12:157–158.

Schuster DJ, Everett PH (1983) Response of *Liriomyza trifolii* (Diptera: Agromyzidae) to insecticides on tomatoes. *J. Econ. Entomol.* 76:1170–1174.

Schuster DJ, Everett PH (1987) Insect control on tomato in Southwest Florida. *Insectic & Acaric Tests* 12:156.

Schuster DJ, Taylor JL (1987) Residual activity of abamectin against *Liriomyza trifolii* (Diptera: Agromyzidae). *Fla. Entomol.* 70:351–354.

Trumble JT (1983a) Pesticidal impact on leafminers and parasites in celery. *Insectic & Acaric Tests* 8:125–126.

Trumble JT (1983b) Suppression of lepidopterous larvae and leafminers on tomato. *Insectic & Acaric. Tests* 8:150.

Trumble JT (1985a) Impact of pesticides and leafminers and their associated parasites on tomatoes. *Insectic & Acaric Tests* 10:166.

Trumble JT (1985b) Integrated pest management of *Liriomyza trifolii:* influence of avermectin, cyromazine, and methomyl on leafminer ecology in celery. *Agric. Ecosystems Environ.* 12:181–188.

Trumble JT, Moar, WJ, Babu JR, Dybas RA (1987) Laboratory bioassay of the acute and antifeedant effects of avermectin B_1. *J. Agric. Entomol.* 4:21–28.

Trumble JT, Nakakihara H (1984) Twospotted spider mite control on strawberries. *Insectic & Acaric Tests* 9:62–63.

Tuttle DM, Mullis CH (1984) Control of carmine spider mite on cotton. *Insectic & Acaric Tests* 9:278.

Waddill V (1982) Evaluation of insecticides for control of insect pests of tomato. *Insectic & Acaric Tests* 7:126.

Williams DF (1983) The development of toxic baits for the control of the red imported fire ant. *Fla. Entomol.* 66:162–171.

Williams DF (1985) Laboratory and field evaluation of avermectin against the imported fire ant. *Southwest Entomol.* (*Suppl.*) No. 7:27–33.

Wright DJ, Loy A, Green A St J, Dybas RA (1985a) The translaminar activity of abamectin (MK-936) against mites and aphids. *Med. Fac. Landbouww.* Rijksuniv. Gent 50/2b:595–601.

Wright DJ, Roberts ITJ, Androher A, Green A St J, Dybas RA (1985b) The residual activity of abamectin (MK-936) against *Tetranychus urticae* (Koch) on cotton. *Med. Fac. Landbouww.* Rijksuniv. Gent 50/2b:633–637.

Wright JE, Jenkins JN, Villavaso, EJ (1985) Evaluation of avermectin B1 (MK-936) against *Heliothis* spp. in the laboratory and in field plots and against the boll weevil in field plots. *Southwest. Entomol.* (Suppl.) No. 7:11–16.

Wynholds PF, Leigh TF (1982) Control of spider mites on cotton. *Insectic & Acaric Tests* 7:165.

Wynholds PF, Leigh TF (1986) Control of spider mites on cotton. *Insectic & Acaric Tests* 11:307–308.

Zehnder GW, Trumble JT (1984) Insect control on celery. *Insectic. & Acaric. Tests* 9:89–90.

CHAPTER 21

Use of Ivermectin in Humans

Bruce M. Greene, Kenneth R. Brown, and Hugh R. Taylor

I. Introduction

Ivermectin (Campbell *et al.* 1983) has been extensively tested in human onchocerciasis, and is now considered the drug of choice. In a single yearly dose, it suppresses microfilariae in the skin and eyes, and in most infected persons prevents disease progression. It also shows considerable promise for treatment of lymphatic filariasis and strongyloidiasis.

II. Treatment of Onchocerciasis

A. Phase I Studies

The first reports of the use of ivermectin against *Onchocerca volvulus* infection in humans were published in 1982 (Aziz *et al.* 1982a; Aziz *et al.* 1982b). In a crossover study on a small number of lightly infected people in Senegal, they found that a single dose of ivermectin exhibited microfilaricidal activity; it was efficacious at remarkably low doses, ranging from 5 to 30μg/kg. This report was followed by further dose-finding studies in Paris (Coulaud *et al.* 1983; Coulaud *et al.* 1984), in which a number of African immigrants, most of whom were also lightly infected, were treated with various doses up to 200 μg/kg. Although microfilariae persisted or reappeared in some people, the drug showed good efficacy overall; doses up to 200 μg/kg were found to be safe and well tolerated.

A third Phase I study was performed in Tamale, Ghana (Awadzi *et al.* 1984; Awadzi *et al.* 1985). Four different doses of ivermectin—50, 100, 150, and 200 μg/kg—were compared for efficacy in an open study. The data suggested that ivermectin was probably safe and effective; 50 μg/kg was less effective than the higher doses. Although some patients exhibited mild transient changes, including postural hypotension, ivermectin showed minimal toxicity. Without an adequate control group, however, the data are difficult to interpret, complicated further by the fact that the study population came from northern Ghana, where there had been 10 years of vector control and the microfilaria counts, even without treatment, were falling.

B. Phase II Studies

The Phase I clinical data made it obvious that ivermectin was a very promising drug (Editorial 1984). This led to a series of Phase II studies, which were conducted as double-blind, controlled clinical trials. They focused particularly on assessing invermectin's safety and efficacy as compared to the standard treatment for onchocerciasis, diethylcarbamazine (DEC); the control group received a placebo. The 4 studies used essentially the same rigorous protocol: subjects were hospitalized, treated with single-dose ivermectin (200 μg/kg) or a 1-week course of DEC, and examined every day—some of the observations being done every 4 to 6 hours. Patients also had detailed eye exams, including fluorescein angiography. Each study had 10 to 15 subjects per group. Phase II studies were conducted in Liberia, Senegal, Ghana, and Mali.

The trial in Liberia (Greene *et al.* 1985) showed that a single dose of ivermectin was at least as effective in reducing the microfilaria counts as DEC given daily for 8 days; also, ivermectin caused very little reaction as compared to DEC. Subsequent results showed that the marked reduction of skin microfilaria counts seen following ivermectin treatment persisted to 12 months (Taylor *et al.* 1986). These results were confirmed in the other 3 Phase II studies (Lariviere *et al.* 1985; Diallo *et al.* 1986; Awadzi *et al.* 1986). Ivermectin was clearly microfilaricidal, but examination of excised nodules showed that it did not kill the adult worms (Greene *et al.* 1985). It did, however, produce a transient interruption of microfilarial release (Schulz-Key *et al.* 1985).

Ivermectin treatment produced either no or a very mild clinical reaction

(Mazzotti reaction). The absence of a Mazzotti reaction is highly significant: this is the limiting factor to widespread use of DEC (Taylor 1984). To quantitate this observation, a clinical grading system, which scores 7 separate clinical signs and then combines them in an aggregate clinical reaction score, was used. The clinical reaction scores of the Liberia Phase II patients treated with DEC were approximately 7.5 on Day 2. Typically, a patient with a score of 5 or 6 felt unwell and would be confined to bed. Ivermectin induced only a mild reaction, and the placebo group had no reaction. The differences between the ivermectin group and the DEC group were statistically significant.

The ocular changes that occur with DEC treatment of onchocerciasis can lead to permanent loss of vision, thus restricting its clinical utility (Taylor 1984; Bird *et al.* 1980). In the Phase II trials, detailed ocular examinations were performed serially over a 12-month period, (Taylor *et al.* 1986; Dadzie *et al.* 1987). DEC treatment caused a marked increase in living and dead microfilariae in the cornea, punctate opacities, and limbitis during the first week of therapy. Ivermectin (200 μg/kg) had no such effect, and resulted in a long-term reduction in intraocular microfilariae comparable to that seen with DEC (Taylor *et al.* 1986). The Phase II trials thus showed that ivermectin appeared to induce few ocular complications, to be better tolerated, and to be more effective than DEC as a microfilaricidal agent in treating onchocerciasis.

C. Phase III Studies

Phase III trials assessed the efficacy of 3 different dosages of the drug (100, 150, and 200 μg/kg) and collected further information on safety. These trials were all double-blind, and, again, patients were followed for 1 year. Each group had at least 50 patients; all Phase III participants were hospitalized for at least 2 days after treatment. At this point, the Liberian study is the only one of the 6 published. Other studies following similar protocols were undertaken in Ghana, Mali, Cote d'Ivore, Togo, and Guatemala.

The 12-month follow-up data of the Liberian study show that, by Day 3, each of the 3 doses of ivermectin produced quite a marked drop in skin microfilaria counts (White *et al.* 1987). This decrease was more marked at Day 3 for the 200 μg/kg group than for the 100 μg/kg dose, suggesting a dose response at this early time point. At 3 months, however, the counts for the 3 different doses were indistinguishable; they were still indistinguishable at 6 months and at 12 months.

In the Phase III trials, the clinical reaction score was assessed as it had been in the Phase II studies. In the Liberian study, each of the 3 treatment groups showed an increase in the clinical reaction score over the first few days following treatment (White *et al.* 1987). Because there were now 50 people in each group (as opposed to only 10 in each group in the Phase II study), this increase was statistically significant for both 200 and 150 μg/kg compared to the placebo group. The reaction score for the 100 μg/kg group was not significantly different from the placebo group. The reaction was relatively mild in each case (except for 1 patient out of 150 who missed 1 day of work) and had essentially resolved by Day 4. Again, no serious ocular lesions were precipitated by treatment, and the ocular status was markedly improved 1 year after treatment (White *et al.* 1987). Similar results from the other Phase III trials have been reported informally (Lariviere *et al.* 1986; Mossinger *et al.* 1987; Hussein, Bird, and Jones 1987; Ranque *et al.* 1986).

The Phase III studies reconfirmed that ivermectin was both safe and effective and induced only a minimal Mazzotti reaction without a significant ocular reaction. These studies suggested that 150 μg/kg was probably the optimal dose, in terms of its antiparasitic activity and lack of side effects.

At the end of the 1-year follow-up in the Liberian Phase III study, participants were reallocated for a dose-interval study. At 12 months, the patients in the 3 treatment groups (100, 150, or 200 μg/kg of ivermectin) were rerandomized so that, in each treatment group, half the persons were retreated with the same dose of ivermectin they had received initially, and the other half were given placebo (Greene *et al.* 1987). The original placebo group received 150 μg/kg on a 6-monthly basis. At 24 months, all patients were again given ivermectin; the dose being the same as they had received initially. This study provided information on 3 different retreatment schedules: 6-monthly treatments with 150 μg/kg with a 1-year follow-up; annual treatment with 100, 150, or 200 μg/kg with a 2-year follow-up; and 2-yearly treatment with the 3 doses, also with a 2-year follow-up.

The 2-year follow-up data suggest that, even 24 months after initial treatment, there is still a marked effect on skin microfilaria counts at each treatment dose (Figure 21.1). Yearly retreatment with 150 μg/kg, however, appears to be an optimal regime for reducing microfilarial counts (Figure 21.2) and for safety. Importantly, the clinical reaction seen after retreatment at 12 months was less than that seen after the initial treatment.

The ocular examination data at 24 months for the 3 different treatment groups are shown in Figure 21.3. There was a marked improvement in the ocular status of each group after treatment (Newland *et al.* 1988). Even without annual retreatment, the ocular status showed marked improvement over conditions prior to the initial treatment, 24 months earlier. Ivermectin was also found to be safe and effective in patients with severe ocular involvement (Taylor *et al.* unpublished). Interestingly, the improvement in ocular disease appeared to be even more prolonged than the effect on the skin snip counts.

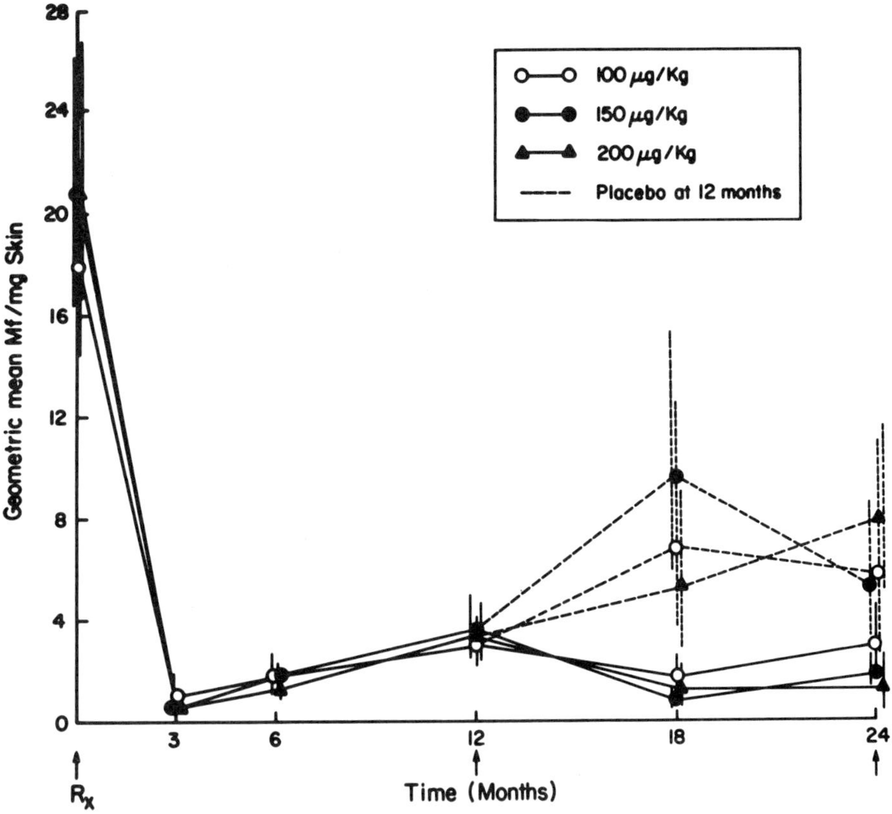

FIGURE 21.1. Skin microfilaria density over 24 months, expressed as microfilariae/mg (mf/mg) skin. The broken line after 12 months shows the response of patients given only a single dose of ivermectin. The solid line shows the response of patients retreated at 12 months. Vertical bars show 95% confidence intervals.

D. Phase IV Studies

Normally, these data, based on treatment of approximately 1400 persons, would be considered sufficient for drug registration. Because ivermectin would be used on a large scale in developing areas and therefore would not be subjected to the normal postmarketing surveillance, however, it was decided that a number of formal Phase IV trials were necessary, involving treating tens of thousands of persons with ivermectin yearly and following them for the occurrence of severe adverse reactions. Such Phase IV studies are currently underway in Liberia (where almost 8000 persons have been treated twice without severe adverse reactions; Pacque *et al.* unpublished), the Volta River Basin Area of West Africa, Cameroon, Nigeria, and Guatemala. Preliminary results from all

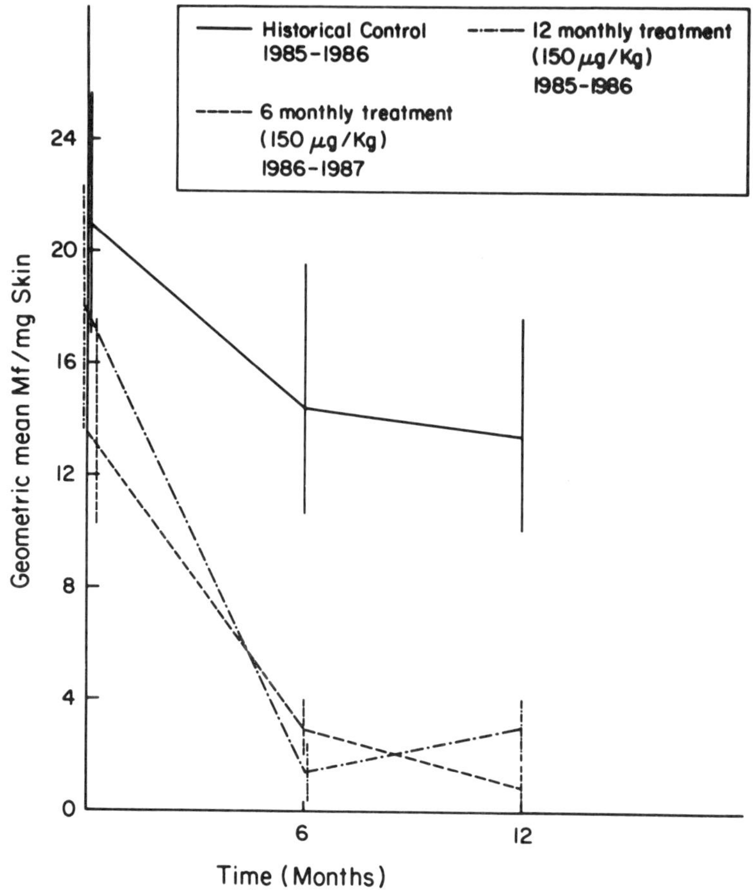

FIGURE 21.2. Comparison of the effect on skin microfilaria density load 6-monthly and 12-monthly treatment with ivermectin 150 μg/kg.

studies—which have now treated more than 70,000 persons—indicate no unexpected major adverse effect of ivermectin (unpublished). Unexplained hypotension did occur in about 1 in 1000 to 1 in 10,000 persons, but this was reversible and also has been reported following DEC administration for *O. volvulus* infection.

E. Ivermectin Effect on the Parasite *O. volvulus*

Ivermectin's effect on the adult worm was examined in detail in both the Phase II and Phase III trials. Ivermectin did not affect the viability of the adult worm—male or female. In some studies, there appeared to be slightly fewer adult males in the ivermectin nodules, but this was not statistically significant (Greene *et al.* 1985; Schulz-Key *et al.* 1985). There

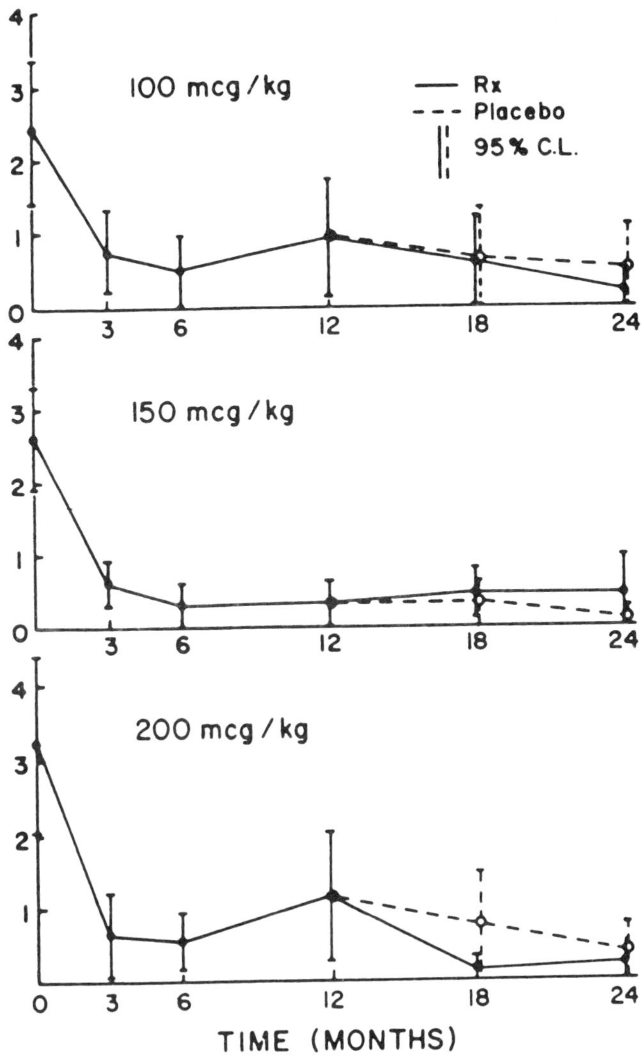

FIGURE 21.3. Ocular reaction index results over 24 months. The broken line after 12 months shows the response of patients given only a single dose of ivermectin. The solid line shows the response of patients retreated at 12 months.

was a dramatic effect on the uterine microfilariae, however; by 2 months, microfilarial production totally ceased, and large numbers of degenerate microfilariae accumulated in the uterus (Schulz-Key *et al.* 1985, 1986). Because microfilariae are not released, they degenerate. By 6 to 12 months, normal production of microfilariae resumes, at least in some of the worms. This effect on the adult female is probably responsible for the delayed reappearance of microfilariae in the skin after ivermectin treatment. In contrast, DEC kills the microfilariae very effectively but has no residual effect on adult worms, which continue to produce microfilariae normally (Albiez *et al.* 1988) The rate of reappearance of microfilariae in the skin after DEC is, therefore, different from that after ivermectin. Pretreatment levels are usually reached 1 to 2 years after DEC (Duke 1968), whereas after treatment with ivermectin, the microfilaria counts in skin snips are still low at 1 or even 2 years.

F. Ivermectin Effect on Transmission and as a Prophylactic Agent

Studies in Liberia (Cupp *et al.* 1986) suggested that ivermectin-treated infected people are much less able to transmit the parasite. Although the study was small and not perfectly controlled, the number of microfilariae taken up by biting black flies was greatly reduced; so was the number of subsequent developing infective larvae. This suggested that community-based treatment with ivermectin might reduce or abolish transmission of new infection. A recent report from the Ivory Coast (Prod'hon *et al.* 1987) confirms and extends these findings.

Because there is no drug available to prevent *O. volvulus* infection, there was considerable interest as to whether ivermectin could be used as a prophylactic agent. A study was undertaken in chimpanzees experimentally infected with infective larvae (Taylor *et al.* 1988). Animals were given ivermectin (200 μg/kg) on the day of inoculation and 28 days later, times selected to coincide with the presence of 3 and 4 larval stages. Unfortunately, the incidence of patent infection in the chimpanzees suggests that ivermectin has no demonstrable effect when given at the 4 larval stage and possibly only a partial effect at the 3 stage, indicating that it will not be effective as a prophylactic drug in humans.

G. Conclusion and Present Clinical Usage

In October 1987, just over 5 years after the first report on ivermectin's use in onchocerciasis was published, the French government approved the drug's use in humans (Lindley 1987). Although not a macrofilaricide—and therefore not a permanent cure for onchocerciasis—ivermectin given as a single oral dose of 150 μg/kg annually shows promise of revolutionizing the treatment of this major disease of humankind, which previously was essentially untreatable.

Ivermectin is now considered the drug of choice for onchocerciasis. It should not be taken during pregnancy nor by lactating females within 3 months of delivery. It induces a minimal reaction (Mazzotti-like) in 5% to 15% of infected adults and a more significant reaction in about 1%. Its safety is unproven in children under the age of 5 and in persons with meningitis, sleeping sickness, and other CNS disorders. Its use was associated with hypotension, usually occurring within 24 hours of administration in about 1 in 1000 persons treated in savannah West Africa. The infrequent problems associated with ivermectin usage do not, however, preclude its widespread use for onchocerciasis control.

III. Ivermectin for Uses in Filarial Infections other than Onchocerciasis

A. Ivermectin in the Treatment of Filariasis Caused by *Wuchereria Bancrofti*

Four studies have been performed in patients with bancroftian filariasis. Diallo and colleagues (1987) studied single-dose ivermectin therapy at a level of either 50 μg/kg (7 patients) or 100 μg/kg (9 patients). Both dose levels cleared microfilariae from the blood within 3 days of therapy; the authors concluded that 100 μg/kg might be the more effective dose.

In a further dose-ranging study of ivermectin in bancroftian filariasis in Polynesia, Roux, Cartel, and Azia (1987) demonstrated the superiority of 100, 150, or 200 μg/kg over a 50 μg/kg single dose, but they were unable to establish superiority of any 1 of the 3 higher doses over the other 2. In a third study, performed in India (Kumaraswami *et al.* 1988), in patients with bancroftian filariasis, all of the dose levels chosen (25, 50, 100, or 200 μg/kg) were efficacious in clearing the blood of all patients treated. This efficacy was evaluated at 5 to 12 days, but in most patients microfilaremia recurred by 3 months after dosing. At 6 months there was no correlation between dose level and efficacy. In this study there appeared to be a good correspondence between high levels of microfilaremia, the higher doses used (100 and 200 μg/kg), and the frequency and severity of adverse reactions. The latter were similar to those frequently seen in patients treated with DEC.

Finally, in a comparative study of DEC and 2 dose levels (1.0 mg or 6.0 mg) of ivermectin reported by Ottesen and colleagues (1987), ivermectin was superior to DEC in rapidly clearing blood microfilaria, and equivalent to DEC in decreasing the microfilaria counts over the first 3 months; ivermectin was inferior to DEC in terms of sustained response at 6 months. Furthermore, adverse reactions reported for ivermectin were qualitatively and quantitatively similar to those for DEC; the higher dose of ivermectin was associated with a higher frequency of adverse reactions and was also correlated with the microfilarial level prior to treatment. Because of the compliance problem with DEC, the investigators conclude that ivermectin given as a single dose would be superior to the standard course of DEC treatment; they propose that it should be considered the best candidate to replace DEC in control programs. Additional dose finding studies are now underway.

B. Ivermectin Use in Patients Infected with More than One Filarial Species

Richard-Lenoble and colleagues (1988) treated patients who were infected with *Loa loa* as well as *O. volvulus;* some of these also had *M. perstans* infection. A single dose of ivermectin at 200 μg/kg had no significant effect on the *M. perstans* in the blood, produced a transitory drop in microfilaremia due to *Loa loa* and, as expected, produced a dramatic drop in counts of *O. volvulus* in the skin. Of greater importance was the high level of safety: no multiply infected patients developed serious adverse reactions related to ivermectin treatment.

C. Ivermectin Treatment for Human Nematodes

Nalin and colleagues (1987) reported efficacy results from studies of 294 infected patients treated with ivermectin. Mean percent cures were: *S. stercoralis,* 82%; *A. lumbricoides,* 100%; *E. vermicularis,* 84%; and *T. trichiuris,* 69%.

Naquira and colleagues (unpublished data on file at Merck Sharp & Dohme Research Laboratories) have studied 100 patients ranging in age from 11 to 74 who were infected with *Strongyloides stercoralis*. Diagnosis was based on the presence of *S. stercoralis* larvae in the stool; ivermectin was given either as a single oral dose (50, 100, 150, or 200 μg/kg) or as a single dose of 100 or 200 μg/kg on each of 2 successive days. Follow-up stool examinations were performed at least once between days 17 to 24 and between days 30 to 38 after dosing.

Patients who received a total of 50 ro 100 μg/kg ivermectin had a response rate which ranged from 69% to 75%, whereas the patients who received a total of 150 μg/kg or more had a cure rate of 88% to 100%. Based on this study, ivermectin in a dose of 150 μg/kg would appear to be highly effective against *S. stercoralis*. Even for patients who were not cured, the change in larval counts in the stool was considered to be very beneficial.

Studies of other parasites in these patients and 131 additional persons without strongyloides were performed; cure rates obtained for human hookworms (either Necator or Ancylostoma) were unsatisfactory even though hookworm egg counts in stools were reduced. Even at 200 μg/kg/day, the 30-day cure rate for patients with hookworm was only 22%; at 30 days patients who were not cured had only a 42% drop in egg counts in the stool. The mean cure rate in all patients at 30 days (regardless of dose) was 85% for *Trichuris trichiura,* 100% for *Ascaris lumbricoides,* and 85% for *Enterobius vermicularis*.

The preceding data demonstrate ivermectin's high degree of efficacy and suggest its possible use as a replacement for thiabendazole in treating *Strongyloides stercoralis*. Ivermectin could not be recommended as a broad-spectrum agent for monotherapy of human roundworm infestation, however, because it fails to effectively control human hookworms.

References

Albiez EJ, Newland HS, White AT, Kaiser A, Greene BM, Taylor HR, Buttner DW (1988) Chemotherapy of onchocerciasis with high doses of diethylcarbamazine or a single dose of ivermectin: microfilaria levels and side effects. *Trop. Med. Parasit.* 39:19–24.

Awadzi K, Dadzie KY, Schulz-Key H, Gilles HM, Fulford AJ, Azia MA (1986) The chemotherapy of onchocerciasis XI. A double-blind comparative study of ivermectin, diethylcarbamazine, and placebo in human onchocerciasis in Northern Ghana. *Ann. Trop. Med. Parasit.* 80:433–442.

Awadzi K, Kadzie KY, Schulz-Key H, Haddock DRW, Gilles HM, Aziz MA (1984) Ivermectin in onchocerciasis (letter). *Lancet* 2:2921.

Awadzi K, Dadzie KY, Schulz-Key H, Haddock DRW, Gilles HM, Aziz MA (1985) The chemotherapy of onchocerciasis X. An assessment of four single dose treatment regimes of MK-933 (ivermectin) in human onchocerciasis. *Ann. Trop. Med. Parasit.* 79:63–78.

Aziz MA, Diallo S, Diop IM, Lariviere M, Porta M (1982a) Efficacy and tolerance of ivermectin in human onchocerciasis. *Lancet* 2:171–173.

Aziz MA, Diallo S, Lariviere M, Diop IM, Porta M, Gaxotte P (1982b) Ivermectin in onchocerciasis. *Lancet* 2:1456–1457.

Bird AC, El-Sheikh H, Anderson J, Fuglsang H (1980) Changes in visual function and in the posterior segment of the eye during treatment of onchocerciasis with diethylcarbamazine citrate. *Brit. J. Ophthalmol.* 64:191–200.

Campbell WC, Fisher MH, Stapley EO, Albers-Schonberg G, Jacob TA (1983) Ivermectin: a potent new antiparasitic agent. *Science* 221:823–828.

Coulaud JP, Lariviere M, Aziz MA, Gervais MC, Gaxotte P, Deluol AM, Cenac J (1984) Ivermectin in onchocerciasis. *Lancet* 2:526–527.

Coulaud JP, Lariviere M, Gervais MC, Gaxotte P, Aziz MA, Deluol AM, Cenac J (1983) Treatment of human onchocerciasis with ivermectin. *Bull. Soc. Pathol. Exot. Filiales* 76:681–688.

Cupp EW, Bernardo MJ, Kiszewski AE, Collins RC, Taylor HR, Aziz MA, Greene BM (1986) The effects of ivermectin on transmission of *Onchocerca volvulus*. *Science* 231:740–742.

Dadzie KY, Bird AC, Awadzi K, Schulz-Key H, Gilles HM, Aziz MA (1987) Ocular findings is a double-blind study of ivermectin versus diethylcarbamazine versus placebo in the treatment of onchocerciasis. *Brit. J. Ophthalmol.* 71:78–85.

Diallo S, Aziz MA, Lariviere M, Diallo JS, Diop-Mar I, N'Dir O, Badiane S, Py D, Schulz-Key H, Gaxotte P, Victorius A (1986) A double-blind comparison of the efficacy and safety of ivermectin and diethylcarbamazine in a placebo controlled study of Senegalese patients with onchocerciasis. *Trans. Roy. Soc. Trop. Med. Hyg.* 80:927–934.

Diallo S, Aziz MA, Ndir O, Badiane S, Bah IB, Gaye O. (1987) Dose-ranging study of ivermectin in treatment of filariasis due to *Wuchereria bancrofti*. *Lancet* 1:1030.

Drummond RO (1985) Effectiveness of ivermectin for control of arthropod pests of livestock. *Southwest. Entomol. (Suppl.)* 7:34–42.

Duke BO (1968) The effects of drugs on *Onchocerca volvulus* I. Methods of assessment, population dynamics of the parasite and the effects of diethylcarbamazine. *Bull. WHO* 39:137–146.

Editorial (1984) Ivermectin in onchocerciasis. *Lancet* 2:1021.

Greene BM, Taylor HR, Cupp EW, Murphy RP, White AT, Aziz MA, Schulz-Key H, D'Anna SA, Newland HS, Goldschmidt LP, Auer C, Hanson AP, Freeman SV, Reber EW, Williams PN (1985) Comparison of ivermectin and diethylcarbamazine in the treatment of onchocerciasis. *New Engl. J. Med.* 313:133–138.

Greene BM, White AT, Newland HS, Keyvan-Larijani E, Dukuly F, Gallin MY, Aziz MA, Williams PN, Taylor HR (1987) Single dose therapy with ivermectin for onchocerciasis. *Trans. Assoc. Amer. Phys.* C:131–138.

Hussein S, Bird A, Jones BR (1987) Ocular lesions seen in phase III trial of ivermectin therapy of onchocerciasis in Togo. *Trop. Med. Parasit.* 38:67.

Kumaraswami V, Ottesen EA, Vijayasekaran MD, Uma Devi S, Sxaminathan M, Aziz MA, Sarma GR, Prabhakar R, Tripathy SP (1988) Ivermectin for the treatment of *Wuchereria bancrofti* filariasis. *JAMA* 259:3150–3153.

Lariviere M, Abelloos J, Aziz M, Beauvais B, Bamba M, Ferly-Therizol M, Basset D, Basset A, Derouin F, Sarfati C, Bosseboeuf C, Toure Y, Song D, Gaxotte P (1986) A double-blind study of ivermectin and placebo in onchocerciasis. Proceedings of the IXth International Congress of Infectious and Parasitic Diseases, Munich, p 548.

Lariviere M, Aziz MA, Weimann D, Ginoux J, Gaxotte P, Vinotain P, Brauvae B, Derouin F, Schulz-Key H, Barret D, Sarfati C (1985) Double-blind study of ivermectin and diethylcarbamazine in African onchocerciasis patients with ocular involvement. *Lancet* 2:174–177.

Lindley D (1987) Merck's new drug free to WHO for river blindness programme. *Nature* 329:752.

Mossinger J, Schulz-Key H, Helling G, Adjamgba A, Klager S (1987) Emergence of *Onchocerca volvulus* microfilariae from skin biopsies of patients treated with ivermectin. *Trop. Med. Parasit.* 38:69.

Nalin D Aziz M, Neu D, Ruiz-Palacios G, Naquira C (1987) Efficacy of ivermectin (MK-933) against intestinal nematode parasites. Abstract A-101. Annual Meeting of the American Society for Microbiology, Atlanta, p 17.

Newland HS, White AT, Greene BM, D'Anna SA, Keyvan-Larijani E, Aziz MA, Williams PN, Taylor HR (1988) The effect of single dose ivermectin therapy on human *O. volvulus* infection with onchocercal ocular involvement. *Brit. J. Ophthalmol.* 72:561–569.

Newland HS, White AT, Greene BM, Keyvan-Larijani E, Taylor HR (in press) The effect of repeated treatment with ivermectin in onchocerciasis. Report of Third General Assembly of the International Agency for Prevention of Blindness.

Ottesen EA, Kumaraswami V, Vijayasekaran MA, Aziz R, Prabhakar R, Tripathy SP (1987) Ivermectin and diethylcarbamazine (DEC) in a blinded, placebo-controlled trial to treat *Wuchereria bancrofti* (Wb) filariasis. Proceedings of the 36th Annual Meeting of the American Society of Tropical Medicine and Hygiene, Los Angeles, p 255.

Prod'hon J, Lardeux P, Bain O, Hebrard G, Prod'hom JM (1987) Ivermectine et modalites de la reduction de l'infection des simulies. *Ann. Parasitol. Hum. Comp.* 68:590–598.

Ranque P, Aziz M, Pichard E, Ginoux J, Cozette P, Rivaud C, Sacko A, Coulibaly S, Gaxotte P (1986) A double-blind study of ivermectin and placebo in onchocerciasis in Mali. Proceedings of the IXth International Congress of Infectious and Parasitic Diseases, Munich, p 140.

Richard-Lenoble D, Kombila M, Rupp EA, Pappaylion ES, Gaxotte P, Njuiri C, Aziz MA (1988) Ivermectin in loiasis and concomitant *O. volvulus* and *M. perstans* infections. Am. J. Trop Med Hyg 39:480–483.

Roux J, Cartel JL, Aziz MA (1987) A dose-ranging study of ivermectin for the treatment of microfilaremic filariasis due to *Wuchereria bancrofti* in French Polynesia. Abstract 395. 36th Annual Meeting of the American Society of Tropical Medicine and Hygiene, Los Angeles.

Schulz-Key H, Greene BM, Awadzi K, Lariviere M, Klager S, Dadzie Y, Aziz MA (1986) Efficacy of ivermectin on the reproductivity of female *Onchocerca volvulus*. *Trop. Med. Parasit.* 37:89.

Schulz-Key H, Klager S, Awadzi K, Diallo S, Greene BM, Lariviere M, Aziz MA (1985) Treatment of human onchocerciasis: the efficacy of ivermectin on the parasite. *Trop. Med. Parasit.* 36:20.

Taylor HR (1984) Recent developments in the treatment of onchocerciasis. Bull. WHO 509–515.

Taylor HR, Murphy RP, Newland HS, White AT, D'Anna SA, Keyvan-Larijani E, Aziz MA, Cupp EW, Greene BM (1986) Comparison of the treatment of ocular onchocerciasis with ivermectin and diethylcarbamazine. *Arch. Ophthalmol.* 104:863–870.

Taylor HR, Trpis M, Cupp EW, Brotman B, Newland HS, Soboslay PT, Greene BM (1988) Ivermectin prophylaxis against experimental *Onchocerca volvulus* infection in chimpanzees. *Am. J. Trop. Med. Hyg* 39:86–90.

White AT, Newland HS, Taylor HR, Erttmann KD, Keyvan-Larijani E, Nara A, Aziz MA, D'Anna SA, Williams PN, Greene BM (1987) Controlled trial and dose-finding study of ivermectin for treatment of onchocerciasis. *J. Infect. Dis.* 156:463–470.

Appendix I

The Determinative Method for Assaying Ivermectin Residues in Tissue and Plasma

G.V. Downing

A. Summary

The tissue sample is homogenized with acetone-water, and dihydro B_{1a} is extracted from the tissue with isooctane. The isooctane is evaporated, and solvent-solvent distributions into acetonitrile out of hexane and into hexane out of acetonitrile-water are performed. Solvent is removed and fluorescence produced by heating at 95° C with the imidazole-derivatizing reagent. After adding chloroform, the reaction mixture is washed through a silica gel SEP-PAK, the solvent is removed, and HPLC analysis (fluorescence detection) on Zorbax C18 is performed on the residue dissolved in methanol. A flow diagram of the assay is shown in Figure AI.1.

Proteins are precipitated from plasma by addition of acetone and then water. The ivermectin dihydro B_{1a} is extracted with ethyl acetate from the acetone-water-plasma mixture. The solvent is removed and fluorescence produced by heating at 95° C with the derivatizing reagent. After adding chloroform, the reaction mixture is washed through a silica gel SEP-PAK, the solvent is removed, and the HPLC analysis (fluorescence detection) on Zorbax C18 is performed on the residue dissolved in methanol.

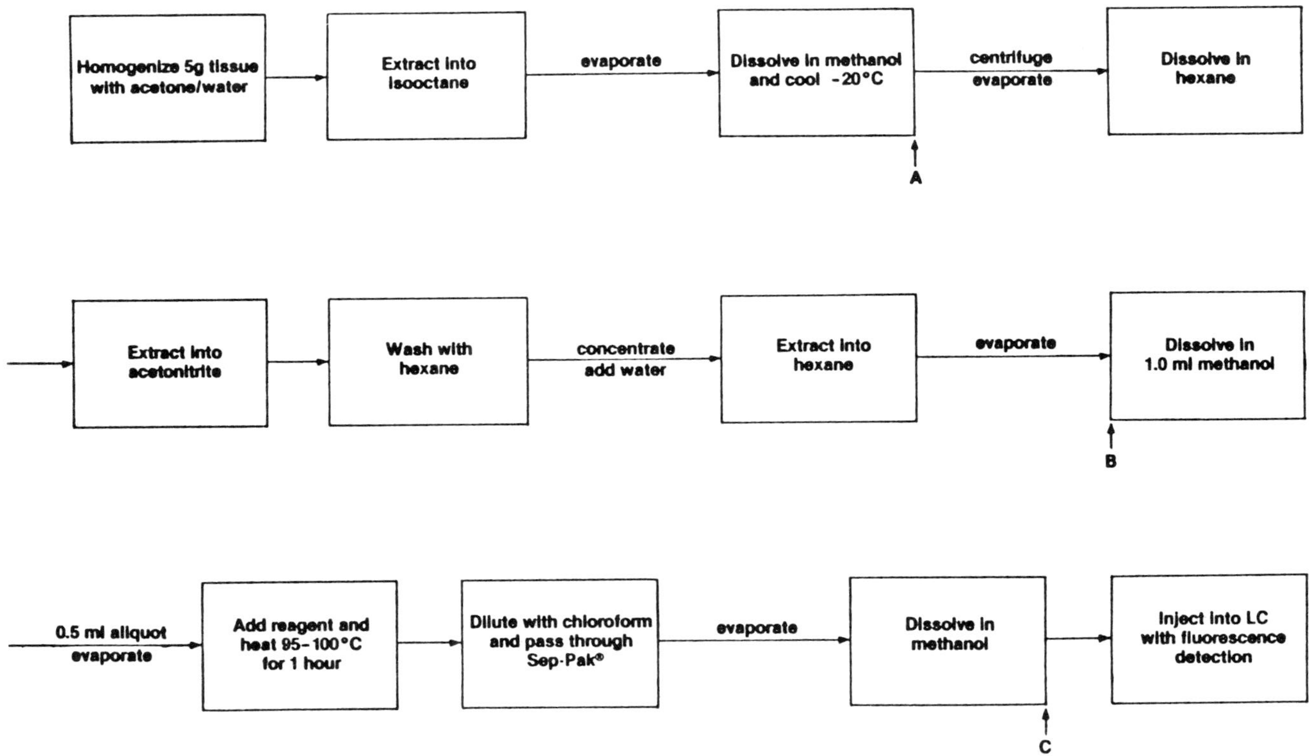

FIGURE AI.1. Flow diagram of determinative assay. A, B and C are possible stopping points during the assay.

B. Reagents

1. Acetic anhydride—Fisher or Baker, reagent grade.
2. Acetone—Mallinckrodt, Nanograde.
3. Acetonitrile—Fisher, HPLC grade; Mallinckrodt, Nanograde; or Burdick & Jackson, distilled in glass.
3. Chloroform—Burdick & Jackson, distilled in glass (1% ethanol preservative).
5. Dimethyl Formamide (DMF)—Baker or Fisher, reagent grade; or Mallinckrodt, AR.
6. Ethyl Acetate—Burdick & Jackson, distilled in glass; or Fisher, pesticide grade.
7. Hexane—Burdick & Jackson, distilled in glass; or Mallinckrodt, Nanograde.
8. Methanol—Burdick & Jackson, distilled in glass; or Mallinckrodt, Nanograde.
9. Methylene Chloride—any grade available.
10. 1-Methylimidazole—99%, Aldrich Chemical Company.
11. Nitrogen—the equivalent of Matheson extra-dry compressed gas.
12. Sodium Chloride—Baker or Fisher, reagent grade.
13. Sylon-CT—Supelco, Inc.
14. 2,2,4-Trimethylpentane—isooctane, Burdick & Jackson, distilled in glass; or Mallinckrodt, Nanograde.
15. Water, Filtered Millipore—Distilled water is treated with a Milli-Q system and then filtered through a Millipore Type HA 0.45μm disc.

C. Solutions

1. Derivatizing Reagent—Mix 0.9 ml of DMF with 0.3 ml of acetic anhydride and 0.2 ml 1-methylimidazole. Make up just before use.
2. Acetone/Water—50% (v/v).
3. 95% Methanol/Water—Make 100 ml of filtered Millipore water to 2 liters with methanol. Mix. With the aid of vacuum, filter mixture through Millipore FH 0.5μm filters. Deaerate by slowly bubbling nitrogen through for 10 minutes.

D. Apparatus

1. Balance—analytical, capable of weighing 1 mg accurately.
2. Balance—capable of weighing 5 g accurately into an approximately 50-g tube.
3. Bath, water—variable temperature 40° to 80° C.
4. Bath, oil—95° to 100° C.
5. Centrifuge, IEC Model HN-S-II, with 6-place rotor IEC #958 and 15-

and 50-ml cups. The centrifuge is run at 2000 to 2500 rpm. The centrifuge used gives ca. 700 to 750 × g maximum centrifugal force (RCF).

6. Centrifuge tubes—glass, 15 to 50 ml with polyethylene stoppers to fit.
7. Centrifuge tubes—50-ml polyproplyene, Corning#25331 (used only for storing standard solutions).
8. Centrifuge tubes, 15 ml, silylated approximately once every 2 months (used only for the derivatization reaction). Tube stoppers must fit tightly. Fill each tube to the top with Sylon-CT. Let stand 20 minutes. Immediately and quickly rinse, first thoroughly with toluene and then with methanol. Fill with methanol. Let stand 20 minutes, rinse thoroughly with acetone, and dry. All glassware used should be *completely* free of all acidic and alkaline residues. (These tubes should be cleaned by hand by first soaking in methylene chloride immediately after use and then in detergent for at least several hours, followed by thorough rinsing with hot water, distilled water, and acetone before thorough drying. Variations in the washing regimen are not recommended, since some analysts have had poor results when the standard washing method was not followed.)
9. Dispensing pipettors—10, 15, and 20 ml.
10. Filtration unit, complete with Millipore FHLP 04700 filter.
11. Freezer—capable of reaching temperatures of −20° C.
12. Gloves—disposable PVC from Fisher Chemical.
13. Graduate cylinder—25 ml, 100ml.
14. Graduate cylinder—2000 ml with ground-glass stopper.
15. Homogenizer, Polytron—Brinkmann Instruments, #27-11-200-5 with PTA 1OS generator #27-11-330-3.
16. Pipets—disposable, Pasteur.
17. Pipets—graduated 1.0 ml and 2.0 ml.
18. Pipets—volumetric 0.5 ml, 1 ml, 2 ml, 3 ml, 4 ml, and 5 ml.
19. Repipet—5 to 10 ml volumes.
20. SEP-PAK—silica cartridge, Part No. 51900—Waters Associates.
21. Spatula—stainless steel.
22. Syringe—50μl, 250μl, and 5 ml and 10 ml.
23. Tape—#13 2956, ½ inch from Ace Scientific.
24. Ultrasonic bath—Sonogen Automatic Cleaner—Branson Model 520 or equivalent.
25. Vortex mixer.

E. Chromatographic Apparatus

A Beckman-Altex Model 110A liquid chromatographic pump complete with Waters Wisp Autosampler and Kratos-Schoeffel Instruments Model FS950 fluorescence detector with a 1-millivolt recorder was used. A

5μm, 4.6-mm ID, C18 standard Brownlee Labs guard column (Spheri-5 RP-18 OD-GU, obtained from Rainin Instrument Co., Inc.) was used before the analytical column. This guard column is replaced monthly unless the pressure reaches 2000 psi, in which case it is replaced immediately.

The ivermectin H_2B1a derivative has a retention time of about 12 to 13 minutes when the indicated conditions are used.

Conditions: 15 cm length × 4.6 mm ID Zorbax ODS-C18 column.
Mobile phase—5% water in methanol (v/v).
Column temperature—30° C.
Flow—1.8 ml/minute (usual pressure 1000 psi, 500 to 2000 psi acceptable).
Detector Settings:
Excitation lamp—FSA 110, standard 365 nm.
Standard Kratos Flowcell—FSA 210.
Excitation filter—FSA 403, 365 nm band filters.
Emission filter—418 nm.
Sensitivity range—0.2 A.
Time constant—about 6.

F. Standards for the Determinative Assay

For tissue assays using the most sensitive scale, accurate aliquots of 50, 100, 150, 200, and 250 μl of ca. 500 ng/ml standard solution of dihydro B_{1a} in methanol (working standard solution) were added to silylated 15-ml centrifuge tubes, and the samples were evaporated to dryness at 60° C with nitrogen purge. For plasma assays, accurate aliquots of 20, 40, 60, 80, and 100 μl of working standard solution were added to silylated tubes and evaporated to dryness. After reaction, SEP-PAK treatment, etc., these derivatized samples are redissolved in 1 ml of methanol to give 25, 50, 75, 100, and 125 ng/ml standard solution equivalents for tissue assays and 10, 20, 30, 40, and 50 ng/ml standard solution for plasma assays.

Starting with solutions of about 0.045% (w/w) dihydro B_{1a} in propylene glycol, stock solutions of about 10 micrograms/ml can be prepared by weighing accurately about 1 gram of the solution into a 50-ml volumetric flask. Methanol is used to dilute to the mark, and the solution is thoroughly mixed. Storage of this stock solution and all dilutions of same should be in polypropylene tubes at −20° C.

Analysts attempting the ivermectin residue analysis for the first time are advised to run a standard curve first before attempting the complete method.

Procedure for the Determinative Assay of Tissues

Homogenization

All Tissues

1. Weigh accurately 5.0 grams of sample into a 50-ml centrifuge tube.

Liver, Muscle, Kidney, and Dose Site

2. Add 15 ml of 50% acetone/water to the tube from a dispensing pipettor.
3. Homogenize for 15 to 20 seconds or shorter time with a Polytron setting of 7. Homogenize until a homogeneous-looking mixture results.
4. Put a clean 50-ml tube in place containing 15 ml of isooctane from a dispensing pipettor.
5. Homogenize 5 to 10 seconds and pour the isooctane into the 50-ml tube with the homogenate. Clean the generator probe between samples with isooctane, distilled water, and acetone.

Fat Only

2. Add 15 ml of the acetone/water and 10 ml of isooctane to the tube and homogenize until a homogeneous mixture results.
3. Rinse probe with 10 ml isooctane in a clean 50-ml tube.
4. Pour isooctance into the 50-ml tube with the homogenate.
5. Add 1 gram of solid sodium chloride to the tube containing the homogenate.

Extractions

All Tissues

6. Stopper the tube, shake well for 1 minute, and centrifuge for 10 minutes.
7. Transfer the upper or isooctane layer to a second 50-ml centrifuge tube with a disposable pipet. Completely avoid the lower layer.
8. Break up the plug by using a vortex mixer and/or shaking; add 15 ml of clean isooctane, repeating the extraction and combining isooctane layers.
9. Evaporate the combined isooctane layers to a small volume (or ca. 5 ml for fat) using an 80° C bath and nitrogen purge.
10. Repeat the extractions with 2 more passes of 15 ml each of isooctane, adding the isooctane in each case to the same tube which had the previous 2 isooctane layers.

11. Again evaporate as far as possible using the 80° C bath and purge.
12. Add 6 ml of methanol to all samples except fat and dissolve or resuspend completely with an ultrasonic bath and/or vortex mixer.
13. Place all samples except fat in a refrigerator until thoroughly cooled (at this point the sample is best left overnight in the refrigerator or freezer).

Fat Only

12. Either add 2 ml of hexane and 5 ml of acetonitrile to the still hot and molten fat or freeze overnight at −20° C. For samples frozen overnight, remelt in a 80° C bath and add the hexane and acetonitrile the next day.
13. Shake the still warm mixture thoroughly for ca. 1 minute and immediately centrifuge.
14. Cool in ice water until the lower or fat layer congeals and the upper or acetonitrile layer can be decanted completely into a fresh 15-ml centrifuge tube.
15. Repeat the melting, extraction with 5 ml of acetonitrile, and transfer into the same 15-ml tube.
16. Add 2 ml of hexane to the 15-ml tube, shake thoroughly, centrifuge, and remove the upper, hexane layer to waste by disposable pipet or by aspiration. Go to Step 22.

Liver, Muscle, Kidney, and Dose Site

14. Centrifuge the cold 50-ml tube for 5 minutes, and decant off the clear supernatant to a clean 15-ml centrifuge tube.
15. Wash the residue in the 50-ml tube with 1 ml of methanol using a vortex mixer, centrifuge, and decant off into same 15-ml tube. (If solids are decanted in either step, recentrifuge the 15-ml tube and decant into a new 15-ml tube to get a clear solution to continue the assay with.)

15a. For muscles and dose sites only, do a 2-ml hexane extraction of the residue solids and add to the combined methanol.

16. Using a 60° C bath and nitrogen purge, evaporate off all the methanol.
17. By repipet add 3 ml of hexane to the tube previously containing the methanol and use an ultrasonic bath to remove all material from the walls of the centrifuge tube.
18. Add by repipet 4 ml of acetonitrile and repeat the ultrasonic treatment briefly.
19. Shake thoroughly, centrifuge 5 minutes, and move the lower or acetonitrile layer to a clean 15-ml tube.
20. Reextract the hexane layer with a second 4 ml of acetonitrile and combine acetonitrile layers.
21. Extract the combined acetonitrile layers with 1 ml of hexane, centri-

fuge to clear the layers, and move the upper, hexane layer to waste by disposable pipet or by aspiration.

All Tissues

22. Evaporate the acetonitrile solution to 1.0 ml using a ca. 60° C bath and nitrogen flush.
23. If the acetonitrile is less than 1 ml, make up to 1 ml with fresh acetonitrile.
24. Use an ultrasonic bath to get a homogeneous mix if necessary.
25. Add 4 ml of distilled water (2 ml for kidney samples) and 5 ml of hexane; shake ca. 1 minute and centrifuge for 5 minutes.
26. Move the upper, hexane layer to a clean 15-ml centrifuge tube using a disposable pipet. Avoid the lower layer.
27. Repeat with 5 ml and, then, 4 ml hexane extractions combining all 3 hexane extracts.
28. Evaporate to dryness (or as near dryness as possible) using a 40° C bath and nitrogen purge. (To get the sample more completely dry, more heat may need to be applied at the end of the evaporation. The bath may go up to ca. 80° C at this point.)
29. Redissolve the residue in exactly 1.0 ml of methanol using a vortex mixer and ultrasonic bath.
30. Mix thoroughly and centrifuge for 5 minutes.

Derivatization

31. Pipet exactly 0.5 ml of the solution from Step 30 into the bottom of a silylated 15-ml centrifuge tube. Use a 0.5-ml volumetric pipet.
32. Completely evaporate the methanol carefully, using at 60° C bath and nitrogen purge. Avoid spattering.
33. With a 1.0-ml graduated pipet, add 0.1 ml of freshly made acetic anhydride-methylimidazole-DMF mix to each tube and a series of standard tubes (see standard section F preceding).
34. Stopper, vortex briefly, and centrifuge for a few seconds.
35. Tape the stoppers in place and put all samples and standards in a well-stirred 95° C oil bath for 1 hour. The bottoms of the tubes should be about 1 inch below the oil surface.
36. Remove the tubes, wash the oil off the outside of the tubes with acetone in a wash bottle, and cool briefly. The residue should be black.
37. Add about 1 ml of chloroform to each tube and vortex to mix.
38. Wash a SEP-PAK cartridge with 3 to 4 ml of chloroform, using a syringe to force the liquid through.
39. Add the sample by disposable pipet to the syringe and force it through the cartridge.

All Tissues

40. Wash the centrifuge tube 3 times with 1 ml each of chloroform into the syringe and through the cartridge.
41. Elute the column with a further 8 to 9 ml of chloroform (with aliquots of 3, 3, 2, or 3 ml).
42. Collect *all* the chloroform eluate from the SEP-PAK in a 15-ml centrifuge tube.
43. Evaporate the chloroform off with a 60° C bath and nitrogen purge. Get the residue completely dry.

HPLC Analysis

44. Pipet 0.5 ml of methanol (or other suitable quantity) into the tube and use a vortex mixer and ultrasonic bath to completely dissolve the residue.
45. Centrifuge briefly and load WISP inserts if autosampler is used.
46. Inject 50 μl of the supernatant of each sample and standard into the HPLC.
47. Measure the peak heights at the retention time of the derivative of dihydro-B_{1a} as indicated by the standards.
48. Generate a standard curve by performing a linear regression analysis of response (peak height) versus concentration (ng/ml) for standards. The curve should be linear with a regression coefficient of 0.97 or better. Use the regression equation to determine the concentration of unknowns with an observed peak height.

    Calculate the sample concentration as follows:

$$\text{ppb} = (\text{ng/ml})\text{s} \times \frac{\text{V1}}{\text{V2}} \times \text{D/G} = \frac{\text{V1}}{\text{V2}} \times (\text{ng/ml})\text{s} \times \text{D/5}$$

Where: (ng/ml)s for the unknown is determined from the standard curve.

V1= ml sample dissolved in at end of assay (Step 44).
V2= ml of sample taken to make derivative (Step 31).
D= dilution of sample at end of assay or 1 if no dilution is made.
G= grams of sample taken = 5.

H. Suitable Stopping Places for Tissue Assays

The following stopping places allow storage for a maximum of 4 days:

1. In a refrigerator at 4° C.
    a. Only in methanol after Step 12.
2. In a freezer at −20° C.
    a. After Step 11 for fat only.
    b. After Step 30, before derivatization.

c. After Step 36, the derivatization.
d. After Step 44, dissolution of the residue in methanol.

If stopping places other than the above are needed, assay stability at said stopping place should be demonstrated first.

I. Analytical Procedure for Assay in Plasma

1. Pipet 5 ml of plasma into a 50-ml centrifuge tube, pipet in 7.5 ml of acetone, shake briefly, and let stand 15 minutes.
2. Pipet 7.5 ml of distilled water and 15 ml of ethyl acetate into the tube and shake by hand moderately for 1 minute. Shaking should be thorough enough to allow extraction but not violent enough to cause emulsions.
3. Centrifuge thoroughly and move the upper, ethyl acetate layer to a second 50-ml tube as completely as possible, using a disposable pipet. Move *absolutely* no lower phase.
4. Thoroughly break up the plug in the bottom of the first tube by shaking or with the wide end of a disposable pipet and repeat the ethyl acetate extraction a second time. Combine the ethyl acetate layers.
5. Evaporate the ethyl acetate completely with a nitrogen purge in a 75° C water bath.
6. Pipet exactly 1 ml of methanol into the dry tube.
7. Dissolve the residue as much as possible by using an ultrasonic bath with intermittent shaking. (The methanol must contact all the tube.)
8. Centrifuge and pour the supernatant solution into a 15-ml centrifuge tube and pipet exactly 0.5 ml of this solution into the bottom of a silylated 15-ml centrifuge tube.
9. Evaporate completely to dryness with a nitrogen purge and 60° C bath.
10. Using a 1-ml graduated pipet, add 0.1 ml of derivatizing reagent to samples and standards, stopper, and use a vortex genie to dissolve the residue.
11. Centrifuge briefly, tape the stoppers, and put unknowns and standards together in a well-stirred 95° C oil bath for 1 hour.
12. Remove tubes and rinse the oil off the outsides with acetone. The residue should be black. (If the residue is not black, the remaining sample from Step 8 can be used to repeat the derivatization with the next set of standards.)
13. Add ca. 1 ml of chloroform to the residue in each tube.
14. Use a vortex genie to thoroughly mix.
15. Wash a silica SEP-PAK cartridge with 3 to 4 ml of chloroform, using a syringe to force the liquid through and discard to waste.
16. Add the chloroform sample to the syringe with a disposable pipet and force the liquid through the cartridge.
17. Wash the centrifuge tube 3 times with ca. 1 ml each of chloroform into

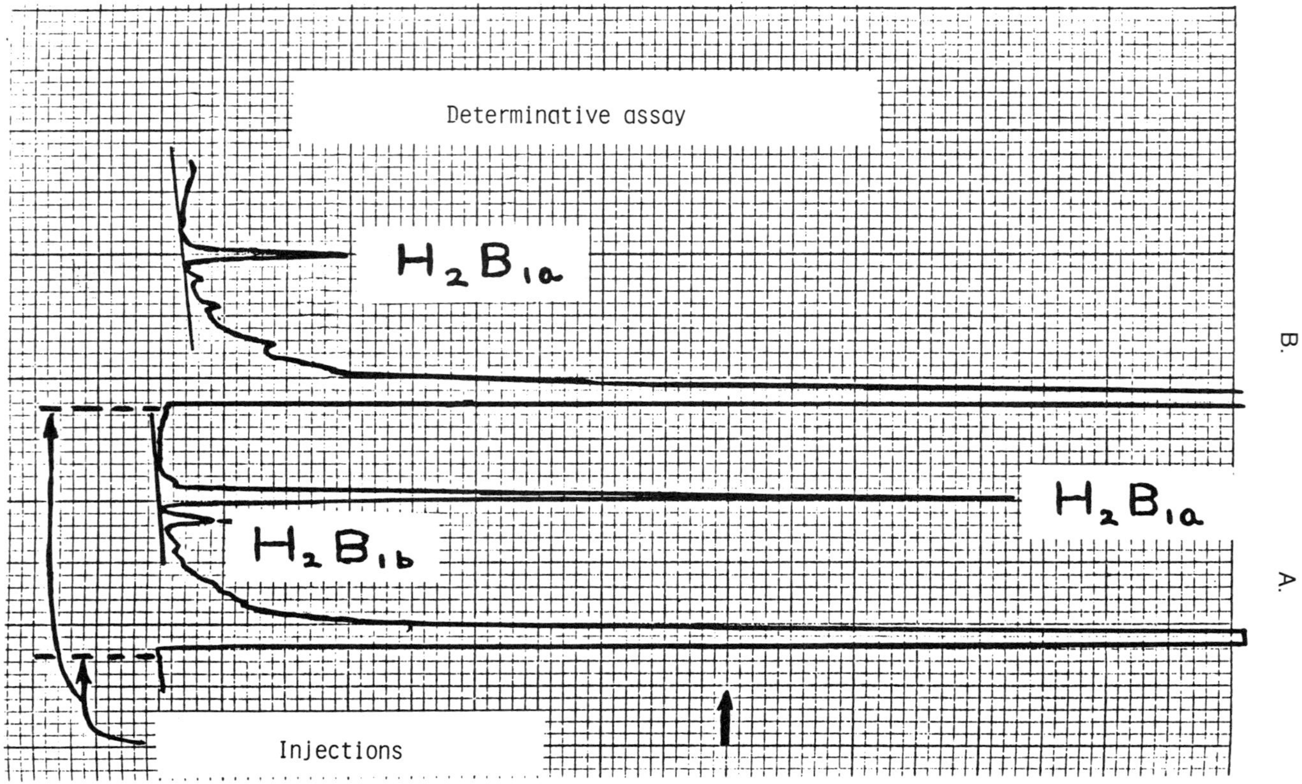

FIGURE AI.2. Chromatographic tracings of (A) standard and (B) plasma sample containing ivermectin.

the syringe and through the cartridge, using the same disposable pipet.

18. Elute the cartridge with a further 8 to 9 ml of chloroform (aliquots of 3, 3, 2, or 3 ml).
19. Collect all the chloroform, leaving the SEP-PAK from Steps 16, 17, and 18 (eluent) in a 15-ml centrifuge tube.
20. Evaporate the chloroform completely off with a 60° C bath and nitrogen purge. The residue must be completely dry.
21. Pipet exactly 0.5 ml of methanol (or other larger volumes for high-assay plasmas) into the tube and use a vortex mixer and ultrasonic bath to completely dissolve the residue.
22. Centrifuge and inject 50 μl of sample from each sample and each standard in turn into the HPLC unit using the WISP Autosampler.
23. Measure the peak heights of the derivative at the retention time indicated by the standards.
24. Calculate results as described in the tissue method starting at Step 48, substituting ng/ml for ppb and 5 ml for G in the equation.

Appendix II

Confirmatory Assay for Assaying Ivermectin Residues in Liver

G.V. Downing

A. Summary of the Confirmatory Residue Method

The tissue is homogenized with acetone-water and the dihydro B_{1a} is extracted with isooctane with the tissue present. Following removal of the isooctane, solvent-solvent distributions into acetonitrile out of hexane and into hexane out of acetonitrile-water are performed. Solvent is removed from aliquots of the resulting solution, and monosaccharide and aglycone derivatives are formed. Extractions into methylene chloride/hexane/isobutyl alcohol out of methanol/water are followed by solvent removal and fluorescence production by heating at 95° C in imidazole reagent. Extractions are performed out of methanol/water into hexane/isobutyl alcohol. Solvent is removed and HPLC analysis performed on Zorbax C18. Confirmation results when peaks are observed at appropriate levels for H_2B_{1a} itself and the monosaccharide and aglycone derivatives.

B. Reagents

1. Acetic anhydride—Baker or Fisher, reagent grade.
2. Acetone—Mallinckrodt, Nanograde.
3. Acetonitrile—Fisher, HPLC grade; or Mallinckrodt, Nanograde.
4. Dimethyl Formamide (DMF)—Baker or Fisher, reagent grade.
5. Hexane—Burdick & Jackson, distilled in glass; or Mallinckrodt, Nanograde.

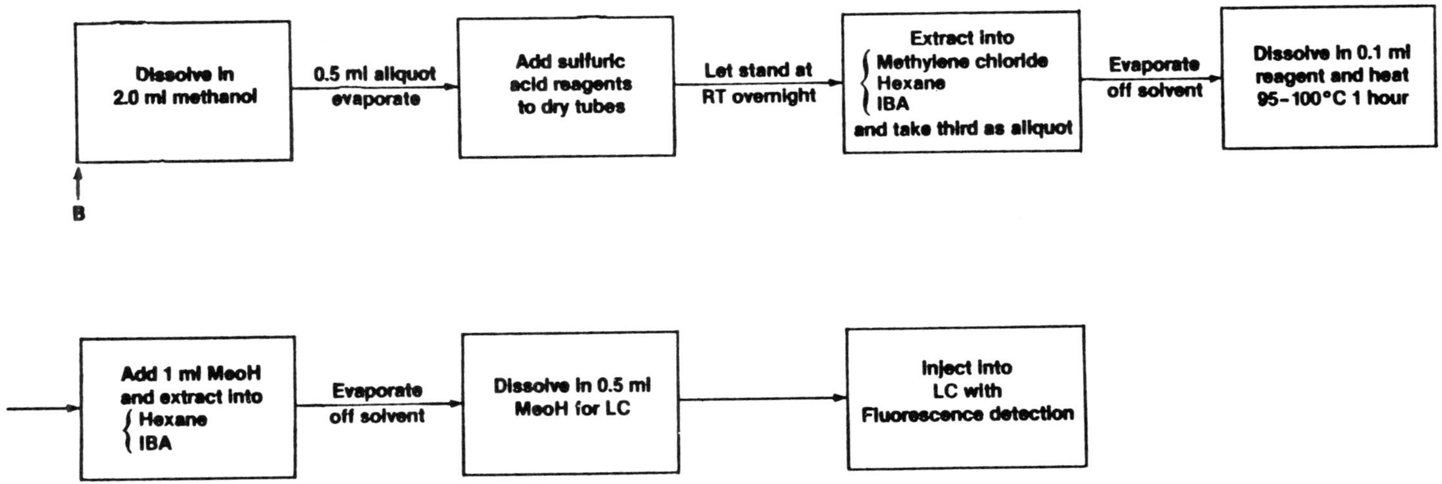

FIGURE AII.1. Flow diagram of confirmatory assay. B is a possible stopping point during the assay.

6. Isobutyl alcohol—Burdick & Jackson, distilled in glass.
7. Isopropanol—Burdick & Jackson, distilled in glass.
8. Methanol—Burdick & Jackson, distilled in glass; or Mallinckrodt, Nanograde.
9. Methylene Chloride—any grade available.
10. Methylene chloride—Burdick & Jackson, distilled in glass.
11. 1-Methylimidazole—99%, Aldrich Chemical Company.
12. Nitrogen—the equivalent of Matheson extra-dry compressed gas.
13. Sylon-CT—Supelco, Inc.
14. 2,2,4-Trimethylpentane—isooctane, Burdick & Jackson, distilled in glass.
15. Water, doubled distilled—Distilled, deionized water is redistilled in an all-glass apparatus.

C. Solutions

1. Derivatizing Reagent—Mix 0.2 ml of 1-methylimidazole with 0.3 ml of acetic anhydride and 0.9 ml of DMF.Make up just before use.
2. Acetone/Water—50% (v/v).
3. Methanol/Water Mobile Phase (90/10)—Make 200 ml of doubly distilled and filtered water to 2 liters with methanol. Deaerate by slowly bubbling nitrogen through for 10 minutes. Make other water content mobile phases correspondingly.
4. 40% Methylene Chloride-Hexane-Isobutyl Alcohol—Fill a 500-ml stoppered graduate to the 200 mark with methylene chloride. Add hexane to the 500-ml mark and, then, 20 ml of isobutyl alcohol. Mix.
5. 1% Isobutyl Alcohol in Hexane—Make 5 ml of isobutyl alcohol to 500 ml in a graduated cylinder. Mix.
6. 1% Sulfuric Acid in Isopropanol—Pipet 0.5 ml of sulfuric acid carefully into about 40 ml of isopropanol in a 50-ml volumetric flask. Mix. Dilute to the mark with isopropanol and thoroughly mix. Make fresh just before use.
7. 1% Sulfuric Acid in Methanol—Pipet 0.5 ml of sulfuric acid carefully into about 40 ml of methanol in a 50-ml volumetric flask. Mix. Dilute to the mark with methanol and thoroughly mix. Make fresh just before use.

D. Apparatus

1. Balance—analytical, capable of weighing 1 mg accurately.
2. Balance—capable of weighing 5 g accurately into an approximately 60-g tube.

3. Bath, water—variable temperature 40° to 80° C.
4. Bath, oil—95° to 100° C.
5. Centrifuge, IEC Model HN-S-II, with 6-place rotor IEC 958 and 15- and 50-ml cups. The centrifuge is run at 2000 to 2500 rpm. The centrifuge used gives ca. 700 to 750 X g maximum centrifugal force (RCF).
6. Centrifuge tubes, glass, 15- and 50-ml with polyethylene stoppers to fit.
7. Centrifuge tubes—50-ml polypropylene, Corning 25331 (used only for storing standard solutions).
8. Centrifuge tubes, 15 ml, silylated approximately once every 2 months (used only for the derivatization reaction). Tube stoppers must fit tightly. Fill each tube to the top with Sylon-CT. Let stand 20 minutes. Immediately and quickly rinse, first thoroughly with toluene and then with methanol. Fill with methanol. Let stand 20 minutes, rinse thoroughly with acetone, and dry. All glassware used should be *completely* free of all acidic and alkaline residues. (These tubes should be cleaned by hand by first soaking in methylene chloride immediately after use and then in detergent for at least several hours each, followed by thorough rinsing with hot water, distilled water, and acetone before thorough drying. Variations in the washing regimen are not recommended, since some analysts have had poor results when the standard washing method was not followed.)
9. Dispensing pipettors—10, 15, and 20 ml.
10. Gloves—disposable PVC from Fisher Chemical.
11. Freezer—capable of reaching temperatures of −20° C.
12. Graduate cylinder—25 ml.
13. Graduate cylinder—500 ml.
14. Homogenizer, Polytron-Brinkmann Instruments, 27-11-200-5 with PTA 10S generator 27-22-330-3.
15. Parafilm—American Can Co.
16. Pipets—disposable.
17. Pipets—graduated 1, 2, 5, and 10 ml.
18. Pipets—volumetric 0.5 ml, 1 ml, 2 ml, 3 ml, 4 ml, and 5 ml.
19. Reciprocating shaker, variable speed—Eberbach, J. T. Baker Catalog 8287-E30 or equivalent.
20. SEP-PAK, silica catridge, Part No. 51900—Waters Associates.
21. Spatula—stainless steel.
22. Syringe—50 μl and 250 μl.
23. Tape—13 2956, 1/2 inch from Ace Scientific.
24. Ultrasonic bath—Sonogen Automatic Cleaner—Branson Model 520 or equivalent.
25. Vortex mixer.

E. Chromatographic Apparatus

A Beckman-Altex Model 110A liquid chromatographic pump complete with Valco sample valve with syringe-loading sample loop or Waters Wisp Autosampler and Kratos-Schoeffel Instruments Model FS950 fluorescence detector with a 1-millivolt recorder is used. A 5μm, 4.6-mm ID, C18 standard Brownlee Labs guard column (Spheri-5 RP-18 OD-G, obtained from Rainin Instrument Co., Inc.) is used before the analytical column. This guard column is replaced monthly unless the pressure reaches 2000 psi, in which case it is replaced immediately.

Conditions: 15 cm length×4.6 mm ID Zorbax ODS-C18 column.
Mobile phase—10% water in methanol (v/v).
Column temperature—43° C.
Flow—1.8 ml/minute (usual pressure 1000 psi, 500 to 2000 psi acceptable).

For FS950:

Excitation Lamp—FSA 110, standard 365 nm.
Standard Kratos Flowcell—FSA 210.
Excitation Filter—FSA 403, 365 nm band filters.
Emission Filter—418 nm.
Sensitivity Range—0.2 A or higher.
Retention Time—14 minutes (or greater with Modifications for I, the parent compound)
Time Constant—about 6.

F. Standards for the Confirmatory Assay

The objective is to have standards for the parent (I), aglycone (A), and monosaccharide (M) at approximately the concentration observed in the determinative assay or at the RM. To achieve this, dilute an aliquot of standard ivermectin solution in methanol with methanol.

The final concentration of the solution should be 10 times the level to be detected (±10%). This results from the following equation:

$$C = 5 \times L$$

where: C= the weight of ivermectin in 2 ml of the diluted standard.
5= number of grams of liver sample used.
L= level of analyst wishes to determine in ppb or ng/g.

Because the unknowns are dissolved in 2 ml before aliquoting into I, M, and A, the standard is figured on the basis of 2 ml. Two 0.5 ml aliquots of the diluted standard solution should be run through each part of the assay (M, A, and I). The M and A standards should start in the procedure at the Step 4 evaporation. The I standard should start at Step 15.

G. Procedure for the Confirmatory Method

1. Follow the method described in the determinative assay procedure up through Step 28.
2. Take the residue up in exactly 2 ml of methanol, using vortex mixer and ultrasonic bath.
3. Mix thoroughly and centrifuge for 5 minutes.
4. Pipet exactly 0.5 ml of the solution from Step 3 into each of 2 fresh 15-ml tubes and blow completely to dryness with nitrogen in a 70° C bath. The dried samples generally look like a small drop of oil. All solvent must be completely removed. Store the remaining 1 ml from Step 3 in a freezer until later.
5. Add 0.1 ml of 1% sulfuric acid in methanol to 1 of the 2 samples (the A sample) and 0.1 ml of 1% sulfuric acid in isopropanol to the second (the M sample).
6. Vortex mix the sample for 10 seconds, thoroughly ultrasound it, and repeat the vortex mixing.
7. Let stand at room temperature for 16–18 hours (overnight in the dark).
8. To all (A) samples and (A) standards at one time, add 0.9 ml of methanol, using a 5-ml graduated pipet.
9. Add the 40% methylene chloride-hexane-isobutyl alcohol solvent mixture to the 7-ml mark and mix.
10. Add 4 ml of distilled water, using a 10-ml graduated pipet, shake for 1 minute, and centrifuge for 5 minutes.
11. Move the mixed solvent upper phase by disposable pipet to a fresh silylated 15-ml tube. Move as much upper phase as possible but absolutely *no* lower phase.
12. Repeate the extraction of the lower phase with a second 6 ml of the mixed solvent and combine the extracts in the silylated tube.
13. Do the same extractions with the (M) samples, except that the shaking must be only moderate and the centrifuging should be for 10 or more minutes (otherwise emulsions may result).
14. Into a third 15-ml silylated tube, pipet another 0.5 ml of the sample from the freezer stored in Step 4 (the I sample).
15. Blow the (M) and (A) extracts and the (I) sample completely to dryness. Again, *all* solvent must be removed and no moisture picked up. A bath temperature of 40° C is suitable for the (M) and (A) samples and temperatures up to 70° C for the (I) sample.
16. Add 0.1 ml of derivatizing reagent to all (M), (A), and (I) dry tubes and all standards, vortex mix 10 seconds, tape the stoppers in place, centrifuge briefly, and place in a 95–100° C oil bath for 1 hour, all at the same time.
17. Cool to room temperature, add 0.9 ml of methanol using a 5-ml graduated pipet, and mix.

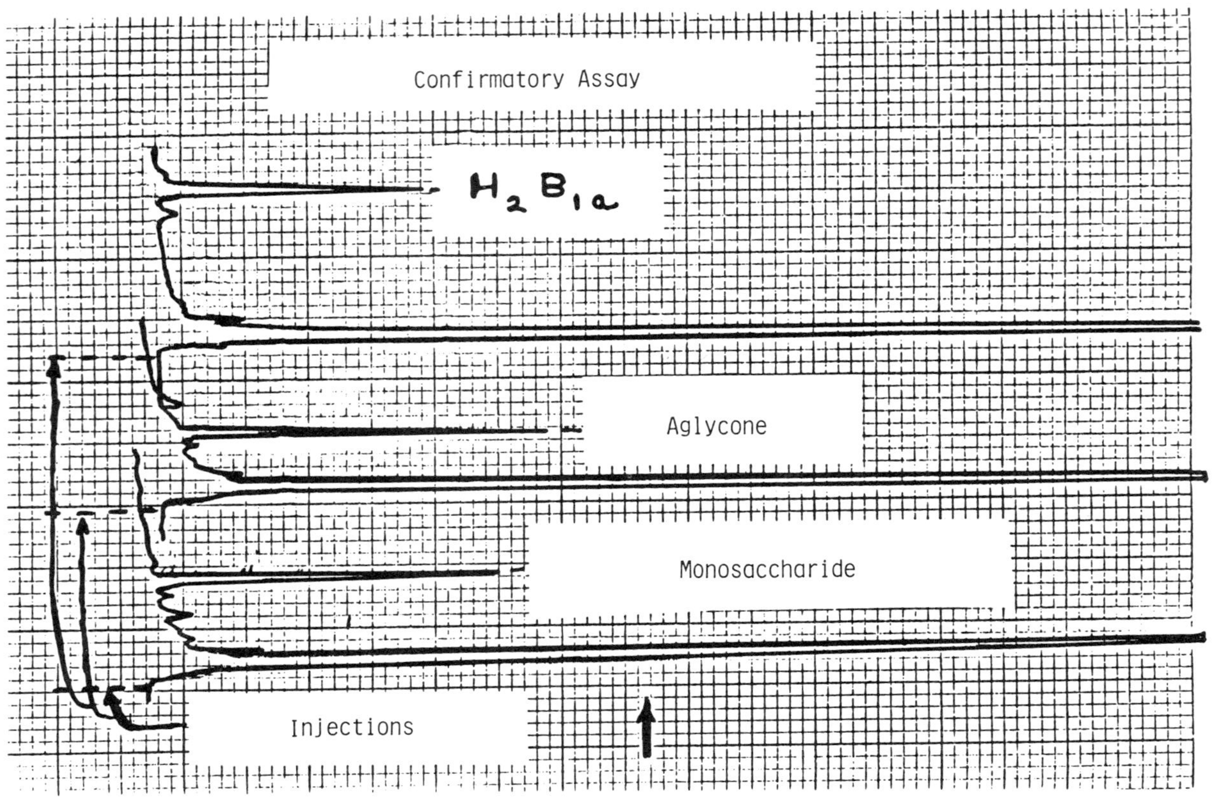

FIGURE AII.2. Chromatographic tracings of standards.

18. Add 1% isobutyl alcohol in hexane to the 7-ml mark and mix.
19. Add 4 ml of water from a graduated pipet, shake 1 minute, and centrifuge for 5 minutes.
20. Move the upper phase as completely as possible to a fresh 15-ml tube. Move *no* lower phase.
21. Repeate the extraction with a second 6 ml and combine extracts.
22. Blow completely to dryness with a nitrogen flush and a 40° C bath. At the end of this evaporation, the temperature can be allowed to rise to 60–70° C.
23. Take up residue in exactly 0.5 ml of methanol, using vortex mixing and ultrasound. In all above (17–23), the (M) samples should be handled first and placed on the LC before handling the (A) or (I) samples. After extraction, protect the (M) samples from light as much as possible. (If the (A) and (I) samples are to be delayed signifcantly, they should be stored in freezer at −20° C before adding the methanol.)
24. Centrifuge and inject 50 μl of the clear phase (M samples) onto the HPLC with the modified mobile phase doing the first standard of a type, the unknowns, and finally the second standard, in that order.
25. Do the same with the (A) and (I) samples.
26. Examine the unknown sample chromatograms for the presence of the (A), (M), and (I) peaks at the same elution time as the standard peak. (That is, compare the unknown (A) to standard (A), etc.)
27. Average the 2 peak heights for each standard (A, M, and I) and calculate each unknown as a precent of that standard average.
28. A value of 60% or more of all 3 (A, M, and I) is proof that that particular level of ivermectin is present in the tissue (liver).

APPENDIX III

List of Registrations

J. Di Netta

Ivermectin was released for registration by Merck & Co., Inc., in 1981 and first registered in France as IVOMEC Injection for Cattle that same year.

Since that time ivermectin has been approved for use in over 60 countries. It is currently registered for use in cattle, sheep, horses, goats, swine, dogs, camels, reindeer, and bison.

The following lists the products and the countries in which ivermectin is registered.

IVERMECTIN APPROVALS

	IVOMEC Injection for Cattle*	
ALGERIA	GUATEMALA	PHILIPPINES
ARGENTINA	HOLLAND	POLAND
AUSTRALIA[1]	HONDURAS	PORTUGAL
AUSTRIA	HUNGARY	ROMANIA
BELGIUM	INDIA	S. AFRICA
BRAZIL	IRELAND	SPAIN
BULGARIA	ISRAEL	SUDAN
CANADA	ITALY	SWEDEN
CHILE	JAMAICA	SWITZERLAND
COLOMBIA	JAPAN	THAILAND
COSTA RICA	JORDAN	TRINIDAD
C.S.S.R	KENYA	TUNISIA
DENMARK	LUXEMBOURG	TURKEY
ECUADOR	MALAYSIA	U.K.
EGYPT	MEXICO	URUGUAY
EL SALVADOR	MOROCCO	U.S.A.
FINLAND	NEW ZEALAND	U.S.S.R.
FRANCE	NORWAY	VENEZUELA
G.D.R.	PANAMA	YUGOSLAVIA
GERMANY	PARAGUAY	ZIMBABWE
GREECE	PERU	
	IVOMEC* Oral Solution for Cattle	
FRANCE	NEW ZEALAND	U.K.
HOLLAND	SOUTHAFRICA	

IVOMEC* Paste for Cattle

CANADA	U.S.A.	

IVOMEC* Pour-On for Cattle

ARGENTINA	HOLLAND	NEW ZEALAND
BRAZIL	MEXICO	U.K.
CANADA		

IVOMEC-F* Injection for Cattle

BRAZIL	IRELAND	SPAIN
FRANCE	MEXICO	U.K.
HOLLAND	PORTUGAL	

IVOMEC* or ORAMEC* Liquid for Goats

BRAZIL	NEW ZEALAND	U.K.
HOLLAND	SOUTH AFRICA	

IVOMEC* or ORAMEC* Liquid for Sheep

ARGENTINA	HOLLAND	MOROCCO
AUSTRALIA	INDIAN	NEW ZEALAND
BELGIUM	IRELAND	SOUTH AFRICA
BRAZIL	JORDAN	SUDAN
CANADA	KENYA	U.K.
FRANCE	LUXEMBOURG	U.S.A.
		URUGUAY
		ZIMBABWE

IVOMEC* Injection for Sheep

ALGERIA	DENMARK	POLAND
ARGENTINA	FRANCE	PORTUGAL
BELGIUM	HOLLAND	ROMANIA
BRAZIL	JORDAN	SOUTH AFRICA
BULGARIA	LUXEMBOURG	SPAIN
C.S.S.R.	MEXICO	SUDAN
CANADA	MOROCCO	TUNISIA
CHINA	PARAGUAY	URUGUAY
		YUGOSLAVIA

IVOMEC* Injection for Swine

AGRENTINA	GERMANY	PORTUGAL
AUSTRIA	HOLLAND	ROMANIA
BELGIUM	HONG KONG	SINGAPORE
BRAZIL	IRELAND	SOUTH AFRICA
BULGARIA	ITALY	SPAIN
CANADA	JAPAN	SWEDEN
CHILE	KOREA	SWITZERLAND
CHINA	LUXEMBOURG	TAIWAN
COLOMBIA	MALAYSIA	THAILAND
C.S.S.R.	MEXICO	U.K.
DENMARK	NEW ZEALAND	U.S.A.
ECUADOR	NORWAY	URUGUAY
FINLAND	PARAGUAY	VENEZUELA
FRANCE	PHILIPPINES	YUGOSLAVIA
G.D.R.	POLAND	ZIMBABWE

IVOMEC* Injection for Young Pigs

HOLLAND	U.S.A.	

HEARTGARD-30* or CARDOMEC* or CARDOTEK-30* Tablets for Dogs		
AUSTRALIA	HOLLAND	SPAIN
CANADA	JAPAN	U.S.A.
FRANCE	MEXICO	

EQVALAN* Paste for Horses		
ALGERIA	HOLLAND	PARAGUAY
ARGENTINA	HONDURAS	PERU
BELGIUM	HONG KONG	PHILIPPINES
BRAZIL	IRELAND	POLAND
CANADA	ITALY	PORTUGAL
CHILE	JAMAICA	SINGAPORE
COLOMBIA	JAPAN	SOUTH AFRICA
COSTA RICA	JORDAN	SPAIN
DENMARK	KENYA	SUDAN
ECUADOR	KOREA	SWEDEN
EGYPT	LEBANON	SWITZERLAND
EL SALVADOR	LUXEMBOURG	THAILAND
FINLAND	MEXICO	TRINIDAD
FRANCE	MOROCCO	U.K.
G.D.R.	NEW ZEALAND	U.S.A.
GERMANY	NORWAY	U.S.S.R.
GUATEMALA	PANAMA	URUGUAY
		VENEZUELA

EQVALAN* Liquid for Horses		
CANADA	MEXICO	U.S.A
HOLLAND		

IVOMEC* Injection for Camels		
ALGERIA	MOROCCO	SUDAN
JORDAN		

[1] AVOMEC

* Trademark of MERCK & CO., Inc., Rahway, New Jersey, U.S.A.

Index

B